THE MEDIEVAL ISLAMIC HOSPITAL

Medicine, Religion, and Charity

The first monograph on the history of Islamic hospitals, this volume focuses on the underexamined Egyptian and Levantine institutions of the twelfth to fourteenth centuries. By the twelfth century, hospitals serving the sick and the poor could be found in nearly every Islamic city. Ahmed Ragab traces the varying origins and development of these institutions, locating them in their urban environments and linking them to charity networks and patrons' political projects. Following the paths of patients inside hospital wards, he investigates who they were and what kinds of experiences they had. *The Medieval Islamic Hospital* explores the medical networks surrounding early hospitals and sheds light on the particular brand of practice-oriented medicine they helped develop. Providing a detailed picture of the effect of religion on medieval medicine, it will be essential reading for those interested in the history of medicine, history of Islamic sciences, or history of the Mediterranean.

AHMED RAGAB is the Richard T. Watson Assistant Professor of Science and Religion at Harvard Divinity School, where he also directs the Science, Religion, and Culture Program. He is a member of the Commission on History of Science and Technology in Islamic Societies and the International Society for Science and Religion.

THE MEDIEVAL ISLAMIC HOSPITAL

Medicine, Religion, and Charity

AHMED RAGAB

Harvard University

CAMBRIDGE
UNIVERSITY PRESS

CAMBRIDGE
UNIVERSITY PRESS

32 Avenue of the Americas, New York NY 10013-2473, USA

Cambridge University Press is part of the University of Cambridge.

It furthers the University's mission by disseminating knowledge in the pursuit of education, learning and research at the highest international levels of excellence.

www.cambridge.org
Information on this title: www.cambridge.org/9781107109605

First published 2015

A catalogue record for this publication is available from the British Library

ISBN 978-1-107-10960-5 Hardback

To Soha and Carmen

Contents

Acknowledgments

I am fortunate that I have many people to acknowledge for their help with this project and that the debts accrued in the making of this book have led to valuable intellectual encounters and the reinforcement of treasured relationships that continue to enrich my life and scholarship after this project has been completed. My friend, mentor, and adviser, Anne-Marie Moulin, watched this project develop from its earliest phases and was present not only as it took shape, but also as I became a historian. Her mentorship, companionship, and friendship will always lie behind my work as a historian of science. I was also so fortunate as to work with Danielle Jacquart, whose work helped shape the history of medieval sciences as we know it; it has been an honor and a privilege to participate in so distinguished a scholarly tradition. Danielle Jacquart's comments, interventions, and advice were integral to my work. I am also grateful to my friend, colleague, co-instructor, and co-author (of another book!), Katharine Park. She remains a mentor and interlocutor to whom I owe much. Katy spent many hours with the draft of this book; thanks to her suggestions, a more coherent story and decisive voice emerged.

I cannot describe my gratitude to Anne Harrington – a central force in my development as a scholar – whose encouragement and mentorship continue to inspire and guide my work. I am deeply indebted, too, to Janet Browne's continued care, advice, and support, and for her investment in my growth as a scholar. Bill Graham's and Janet Gyatso's counsel and guidance bore tremendous impact on my scholarship, as well as on the development of this project over the past years. I am also much obliged to David Hempton for all he has done to facilitate my work and scholarship.

Faye Bodley-Dangelo edited the book and helped guide it to its current state. Joseph Vignone and Hadel Jarada helped me revise the transliterations. Anna Attaway, Lewis West, and Will Morningstar patiently and carefully copyedited and proofread the final version of the book, with Anna and Lewis making sure that the narrative was lucid and unencumbered by errors or oversights. Alex Chen helped me with the preparation of the maps and illustrations. I am beholden to them all.

The comments of my anonymous reviewers were integral to the development of this project and the execution of the book; their insights and views were very beneficial and are much appreciated. I have also been grateful, throughout this process, for the sure hands of Laura Morris – my editor at Cambridge University Press – and for her care of the manuscript and project as a whole, which were a major force in bringing it to completion.

It is hard to imagine being here without the care, support, encouragement, and doubts of my parents. Their love and dedication to the education and well-being of my siblings and myself are at the heart of all that I do.

Throughout the years of working on this project and of writing this book, there has been one person, especially, who stood by me through it all: my love, partner, wife, and friend, Soha Bayoumi. Her insights and opinions helped move this research on to more interesting, more innovative grounds. Her patience with the emotional and psychological toll that this work exacts allowed the book to come to life. As the book was slowly coming together, our little one, Carmen, arrived in our family. It is not possible to describe the joy that she brought, and continues to bring, to our lives. No words can describe my gratitude for all that Soha did at that time to allow this book to come to life and how she did so with such grace, love, care, and personal investment. This book is as much hers as it is mine.

Preface

For a long time, the study of the history of Islamic hospitals has focused on what Michael Dols called "their apparent modernity."[1] Earlier historians of Islamic medicine were attracted to what seemed to be a premodern ancestor of modern hospitals: Islamic hospitals were seen as "relatively secular" (to use Dols's terms again) because they were run by physicians or state officials – and not by religious scholars – and also because they had non-Muslim physicians working in them. This "medical" nature of the Islamic hospital was embodied in a number of qualities, namely, that it was designed and managed by educated Galenic physicians; furthermore, the hospital focused on the sick with the intention of curing rather than isolating them (and, because of this, hospitals were built in the centers of cities and not on their outskirts) and sponsored medical education and training.

As such, the Islamic hospital stood in contrast to earlier and contemporary charitable institutions, where physicians had little role or control and care was generally focused either on the needy – such as paupers, the hungry, crippled, blind, and the like – or on a specific group of diseased people that the institution cared for but isolated, like lepers. The Islamic institution was thus medicalized in that it was not a hospice, an orphanage, or a leprosarium. This focus on medicalization as a distinctive characteristic of hospitals in general, and of Islamic hospitals in particular, legitimized and prompted investigations into the origins of these hospitals. When did the first (true) Islamic hospital appear? What are the premedicalized, prehospital origins of these practices? And how did they become medicalized over time? Finally, how and when did the hospital deteriorate, or lose its medical nature by allowing religious scholars to dominate the field and the institution?

[1] Dols, "The Origins of the Islamic Hospital."

At the same time, the study of Islamic hospitals followed in the footsteps of the historiography of Islamic medicine and sciences in how the field was delimited and organized temporally and geographically. On one hand, all institutions throughout the expanses of Islamdom, much like all medical practice, were seen as part of a larger whole. Although changes and developments were admittedly explored and explained, the "Islamic hospital" was reduced to a singular, if multifaceted, unifying category, with different examples from anywhere between Iran and Andalusia. On the other hand, the perceived coherence of this category served to alienate and negate influences from neighboring charitable institutions, which belonged to a different religio-cultural realm – such as Crusader hospitals – or which belonged to different intellectual or professional environs – such as khānaqāhs and madrasas. Islamic hospitals were thus perceived as a rarified category stretching across time and space; their historians limited themselves to searching for the origins and developments of medicalization, as well as to attempts to chart the stages in which the Islamic hospital had consolidated or rejected its medical nature.

Recently, the works of Peter Pormann and Peregrine Horden began to challenge these assumptions and to ask more nuanced questions about the history and impact of these institutions.[2] This book continues their lines of inquiry, arguing against the previously mentioned two assumptions: first, the medicalized nature of the Islamic hospital, and second, the unity and coherence of the "Islamic hospital" itself, but arguing against them in reverse order. First, the book argues that the analytical category of "Islamic hospital" is far from coherent or discrete. Not only did these institutions develop from different origins and on different trajectories, they also served different audiences and purposes and had different raisons-d'etre. The book identifies two major models or prototypes of Islamic hospitals: one that was most common in Iraq and Iran, and another in the Levant and Egypt. I argue that these institutions need to be considered not from within a rarified medical category, but rather as part of local and embodied networks of charity and as institutions that served specific audiences and specific goals, some historical and some contemporaneous with their particular context.

This focus on the physical and embodied entails two major commitments. The first is to locate any given Islamic hospital within its local environment and landscape. This means that one must consider seriously

[2] See Pormann, "Medical Methodology and Hospital Practice," and "Islamic Hospitals"; Horden, "The Earliest Hospitals in Byzantium," and *Hospitals and Healing*.

the local encounters and influences (such as Crusader hospitals in the case of the Levantine and Egyptian institutions). Although these influences may not be represented in our written sources – which were produced by scholarly elites with specific religio-cultural and professional commitments – they may be observed in physical, architectural, and administrative arrangements and through the expectations of institutions' audiences. These influences may also be seen animated by artisanal knowledge as by elite, interpolity religio-cultural and military competition. Similarly, this commitment requires a focus on other institutions that shared physical space with a given hospital – be they madrasas, mausoleums, sabils, or khānaqāhs – and on other institutions that shared the imaginary discursive spaces of a particular patronage project or built heritage. These institutions and establishments played a significant role in shaping how a given hospital was imagined and created, as well as in shaping the hospital's functions throughout its history.

Second, this emphasis on material history entails a commitment to the physical experience of patients and practitioners. In this vein, the architectural design of a given hospital, the decorations on the walls, and even the amulets hanging from its roof need to be taken into consideration, as do the lines of movement people traced through their cities and inside the institutions at hand. Such physical experience is part and parcel of how these institutions passed their lives and their histories and, as such, merit our careful analysis. Here, I explicitly argue for integrating as much architectural and urban history as possible into the study of medical institutions and medical practice. In this regard, the excellent work done by many historians of art and architecture serves as a tremendous resource.

I will also argue in this book that the historiography of Islamic hospitals needs to dispense with preconceived considerations of medicalization, beginning with the term "hospital" itself. Bīmāristāns were certainly institutions that cared for the sick and were undeniably suffused with medical intellectual, social, and professional priorities, but they were primarily charitable institutions, aimed at serving the poor as part of a patron's charitable and pietistic endeavors. The focus on the sick was not an exclusionary function, wherein the bīmāristān refused to care for those who did not fit the paradigmatic definition of "the sick." It was, rather, inclusionary: the focus on the sick located the bīmāristān within a wider network of charity and allowed it to better serve particular populations as other institutions better served others. The bīmāristān was not a "secular" institution – not least because "secularism" is an anachronism and thus is not useful as a category here, but also because the bīmāristān was deeply rooted in charitable and pietistic endeavors that were, in turn, embedded in religio-social traditions and conventions. Even the medical education that eventually became a role played by most bīmāristāns was part of a charitable commitment to teaching and learning, a commitment that animated medical learning as it did legal and religious learning in madrasas and mosques. However, this understanding of the bīmāristān's charitable role should be tempered by the commitment – stated earlier – to the incoherence of the category of the "bīmāristān" or "Islamic hospital" in light of the institution's variable histories, roles, and genealogies. This book explains that bīmāristāns' pietistic and charitable characteristics performed and manifested in unique and various ways throughout different regions and time periods.

That said, this book also takes care to understand the role of medical elites and medical practitioners in the bīmāristān. It is also deeply concerned with exploring patients' experiences of their patienthood; these experiences were defined by medical expertise, by preexisting medical paradigms, by nonlearned healing practices, and by embodied physical and pietistic performances. As a professional group, physicians had highly adaptable relationships to their various bīmāristāns. They were entrusted with much of the bīmāristān's functions, were sometimes invested in the project's construction and development, and were part of the same patronage networks that gave birth to bīmāristāns; as such, physicians were as connected to patrons and to their projects as were the bīmāristāns themselves. This book takes seriously the professional and intellectual commitments of physicians working in bīmāristāns but is careful not to see them as a single coherent group (the "Islamic Galenic physician") but as descendants of various intellectual genealogies and commitments. At the same time, this book's focus on materiality allows for the consideration of medical practice qua practices rooted in the physical building of the bīmāristān and in its financial and institutional commitments; all of these impacted medical practice and shaped what might be called bīmāristān-specific medical priorities and traditions.

In short, this book is a study of the material and embodied histories of bīmāristāns. It proposes to study bīmāristāns as physical institutions that were part of charitable networks and specific physical and architectural environments. These institutions will be investigated as variable historical occurrences that differed from one another based on locality and on regional and historical specificities; they will be explored as projects that animated, were engaged in, and were influenced by medical and bureaucratic elites and their particular priorities.

In this vein, this study is indebted to the work of new generations of historians of Islamic medicine, as well as to historians of hospitals in different regions and periods, particularly John Hendersen and Charles Rosenberg. It relies also on the work of a number of historians of science who – with Katharine Park, Joan Cadden, and Lorraine Daston as exemplars – have highlighted the importance of the physical, the embodied, and the gendered. Finally, this study has served to show me, as I hope it will show you, that there is much more work to be done.

Note on Transliteration

I followed the Library of Congress conventions with some modifications, as outlined below:

ء	ʾ	ط	ṭ	َ	a
ب	b	ظ	ẓ	ُ	U
ت	t	ع	ʿ	ِ	I
ث	th	غ	gh	ّ	Double consonant
ج	j	ف	f	آ	ā
ح	ḥ	ق	q	أ	ā
خ	kh	ك	k	وُ	ū
د	d	ل	l	يِ	ī
ذ	dh	م	m		
ر	r	ن	n		
ز	z	ه	h		
س	s	و	w		
ش	sh	ي	y		
ص	ṣ	ة	h t (in construct)		
ض	ḍ	ال	al-		

- *Ibn* and *bint* were rendered "b." and "bt." when between two proper names. They were kept as *Ibn* and *bint* when part of a known *Kunya.* For instance: Muḥammad *b.* Qalāwūn, *Ibn* Sīnā, Muḥammad *b.* Abī Bakr *ibn* al-Qayyim.
- The *lam* of the definite article before "sun" letters was not assimilated.
- A hyphen was used with the definite article and inseparable propositions except for the proposition *li-* followed by the definite article as in *lil-sultan.* The proposition *wa* was not linked to subsequent words.

- Final inflictions were represented only in verbs and adverbs (*ḥāl*).
- Diacritics were not used in dynastic names (Abbasid, not ʿAbbāsid) or Arabic words that have entered English (mufti, not muftī).
- English spelling was given to known English place names (Cairo, not Qāhirah; Homs, not Ḥimṣ)
- Transliterations in cited non-Arabic works were left as found in their original source.
- All proper names were transliterated according to previous rules except for modern names when a preferable spelling is known (Maqrīzī, not Maqrizi; Ragab not Rajab)
- *The* was not added to nouns in *Iḍāfah* constructions or nouns starting with *al-* (Bīmāristān al-Sayyidah, not *the* Bīmāristān al-Sayyidah; Bīmāristān Badr, not *the* Bīmāristān Badr; al-Bīmāristān al-Manṣūrī, not *The* al-Bīmāristān al-Manṣūrī).
- An exception to the above rule is when *Iḍāfah* constructions refer to generic institutions. (*the* Dār al-ʿAdl, and *a* Dār al-ʿAdl)
- Unless explicitly mentioned, plural of arabic nouns was created by adding *s*.
- *yāʾ al-nasab* was transliterated as double *yāʾ* (al-ṣāliḥiyyah, not al-ṣālihīyah)

Introduction

> When the Sultan ... al-Manṣūr [Qalāwūn] observed (*ra'ā*) the mausoleum [of al-Ṣāliḥ Ayyūb], he ordered that a mausoleum for himself be built [with] a *madrasa*, a bīmāristān and a *maktab*.[1] So the Quṭbī palace (*al-dār al-Quṭbiyyah*) and [the buildings] beside it were bought from the Sultan's own money (*min khāliṣ māl al-sulṭān*). [The Sultan] appointed the emir ʿAlam al-Dīn al-Shujāʿī to supervise the construction (*mashadan ʿalā al-ʿimārah*). [Al-Shujāʿī] showed unheard of interest and dedication and [the construction] was completed in the shortest time ... in the months of the year 638 [1285 CE]. If one saw this huge construction and heard that it was completed in this short time, he may reject it as false. When the construction was completed, the Sultan endowed (*waqafa*) property, shops, bath-houses, hotels, etc. ..., and dedicated the majority of [the revenue] to the bīmāristān, then to the mausoleum.[2]

Shihāb al-Dīn al-Nuwayrī (d. 1333) placed this account at the opening of his more extensive description of al-Bīmāristān al-Manṣūrī, thus highlighting the significant political and symbolic role of this new complex, erected in the center of the Mamluk empire's capital in 1285. Al-Nuwayrī suggested that it was the mausoleum of al-Ṣāliḥ Ayyūb (r. 1240–1249), the last sovereign of the previous Ayyubid dynasty, that motivated al-Manṣūr Qalāwūn (r. 1279–1290) to build his own. Qalāwūn's complex was built

[1] *Maktab* is usually used to refer to a children's school, where they would learn Quran in addition to reading and writing. The Egyptian historian and scholar Ibn al-Furāt (1334–1405) explained that "al-Manṣūr [Qalāwūn] appointed [in the *maktab*] two scholars (*faqīh*) to teach sixty orphan children ... the Book of God [the Quran]. [He gave them] an appropriate salary and [food] ration for each of them; thirty dirhams a month [as salary] and three pounds of bread a day [as food ration], in addition to a garment in the winter and a garment in the summer. He appropriated for each of the orphans two pounds of bread a day, a garment in the winter and a garment in the summer" (Al-Furāt, *Tārīkh Ibn al-Furāt*, 8:10). The *maktab* was probably the least endowed among the different parts of the Qalawunid complex and is hardly mentioned in the majority of contemporaneous or later sources, but it does give us an idea, by contradistinction, of the size and impact of the other parts of the complex. On *Maktab al-Aytām* (school for orphans), see Little, "Notes on Mamluk Madrasahs," 13.

[2] Al-Nuwayrī, *Nihāyat al-Arab*, 31: 105–06.

just across the street from the Ayyubid mausoleum, rising to literally overshadow the latter as they flanked the most important boulevard in the center of Cairo.[3] Although Qalāwūn's mausoleum was the discursive center of the complex in al-Nuwayrī's account, the bīmāristān was the effective one: it was the most richly endowed of all the different parts of the complex,[4] was the largest in size, and was situated at the physical heart of the complex.[5] In fact, many Mamluk historians, when discussing different events or issues attached to the complex, referred to the entire complex as the Bīmāristān.[6] The complex was built at the height of al-Manṣūr Qalāwūn's career and symbolized the stability of his rule,[7] and, soon enough, the new mausoleum would replace al-Ṣāliḥ Ayyūb's as the center of political and religious events and the bīmāristān would become the heart of an expanding network of charitable institutions that served the growing population of Cairo and its suburb al-Fusṭāṭ.[8]

In building a bīmāristān, al-Manṣūr Qalāwūn was reenacting an old tradition; for centuries, sovereigns had built hospitals as part of their charitable endeavors and also as symbols of their political power and control. An earlier bīmāristān, built ca. 872 by the Abbasid governor of Egypt, Aḥmad b. Ṭūlūn (r. 868–884), was thought to be the first bīmāristān built in Egypt.[9] The ambitious Abbasid governor, aiming to build a dynastic kingdom out of his prized province of Egypt, built a new capital, al-Qaṭāʿiʿ, at the center of which stood the governor's palace, his mosque, and his bīmāristān.[10] The emir and his offspring ruled over Egypt and regions of the Levant from their capital until the Abbasids reconquered the region in 905. In 935, Muḥammad b.Ṭughj al-Ikhshīd was appointed governor of Egypt by the Abbasid caliph and was given the province to rule with his descendants for thirty years. Al-Ikhshīd moved the center of his realm back to the old city of al-Fusṭāṭ and built Bīmāristān al-Ikhshīd there.[11] Medical supplies and

[3] More details on the political significance of the complex and its architecture will be explained in the third chapter of this book. See also al-Harithy, "Space in Mamluk Architecture" and "Urban Form and Meaning."
[4] Al-Furāt, *Tārīkh Ibn al-Furāt*, 8: 9.
[5] Al-Harithy, "Space in Mamluk Architecture."
[6] See, for instance, al-Maqrīzī, *al-Sulūk*.
[7] See Northrup, *From Slave to Sultan*.
[8] For more information on charitable institutions, see Sabra, *Poverty and Charity in Medieval Islam*; Cohen, *Poverty and Charity*; Borgolte and Lohse, *Stiftungen in Christentum, Judentum Und Islam Vor Der Moderne*; Frenkel and Lev (eds.), *Charity and Giving in Monotheistic Religions*.
[9] Al-Maqrīzī, *al-Khiṭaṭ*, 4: 405.
[10] Al-Kindī, *Al-Wulāh wa al-Quḍāh*; al-Balawī, *Sīrat Aḥmad Ibn Ṭūlūn*.
[11] Al-Maqrīzī reported that Bīmāristān al-Ikhshīd was not, in fact, built by Muḥammad b. Ṭughj (the dynasty's patriarch) himself, but rather by his son in 957. See al-Maqrīzī, *al-Khiṭaṭ*, 4: 407.

equipment, including cookware and tools to make medications, were moved from al-Bīmāristān al-Ṭūlūnī to the new bīmāristān, a move symbolic of the change from an older to a newer dynasty.[12] Similarly, when the Fatimids conquered Egypt and removed the Ikhshīdids from power, their victorious general Jawhar al-Ṣiqillī laid the foundation for their new capital Cairo in 969. In their new capital, the Fatimids established a bīmāristān as well, one that – alongside the Caliph's palace and the huge new mosque and college, al-Azhar – represented the new rule.[13] Ultimately, however, Ṣalāḥ al-Dīn (d. 1193), the famous founder of the Ayyubid dynasty and warrior against the Crusaders, dealt the coup de grace to the ailing Fatimid Caliphate (ca. 1171), establishing his own dynasty under nominal Abbasid control. Ṣalāḥ al-Dīn revamped and remodeled Fatimid Cairo by adding a huge citadel and by expanding its walls. At the heart of his remodeled capital, Ṣalāḥ al-Dīn built al-Bīmāristān al-Nāṣirī (named after his honorific title: al-Nāṣir) in 1181 to replace a Fatimid palace built in 994.[14] In the Levent, Nūr al-Dīn Zankī (d. 1174), another warrior against the Crusaders – the true founder of the Zangid dynasty in the Levant and, by turns, Ṣalāḥ al-Dīn's master then enemy, built al-Bīmāristān al-Nūrī in the heart of Damascus, the capital of his growing dominion. In turn, al-Manṣūr Qalāwūn, one of the stronger sovereigns in the new Mamluk empire, built his own bīmāristān that overshadowed his predecessors' monuments.

In all these examples, bīmāristāns were integral parts of a new sovereign's plan. The size of these endeavors and the investments of time, money, and influence needed to make them, made these bīmāristāns political and social edifices that symbolized a ruler's wealth, power, and magnanimity, as well as the stability of his rule and his control over his realm. Their charitable mission symbolized his generosity, piety, and care for his flock and gained him immortality as well as Divine reward. Although many of these bīmāristāns continued to exist alongside their predecessors, newer bīmāristāns were generally envisioned as replacing the old – whether by literally moving supplies and tools from the old to the new (as in the case of Bīmāristān al-Ikhshīd in relation to al-Bīmāristān al-Ṭūlūnī) or by effectively diverting attention and care to

[12] Al-Quḍāʿī, *Tārīkh al-Quḍāʿī*, cited in ʿĪsá, *Tārīkh al-Bīmāristānāt fī al-Islām*, 51. Al-Ikhshīd's bīmāristān was also known as the Lower Bīmāristān (*al-Bīmāristān al-Asfal*) compared to al-Bīmāristān al-Ṭūlūnī (known as *al-Bīmāristān al-Aʿlā* because it was located on higher ground, close to al-Muqattam Hill).

[13] See also Behrens-Abouseif, *Islamic Architecture in Cairo*.

[14] Ibn Jubayr, *Riḥlat Ibn Jubayr*, 21.

the new bīmāristān as the old fell into oblivion (as with al-Bīmāristān al-Manṣūrī in relation to al-Bīmāristān al-Nāṣirī).

Origins and Identities

Since Michael Dols's monumental work on the history of Islamic hospitals, historians of medieval Islamic medicine have continued to regard the "Islamic hospital" as a singular institution that developed sometime in the late ninth or early tenth century in Baghdad and was replicated throughout Islamdom in a basically identical fashion.[15] Moreover, and with few exceptions, hospital historiography has taken the Eastern regions of Islamdom, such as Iraq and Iran, as the major loci for the development of these institutions, tracing the development of hospitals there but overlooking important evidence from the Levant and Egypt because it fell outside the usual scope of analysis. Modern scholarship on medieval Islamic hospitals has also sought to isolate the bīmāristān from other institutions of care and to identify the specific moment at which these institutions became "hospitals." This emphasis on medicalization as a distinguishing factor of the quintessential bīmāristān has led to historians' neglect of an array of institutional developments across Islamdom, as well as – because of perceived similarities attributable to their medical nature – their neglect of many differences between various medical institutions.

Much attention has also been paid to the question of the origin of Islamic hospitals: when was the first hospital built? Can we even call it a hospital? How medicalized was it? And how were these institutions connected to (or disconnected from) a Byzantine and Syriac heritage? As Peter Pormann has recently shown, there is no conclusive contemporaneous evidence confirming later reports that the first "Islamic hospital" was founded by Harūn al-Rashīd (r. 786–809). However, there are clear references to the Bīmāristān in ninth-century writings, such as those by al-Jāḥiẓ (767–868), indicating the existence of an audience aware of and familiar with bimāristāns, probably since the early or mid-ninth century.[16] Similarly, Ibn Ṭūlūn built his bīmāristān in Egypt ca. 872, clearly

[15] See, for instance (before Michael Dols's work), ʿIsá, *Tārīkh al-Bīmāristānāt fī al-Islām*; see also (after Dols) Dunlop, Colin, and Sehsuvaroglu, "Bīmāristān," in *Encyclopedia of Islam*; Pormann, "Islamic Hospitals" and "Medical Methodology and Hospital Practice"; Khafipoor, "A Hospital in Ilkhanid Iran"; Horden, *Hospitals and Healing* and "The Earliest Hospitals"; Hamarneh, "Development of Hospitals in Islam"; Conrad, "Did al-Walid I Found the First Islamic Hospital?"; Baqué, "Du Bimaristan À l'Asile Moderne."

[16] Pormann, "Islamic Hospitals," 352–55.

emulating a model with which he became familiar in the Abbasid capital and major Iraqi cities. All this suggests that the first bīmāristāns were built in the first decades of the ninth century in Baghdad, whether by al-Rashīd, his Persian vizirs the Barmakids, or one of al-Rashīd's sons and successors. Also, the use of the term "bīmāristān" to refer to these institutions suggests an Eastern origin, somewhere in the major Iraqi and Iranian centers.

Despite such inconclusive evidence regarding the origins of the bīmāristān, there is no doubt that, by the tenth century, many of the cities and urban centers in Islamdom knew of this institution. Most Arabophone authors and audiences were able to understand and identify this institution, referring to it as a distinguishable institution within their own social fabric – despite the differences between bīmāristāns in different times and locales. By the end of the twelfth century, Ibn Jubayr (d. 1217), during his pilgrimage from 1183 to 1185, expected to see a bīmāristān in each town he visited, inquiring when he could not find one.[17] The question of the origin of the bīmāristān, or of the date on which the first one was built, has proved itself unanswerable with any accuracy. More significant questions, then, concern what makes a bīmāristān and what role this institution played in society.

When Ibn Jubayr asked about a bīmāristān in Homs, he was told by an older man that the entirety of Homs was a bīmāristān. Undoubtedly, then, neither Ibn Jubayr nor his interlocutor understood the "bīmāristān" in this statement as simply a place for the sick. Instead, both men, as well as Ibn Jubayr's readers, understood the bīmāristān primarily as a site of charitable care and support, as part of the growing network of charitable institutions at the heart of the medieval Islamicate urban center that were very helpful to travelers like Ibn Jubayr himself.[18] Although bīmāristāns stood out from other charitable institutions because of their ostensible concern for health and disease, it seems that their fundamental character was found in their charitable mission, their role within a network of support for the poor, travelers, the sick, and the disabled. In this view, its "specialization" in caring for the sick and tired or its ostensible commitment to medicine should not be seen as an exclusionary function (as if a particular bīmāristān

[17] Ibn Jubayr, *Riḥlat Ibn Jubayr*, 246.

[18] See Frenkel and Lev (eds.), *Charity and Giving in Monotheistic Religions*; Pahlitzsch, "Christian Pious Foundations"; Lev, "Ethics of Islamic Medieval Charity"; Borgolte and Lohse, *Stiftungen in Christentum, Judentum Und Islam Vor Der Moderne*; Sabra, *Poverty and Charity in Medieval Islam*; Bonner, Ener, and Singer (eds.), *Poverty and Charity in Middle Eastern Contexts*. For the non-Islamic context of the region, see Cohen, *Poverty and Charity*; Galinsky, "Jewish Charitable Bequests." See also Brodman, *Hospitals and the Poor in Medieval Catalonia*.

would not accept anyone who was not clearly identifiable as "sick"). Rather, this care was inclusionary in its institutional scope, as one among a number of other sites of charitable care. That is, the bīmāristān would welcome anyone, but would have a specific advantage in supporting populations with specific needs. In a similar way, sabils were better suited to care for the thirsty, hostels in providing housing, and khānaqāhs as a place for Sufis, and so forth. The bīmāristān, thus, would have been approached by those it could serve best.

This approach makes the question of medicalization redundant. It suggests a gradual, nonlinear, and inconsistent medicalization. It also does not trace a progressive trajectory, does not ask how "developed" these institutions were, or whether they might legitimately be recognized as "hospitals." Rather, this approach argues that bīmāristāns acquired their social identity through their charitable existence and attention to the sick and tired – regardless of how effectively this attention was mediated by learned medical practitioners and regardless of the extent to which these practitioners controlled the institution or determined its trajectory.[19] That being said, there is no doubt that certain bīmāristāns could boast of the services of some of the most highly recognized Galenists in the region. However, there is little evidence that bīmāristāns grew consistently more medicalized with time or that these institutions based their identities on how medicalized they were.

That being said, bīmāristāns played a significant role in medical education and training, which was in fact part of their charitable role as well. For instance, al-Bīmāristān al-Manṣūrī required the chief physician of the Mamluk capital to give public medical lectures that would be available to those seeking medical education but who did not have access to the more exclusive relations of apprenticeship.[20] Ibn Abī Uṣaybiʿah, similar to other physicians, discussed the details of his own training at al-Bīmāristān al-Nūrī in Damascus, where a student or a young physician would accompany a master as the latter practiced in the bīmāristān and examined

[19] The emphasis on the charitable role of the bīmāristān can be seen in other regions and other periods as well. See, for instance, Pormann's discussion of Abbasid Bīmāristāns, in which a charitable role is equally evident ("Medical Methodology and Hospital Practice"). Contemporaneous institutions in Europe maintained a similar focus on charity and care for the poor; see Henderson, *The Renaissance Hospital*.

[20] Ibn Ḥabīb, *Tadhkirat al-Nabīh*, 1: 366. According to the *OED*, a *waqf* is, "[i]n Islamic countries, the custom of giving a piece of land [or other property], etc., to a religious institution, so that the revenue can be used for pious or charitable purposes; also, the property given in this way" (for full reference list: "wakf | waqf, n."). OED Online. September 2014. www.oed.com/view/Entry/225194?redirectedFrom=waqf (accessed November 20, 2014).

patients. Students and young physicians were often given the opportunity to read and discuss medical texts with their masters after a day of examining patients. Ibn Abī Uṣaybiʿah seemed to have particularly valued attending discussions among the masters of the profession serving together in al-Bīmāristān al-Nūrī.[21] Here, we find what appear to be two distinct methods of medical education. The first method is reminiscent of public lectures in mosques and madrasa, which were ostensibly open to everyone. There were other public lectures on medicine, such as the one in the Tūlūnid mosque, that continued to exist well into the fifteenth century. This practice was not concerned with the actual education of attendees (since much of medical education required an apprenticeship), but rather with disseminating medical knowledge and with opening spaces for more Muslim students to join the ranks of the profession, as will be shown later.[22] These lectures were also part of the patron's pietistic and charitable endeavor, where the bīmāristān resembled madrasas as sites for education.[23] The second method, described by Ibn Abī Uṣaybiʿah and other physicians, is similar to Vivian Nutton's portrayal of medical training in Byzantine Nosokomeia, where the main method was apprenticeship: students followed their masters in the Nosokomeion as they did elsewhere.[24] Similar apprenticeship procedures are described in Ibn Abī Uṣaybiʿah's biographies of some of his masters and contemporaries whose education appears to have been connected to their masters, each of whom worked in a bīmāristān; students trained where their masters worked, but the bīmāristān itself was not an independent site of medical education.

Finally, bīmāristāns were largely urban institutions, found in different cities and urban centers to serve the growing population of urban poor.[25] These structures, whether built de novo, from other repurposed structures, or from renovated older bīmāristāns, played a significant role in shaping the local urban environment. For instance, the mere physical existence of al-Bīmāristān al-Manṣūrī altered the structure of Cairo's central corridor and influenced the movement of people in what were Cairo's busiest avenues.[26] A century earlier, when Ṣalāḥ al-Dīn decided to build al-Bīmāristān al-Nāṣirī in Cairo, he chose to convert one of the more

[21] See Ibn Abī Usaybiʿah, *ʿUyūn al-Anbāʾ*, 3: 189–95. Pormann's analysis of al-Kaskari's *kannash* and the bīmāristāns mentioned there shows the presence of libraries, books, and also lessons of medicine. See Pormann, "Islamic Hospitals," 345–52.

[22] Lewicka, *Medicine for Muslims?*

[23] Northrup, "Qalawun's Patronage."

[24] Nutton, " 'Birth of the Hospital,' Essay Review."

[25] Bonner, "Rise of the Muslim Urban Poor."

[26] Al-Harithy, "Space in Mamluk Architecture."

luxurious pavilions in the Fatimid Caliphal Palace in the center of Fatimid Cairo into a bīmāristān to serve the poor. This new bīmāristān opened up to the public the center of the Fatimid city and its most sacred and revered site – the seat of the Caliphs and the sacred cemetery of the Imams who were buried inside the palace complex – transforming a seat of government into a site for the poor. Although Ṣalāḥ al-Dīn's repurposed structure did not alter the physical appearance of the city, it dramatically changed its population traffic by bringing travelers, students, the sick, and the poor into what had originally been a closed-off quarter of the royal city.

In these cases – al-Bīmāristān al-Manṣūrī, al-Nāṣirī, and many others – the location of the bīmāristān was directly connected to the specific population it intended to serve: either that population already frequented the city, as in al-Manṣūrī's case, or the bīmāristān purposefully attracted its population to its locale, as in al-Nāṣirī's case. Alternatively, Crusader hospitals, along with other charitable structures intended for pilgrims of different traditions, were not necessarily intended to serve local residing urban populations (although they probably did so as well). Instead, they focused on serving the potential population of those traveling for pilgrimage. Their locations on pilgrimage routes and their sizes, which sometimes exceeded the needs of residing populations, were directly related to their imagined and intended audiences. In these different iterations, bīmāristāns were social institutions, performing a number of functions in medieval Islamicate cities whose stories cannot be reduced simply to their medical, charitable, or political roles. More importantly, the complex identity of this institution requires that special attention be paid to regional variations, different trajectories, and local traditions that may have played a role in their development.

Book Organization

Focusing on al-Bīmāristān al-Manṣūrī (built ca. 1285), this book attempts to address several aspects of the history of Islamic hospitals in Egypt and the Levant from the twelfth to fourteenth centuries. This period witnessed the creation of large bīmāristāns in this region, ranging from al-Bīmāristān al-Nūrī in Damascus and al-Ṣalāḥī in Jerusalem, to al-Nāṣirī and al-Manṣūrī in Cairo. During the same time period, the region witnessed the rise of Crusader Xenodocheia, with the Jerusalem Xenodocheion and House of the Hospitaller Order located at the center of a constellation of houses spreading across pilgrimage routes from Latin Europe to Jerusalem. Whereas Islamic literary sources hardly describe any influence or interaction between these Crusader institutions and the Islamicate ones, it is hard to imagine how al-Bīmāristān al-Ṣalāḥī in Jerusalem, built in part on the grounds of the House of the Hospitallers, could fail to be influenced by such an institution or by the century-long practices that prevailed in the city throughout Crusader rule. It is also safe to assume that Crusader institutions were influenced by neighboring Islamic institutions – including the bīmāristān, which functioned in Jerusalem before the Crusades and that Nāṣir-i Khusraw (d. 1088) saw in his visit to Jerusalem in 1047.[27] Although this book tries to highlight these connections, there is much work to be done in writing an integrated history of these charitable institutions in the Levant.

The prologue analyzes institutions of charitable and collective care in late antiquity, thus providing a historical background for charitable practice in the twelfth to fourteenth centuries. It discusses Byzantine and Syriac Xenodocheia, as well as the Islamicate institutions that developed in the eighth and ninth centuries in a manner consistent with pre-Islamic traditions. It analyzes the accounts of Gundisapur, which represent a significant chapter in the historiography of bīmāristāns but have recently raised much doubt. The prologue traces the origins of these narratives about the Syriac-Sassanid-Abbasid center. Finally, the prologue compares near-contemporary bīmāristāns in Iraq and Egypt in an attempt to discern possible differences among these institutions in these different regions.

Part I of the book, composed of three chapters, looks at al-Bīmāristān al-Manṣūrī as a story of royal patronage, seeking this institution's location within the history of its patron and within the precedents established by earlier sovereigns. This part of the book also draws special attention to the bīmāristān as an architectural monument symbolic of its patron's power and piety[28] and illustrates how earlier bīmāristāns in Egypt and the Levant functioned in the same manner. Chapter 1 will address the Levantine precedents: in particular, al-Bīmāristān al-Nūrī (seen within Nūr al-Dīn Zankī's program of architectural patronage), the Crusader Xenodocheion of Jerusalem, and Ṣalāḥ al-Dīn's al-Bīmāristān al-Ṣalāḥī in the city. The connections between al-Manṣūr Qalāwūn and Nūr al-Dīn, and between their two bīmāristāns, were referenced many times by historians contemporary to al-Bīmāristān al-Manṣūrī; these references indicate that Qalāwūn and his elites were deeply impressed and influenced by the Zangid ruler.

[27] Khusraw, *Nāṣer-E Khosraw's Book of Travels (Safarnāma)*, 23.

[28] See Pruitt, "Fatimid Architectural Patronage and Changing Sectarian Identities (969–1021)"; O'Kane, "Monumentality in Mamluk and Mongol Art and Architecture"; Williams, "Urbanization and Monument Construction in Mamluk Cairo."

Moreover, Qalāwūn renovated al-Bīmāristān al-Nūrī early in his reign, adding on new wings and new *waqfs*, thus further demonstrating his connection to the Zangid ruler and to his bīmāristān. In Jerusalem, where both al-Bīmāristān al-Ṣalāḥī and the Crusader Xenodocheion continued to function into the thirteenth and fourteenth centuries, Qalāwūn was also interested in creating a number of establishments of his own. These included a bīmāristān (also called al-Bīmāristān al-Manṣūrī) located in the city of Hebron, which was connected to Jerusalem, as will be discussed later. In all these cases, the earlier bīmāristāns of the Levant constituted points of inspiration, forming the historical and architectural backdrop of al-Bīmāristān al-Manṣūrī.

Chapter 2 moves to Cairo, opening with a background discussion of the city and the formation of its politico-architectural landscape over time, ending with the Ayyubid-Mamluk city. The chapter then discusses the works of Ṣalāḥ al-Dīn in Cairo, focusing on al-Bīmāristān al-Nāṣirī, which was located only some hundred meters from al-Bīmāristān al-Manṣūrī. This is followed by an examination of Qalāwūn's architectural patronage throughout his ten-year reign, as well as the place of al-Bīmāristān al-Manṣūrī within this larger plan of architectural patronage, and addresses the bīmāristān's location, its planning, and its inauguration. Chapter 3 begins with a discussion of Qalāwūn's medical patronage via an analysis of the three main documents of his medical patronage surviving from the period: namely, the bīmāristān's *waqf* document, as well as the two decrees appointing the chief physician and the lecturer in medicine to the bīmāristān. These documents help us further understand the process of medical patronage in this period. This chapter's analysis of the *waqf* document sheds light on the bīmāristān's administration, its finances, and the different rules by which it was governed. It is important to remember that the *waqf* document does not represent a statement of actuality but rather a statement of legality; it outlined how the bīmāristān was *supposed* to function rather than describing how it actually did so. The discussion will be supplemented by some contemporaneous accounts that help us discern some of the details of the bīmāristān's functioning.

The book's second part focuses on medical practice in al-Bīmāristān al-Manṣūrī and other bīmāristāns in Egypt and the Levant. The first chapter in this part attempts to paint an intellectual landscape for medical practice at that time. It traces a circle of physicians and medical authors who gathered around a Baghdadi emigre named Muhadhdhab al-Dīn al-Naqqāsh (d. 1178). Al-Naqqāsh came to Damascus, worked for Nūr al-Dīn, and contributed to the foundation of al-Bīmāristān al-Nūrī; he was himself a student of the famous Baghdadi physician Amīn al-Dawlah ibn al-Tilmīdh, and together they worked in al-Bīmāristān al-ʿAḍudī, one of Baghdad's largest and most celebrated bīmāristāns. Al-Naqqāsh's students – Ibn al-Muṭrān, al-Raḥbī, and Ibn al-Muṭrān's student al-Dakhwār among others – would become the major medical figures in the Ayyubid context. Their own students would, furthermore, come to dominate the medical scene under the Mamluks and would include among their number those who presided over the medical practitioners at al-Bīmāristān al-Manṣūrī. The chapter analyzes their writings, the books they read, and their approach to practice, ultimately arguing that they represented an important shift in medical thought and practice that impacted the major bīmāristāns of those regions – namely al-Nūrī and al-Manṣūrī – up through the fourteenth century.

The final chapter in Part II describes medical practice and patients' experiences at al-Bīmāristān al-Manṣūrī. Using medical texts and accounts of patients from various sources, the chapter addresses medical examination and medical thinking, describes how physicians and medical practitioners thought in the bīmāristān, and questions whether the bīmāristān required different types of medical thinking. The chapter "walks through" the physical structure of al-Bīmāristān al-Manṣūrī and attempts to describe the patient's experience, the different interactions he or she might have had, and the system for classifying patients in the bīmāristān. Finally, the chapter analyzes *al-Dustūr al-Bīmāristānī* – a drug formulary used at al-Bīmāristān al-Nāṣirī and then at al-Manṣūrī – and ends by comparing it to market formularies known at that time.

Prologue: A Tale of Two Bīmāristāns

A Deep Inquiry: Care and Cure in Late Antiquity

The history of institutions providing collective (medical) care in the Middle East can be traced back to the middle of the fourth century, when St. Leontius of Antioch (d. 358) built his xenodochion. "A little later, in the late 350s or 360s, Eustathius of Sebaste (or Sivas, in northern Turkey) built a ptochotropheion: literally, a place in which beggars were nourished. Shortly thereafter, St. Basil established his charitable 'multiplex' for the sick, the paralyzed, lepers, and strangers, a 'new city.' "[1] Saint John Chrysostom (d. 404), bishop of Constantinople, built a similar institution in the capital, which his biographer called "Nosokomion."[2] These early examples of Byzantine hospitals were closely connected to the Church and represented part of an emergent philanthropic tendency that would come to characterize Byzantine society for centuries.[3] In this context, philanthropy was not perceived as an individual or even as a simple collective act; rather, it signified belonging to the growing Byzantine Church – an institution now embraced by the imperial throne – and thus became a governing characteristic in the Byzantine performance of piety. Peter Brown argues that the early Church, especially in the Eastern Roman and Byzantine provinces, attempted to replace the earlier model of Roman civic belonging with a universal belonging to Christ and to the Church. In doing so it introduced novel institutions that established the bishop's position at the top of this new mode of belonging and, in so doing, replaced the nobleman of antiquity who protected the Roman civic structure and provided care and support for its citizens. Brown argues that "the

[1] Horden, "The Earliest Hospitals," 366.

[2] Miller, "Byzantine Hospitals," 54–55. Miller's work eventually came under attack because of his interpretation of sources and his anachronistic views regarding the medicalization of Byzantine institutions of care. See Nutton, " 'The Birth of the Hospital in the Byzantine Empire,' Essay Review."

[3] Constantelos, *Byzantine Philanthropy.*

poor," a concept signifying a group of people deserving charity, was at many levels the invention of the bishops.[4] The examples of "hospitals" cited here were only part of an expanding array of philanthropic institutions that aimed not only to exemplify Christian, Eastern Roman/Byzantine ideals, but also created and defined "the poor" as a category carrying social and pietistic significance.[5]

Xenodocheia continued to arise in different cities, towns, and other political and commercial centers: "Between 400 and 600, several xenons were built in Constantinople. The Sampson, the Euboulos, and the St. Irene in Perama were established before 500. The St. Panteleimon and probably the Christodotes were added before 600 . . . The great commercial cities of Antioch and Alexandria possessed a number of hospitals by the sixth century."[6] This Byzantine institution was an urban phenomenon par excellence and was as much a part of the new urban Christian environment as it was a tool for its Christianization: the *xenodocheion* provided a locus of care for the weak, the sick, and the foreigner, each of whom could be defined and identified only in relation to the strong, the healthy, and the local. In the course of the development of the new Byzantine Christian community, the institution of the Xenon and/or Nosokomion functioned as a cornerstone in how that community constructed both "the self" and "the other," serving also to justify and symbolize the new society's values. "In major cases, such as St. Basil's cluster of philanthropic foundations outside Caesarea in the early 370s, hospitals can even provide new focuses for urban or sub-urban space. The 'Basileias' was lauded as a 'new city' not only because, in Brown's terms, it exemplified the novel significance of episcopal 'love of the poor' but also because, like some extramural shrine or new church building, the hospital complex offered a topographical challenge to the established center of Caesarea."[7]

The roles *xenodocheia* played in the urban environment also influenced how Byzantine elite societies – both clerical and imperial – imagined their own philanthropic responsibilities. With precedents having been set by some of the Church fathers, the Byzantine Church and the Emperor became the most important patrons of these institutions, establishing iterations of *xenodocheia* in different urban areas in order to illustrate their generosity, piety, and care for the poor. Whereas the

[4] Brown, *Authority and the Sacred*. On the role of charity in constructing the relationship between the Church and the poor, see also Grey, *Constructing Communities*; Mayer, "Patronage, Pastoral Care."

[5] Horden, "The Earliest Hospitals," 362–63.

[6] Miller, "Byzantine Hospitals," 56.

[7] Horden, "The Earliest Hospitals," 364.

first *xenodocheion* in Constantinople was established by Saint John Chrysostom, the capital's bishop, emperors also appeared to have embraced the tradition, constructing more hospitals in the capital city and elsewhere. Emperor Maurice (d. 602) built a hospital in his native town of Arabissi in Cappadocia. Empress Irene (d. 803), who ruled over the empire in the wake of the iconoclasm controversy, built a new hospital in her name in Constantinople. Emperor Theophilos (d. 842) followed Irene's example and established another large hospital. And so the tradition continued, culminating in the famous Pantokrator Xenon built by John II Komnenos (d. 1143).[8]

Historians disagree on the degree of medicalization of these different Byzantine institutions. Whereas Miller argues that Byzantine hospitals were highly medicalized institutions that employed expanding medical staffs and were eventually run by medical practitioners,[9] Vivian Nutton and others question Miller's conclusions and argue that these Byzantine institutions were largely institutions of collective care that provided support to the poor.[10] Horden, too, argues that although they may have employed medical practitioners, it is unlikely that they were as medicalized as Miller suggests.[11] By the seventh century, the major urban centers of the Byzantine Levant and Egypt probably enjoyed a host of charitable institutions that were largely affiliated with and patronized by the Church and by the empire and that served the poor and the sick, as well as travelers, strangers, and pilgrims, with little distinction among these categories. These establishments included leprosaria, hospices, and other institutions that served beggars as well as the crippled and the old. When Damascus, the capital of Byzantine Syria, was conquered by the Arabs in September 635, a host of these institutions existed alongside its famous Basilica of Saint John the Baptist at the city's center. The Basilica – seat of the Bishop of Damascus, who ranked second in the patriarchate of Antioch following the Patriarch – continued to serve the Christian population of Damascus under Muslim rule until the Umayyad mosque was built in its place, repurposing much of its material and architecture, in 706. Like other important Byzantine cities and dioceses, Damascus enjoyed various

[8] Miller, "Byzantine Hospitals," 57. However, as Vivian Nutton explained, although "the hospital was an important institution in Byzantium . . ., it took very much a second place to treatment in the home by a privately engaged and self-employed physician" (Nutton, " 'Birth of the Hospital,' Essay Review," 221).

[9] See Miller, "Byzantine Hospitals."

[10] Nutton, "'Birth of the Hospital,' Essay Review."

[11] Horden, *Hospitals and Healing*.

Church-related charitable institutions, including those serving the sick, the poor, the old, crippled, and also lepers.[12]

In the Eastern Levant, Syriac communities, located in the borderlands between the Byzantines and the Sassanids, continued church traditions of providing support and care for the poor and for travelers. In 370, during a famine, Saint Ephrem the Syrian (c. 306–373) "set up a hospice with three hundred beds for the poor and the homeless."[13] Saint Ephrem, who was born and lived his early life in Nisbis, had moved by that time to Diyarbakir and then to Edessa, where he established his hospice; evidence also suggests the existence of a *nosokomeion* fifty years later. "Rabulla, bishop of [Edessa] from about AD 411 to 435, founded permanent hospitals, one for men and one for women, and he endowed them with an annual income of about one thousand denarii. The beds were reportedly soft and clean, and the bishop used ascetics of both sexes as attendants. He saw it as his highest duty to supervise the hospices: to visit the sick, to respect them, and to greet them with a kiss."[14] Edessa continued to be an important center for Syriac-speaking Christianity for years to come until it was effectively eclipsed by the school of Nisbis.[15] Although St. Ephrem's three hundred-bed hospice was huge, its size might have been related to the famine in Edessa. However, the presence of this hospice suggests clearly that the Church's tradition of establishing different institutions of care for the strangers, the poor, and the sick, along with leprosaria, was alive and well in older centers of Syriac Christianity around Diyarbakir, Edessa, and Nisbis – and this was well before the Nestorian Schism and the separation of these centers from the Byzantine Church.

Following Rabbula's death in 435, his successor to the bishopric, Ibas of Edessa (d. 457), reversed Rabbula's teachings and policies – antagonistic to Nestorian teachings – thereby further deepening the rift caused by Nestorianism.[16] In 489, Emperor Zeno (d. 491) ordered the closure of

[12] See Khalek, *Damascus after the Muslim Conquest.*

[13] Dols, "The Origins of the Islamic Hospital," 372.

[14] Ibid.

[15] The accounts of the school of Nisbis "replacing" the School of the Persians in Edessa originate in Barḥadbeshabbā's writings from the sixth century (Barḥadbeshabbā and Scher, *Cause de la Fondation des Écoles*). Recently, Adam Becker has attempted to add more nuance to the connection between the two schools and argued that the school of Nisbis was not the "successor" of the School of the Persians in Edessa and that more innovation in the administration and organization of the School of Nisbis could be detected in the sources than previously thought (Becker, *Fear of God*, 77–97).

[16] Ibas of Edessa was fiercely attacked for his perceived Nestorian sympathies and was put to trial first in Tyre and then in Beirut, removed from office, and jailed. He was later acquitted and returned to his position in Edessa until his death. In spite of his anathematizing Nestorius, the Syrian Orthodox Church anathematized Ibas as a Nestorian. The events of Ibas's reign are evidence of the strong

the School of the Persians in Edessa on account of its Nestorian sympathies. Many of the scholars in Edessa immigrated to Nisbis, which was then under Sassanid Persian control.[17] The growth of Nestorian teachings and the growing tensions in Edessa – as well as in other centers of Syriac Christianity – during the second half of the fifth century did not impact the continuity of the Byzantine Church's charitable traditions. In fact, St. Nonnus (d. 471), who succeeded Ibas as bishop of Edessa, built a hospital and a leper house close to his monastery.[18] However, the Nestorian Schism, accompanied by the rise of the school of Nisbis (which was under Sassanid control), allowed for the development of a variation on these charitable initiatives and projects in the new Syriac-Sassanid urban centers. Deprived of state sponsorship and support, and relying heavily on the Syriac Church, these establishments would acquire a new identity. An anonymous author wrote in the Syriac chronicle known as the "Chronicle of Zachariah of Mitylene" (also Zachariah the Rhetor) – the composition of which was possibly completed in the city of Diyarbakir (Syriac: Amida) in 569 – about the Sassanid emperor Khusraw (Chosroes) I (r. 531–579) in the context of the years 553–556:

> Out of kindness towards the captives and the holy men he has now by the advice of the Christian physicians attached to him made a hospital, a thing not previously known, and has given 100 mules and 50 camels laden with goods (?) 10 from the royal stores, and 12 physicians, and whatever is required is given.[19]

The report also mentions Catholicos Joseph, who was the Patriarch of the Church of the East in Selecucia-Ctesiphon (the Sassanid capital) from 552 to 567. Joseph was Chosroes I's physician, and was apparently close to the emperor: "Joseph . . ., the Catholic of the Christians, is high in his [Chosroes I's] confidence, and is closely attached to him, because he is a physician, and he sits before him on the first seat after the chief of the Magians, and whatever he asks of him he receives."[20] Joseph, however, was hated and despised by his own bishops because his appointment appeared to have come from the Sassanid emperor rather than from the Church's

tensions in this part of the Byzantine world, which would eventually result in the migration of many Nestorians (back) to Nisbis while it was under Sassanid control. See Becker, *Sources for the History of the School of Nisibis.*

[17] Hunter, "The Transmission of Greek Philosophy." See also Drijvers, *The School of Edessa.*

[18] Dols, "The Origins of the Islamic Hospital," 472.

[19] Bishop of Mytilene Zacharias et al., *The Syriac Chronicle Known as That of Zachariah of Mitylene*, 336–37.

[20] Zacharias et al., *The Syriac Chronicle Known as That of Zachariah of Mitylene*, 336.

hierarchy. The bishops even deposed him, but did not replace him because they feared Chosroes's wrath. Joseph spent the last three years of his life as the official Catholicos and Patriarch of the Church in the eyes of the Sassanid empire, but as a deposed Patriarch in the eyes of his own bishops.[21] What is significant in this story is that the new hospital mentioned in the chronicle seems to have been an innovation in the Sassanid context and that it was a gift from the emperor to his favorite physician(s), whom he trusted and whose instructions he followed leading him to change his diet and his regular habits.[22]

A few decades earlier, in the beginning of the sixth century, another influential Syriac physician named Qashwi had influenced the Sassanid court to help the school of Nisbis establish a *xenodocheion* for the students: "The School was expanded in the early sixth century with the help of Qashwi, an influential physician at the Sasanian court. The director of the School, Abraham de-Bet Rabban, first built for [the students] a hospice [*xenodocheion*] in order that they would not need to roam in the town and be plundered and dishonored."[23] In addition to the *xenodocheion*, two bathhouses were also built to serve the students. The Xenodocheion of Nisbis also figures in the biography of Mar Babai (d. 628), who learned medicine in the Xenodocheion before embarking on his trips of miraculous healings and conversions.[24] Joseph's Xenodocheion, too, was probably built for students, monks, and other clergymen; our chronicler explained that it was built for the "captives and the holy men"–"captives" is the term the chronicler used to describe clergymen and other educated people captured by the Sassanids from Byzantine territories. The two *xenodocheia*, both Nisbis's (ca. 510) and Joseph's (between 552 and 567), were not new in the Syriac context and were simply contemporary iterations of older

[21] Bar Hebraeus, *Chronography*.

[22] Zacharias et al., *The Syriac Chronicle Known as That of Zachariah of Mitylene*, 336. The chronicler explained how the (Syriac Christian) physicians advised the king to change his diet and move away from dead animals and from blood. "For one week of years [seven years] the king of Persia also, as those who know relate, has separated himself from the eating of things strangled and blood, and from the flesh of unclean beasts and birds, from the time when Tribonian the archiatros came down to him, who was taken captive at that time . . . From that time he has understood his food, and his food is not polluted according to the former practice, but rather it is blessed, and then he eats." It is noteworthy to consider the title "archiatros" that the chronicler gave to the Christian Syriac physician who accompanied the Sassanid Emperor.

[23] Dols, "The Origins of the Islamic Hospital," 374.

[24] Scher, *Histoire Nestorienne Inédite*. This Syriac chronicle survived only in Arabic translation from the tenth century. Here, the term *xenodocheion* is translated as "bīmāristān," showing how the earlier Syriac institution was converted to the Arabic/Islamic term. It is important to note that the word bīmāristān (lit. house of the sick) comes from Middle Persian and may have been used by the multilingual Syriacs (like Mar Babai himself) as a Persian equivalent to *xenodocheion*.

Byzantine practices. However, they were new to the Sassanid context and had no local precedents.

These *xenodocheia* stand out on another level as well: they indicate that these Syriac elite physicians within the Sassanid court viewed the Xenodocheion as an institution they ought to support and also that the Sassanid emperor considered this construction a gift to his physician(s). Our chronicler clearly linked this establishment to the physicians, their presence in the court, and their closeness to the emperor, since he located the account within a discussion of medicine, diet, and the physicians' proximity to the emperor. Dols adds, "The passage is also important for defining the Syriac Xenodocheion as a medical institution, that is, an institution with medical personnel."[25] Although there is no reason to assume a much higher degree of "medicalization" in the Syriac *xenodocheion* than in its Byzantine contemporaries, the Syriac institution was more closely linked to physicians, who were among the more distinguished members of the community and the closest to Sassanid elites. For this Syriac elite, the *xenodocheion* was becoming a more natural avenue for charity. For their patrons, building a *xenodocheion* was not only an act of patronizing the Church but, possibly more significantly, an act of patronizing their own physicians and clients.

The next main account of Syriac *xenodocheia* comes from the late eighth to early ninth century in the letters of Timothy I, the Patriarch of the Church of the East from 780 to 823. Timothy I, who was close to the Abbasid court, moved the Patriarchate from the old Sassanid capital to Baghdad, signaling a new chapter in the life of the Syriac Church. In his letters to Sergius – a physician and the metropolitan of Khuzistan (in the southeast of modern Iran, bordering Iraq and the Persian Gulf) – Timothy explained that he was sending one of his students to learn medicine with Sergius in Gundeshapur, which was the metropole of Khuzistan.[26] Timothy also raised funds to build a "bīmāristān" in Selecucia-Ctesiphon.[27] This bīmāristān may have simply been a renovation of the old fifth-century *xenodocheion*, which may have continued to serve the seat of the Patriarchate in different capacities until then. Most remaining accounts of Syriac institutions come from Arabic sources and focus on Gundisapur as a city where a major academy and hospital had existed for centuries; as Dols explains, there are no Syriac or Sassanid sources proving

[25] Dols, "The Origins of the Islamic Hospital: Myth and Reality," 373.

[26] Macdonald, Twomey, and Reinink, *Learned Antiquity*, 165.

[27] Ibid.

the existence of such a large establishment in Gundisapur prior to Islamic control of the Sassanid empire in the seventh century.

The story of Islamic hospitals has always been connected to Gundisapur, following many of the accounts of the hospital found in Abbasid sources; these accounts cannot, however, be supported by other contemporary or older non-Islamic accounts.[28] Whereas Nisbis was clearly an important school in the Syriac Christian environment, and evidence suggests the existence of a *xenodocheion* there, there is little evidence that the theological school in Gundisapur enjoyed similar repute or influence. However, Gundisapur was not an obscure city; rather, it was the metropole of the Syriac Church's oldest metropolitan seat in Khuzistan and had boasted a theological school since the sixth century, which was supervised by the metropolitan. As in Nisbis and other major Syriac centers, Gundisapur's school and church establishments included a small *xenodocheion* that served the metropole's church subjects – and which may have provided some form of medical education similar to what we saw in Nisbis,[29] thus explaining Timothy's letters. As will be explained later, the exaggerated claims about Gundisapur can be traced to the major medical families from that city who immigrated to Baghdad under the Abbasids. These families, such as Banū Bakhtīshūʿ, propagated an elaborate narrative of the greatness of the old Syriac-Sassanid city, which may not have been accurate. Yet, the actual presence of these medical families, with their students, clients, and protégés, proves that Gundisapur enjoyed a Syriac medical community during the eighth and ninth centuries that was closely connected to a *xenodocheion* (although it may have been much smaller than Islamic sources suggest).

In the previous pages, we witnessed the gradual development of Christian charitable institutions – such as *xenodocheia* and *nosokomeia* – in the Byzantine Levant and Asia Minor, beginning in the late fourth century and progressing into the seventh. These institutions were largely supported by the Byzantine Church and gradually became part of the Imperial structure as well, prompting a number of Byzantine emperors to sponsor their own institutions. There is little evidence to suggest that these institutions were highly medicalized or were exclusively concerned with sick people. Instead, they appear to have been focused on the service of the poor and needy, even though many were more populated with the sick, the crippled, or the leper. In any case, these institutions were part of a

[28] See Pormann, "Islamic Hospitals in the Time of al-Muqtadir."
[29] Dols, "The Origins of the Islamic Hospital," 377.

widespread philanthropy that originated in the "centralized" Byzantine Church and Empire and eventually was extended to the new "citizens" of the Church-Empire. Institutions were unmistakably connected to cathedrals and monasteries and were located in the urban centers whose populations they aimed to serve.

Syriac institutions were originally an extension of these Byzantine institutions and were built in the same manner under the sponsorship of bishops and metropoles. However, the nature of the *xenodocheia* changed over time with the gradual isolation of the Church of the East from the Byzantine Church; these Eastern institutions were also influenced by their location in Sassanid domains, where other forms of charity already existed and where the major centralized forms of charity came from Zoroastrian institutions.[30] The *xenodocheia* eventually came to be confined within the walls of monasteries and academies, did not offer substantive support to the neighboring population, and were probably built by different metropolitans and bishops with little, if any, aid from the Sassanid elites to support students and clergymen. The only connections between the Sassanid elites and the *xenodochia* arose through the Syriac physicians, who were becoming the most influential Syriac Christians in the Sassanid court. Sassanid patrons provided support to their physicians with the construction of the *xenodocheia*, which had become deeply connected to the physicians' careers and lives. It is safe to assume that these physicians, and probably their students and protégés, were serving and teaching their art (to varying degrees) in these infirmaries and that they saw these infirmaries as an important part of their practice.

Byzantine *xenodochia* continued primarily as charitable institutions intended to symbolize the Church's and the Emperor's philanthropy and care for their subjects. They were commonplace in Byzantine urban life; the emergence of "the poor" necessitated philanthropic care for the weak, the hungry, the pilgrim, the crippled, the sick, the leper, and the like. Syriac *xenodochia*, however, served a narrower population; they were often restricted to students and clergymen, seeking to protect them from being "plundered and dishonored" in the city.[31] Their impact on their urban surroundings, then, was less than that of their Byzantine counterparts. The differences in institutional priorities and intended audience, size, and the perceived roles of physicians and medical practitioners played a significant role in defining the

[30] On charity in the Zoroastrian context, see Boyce, "The Pious Foundations of the Zoroastrians"; Stewart, "The Politics of Zoroastrian Philanthropy."

[31] Dols, "The Origins of the Islamic Hospital: Myth and Reality," 374.

different Islamic institutions that eventually inherited both these variants on institutions of care, as will be shown in the following sections.

The (New) Islamicate Story

Over the first half of the seventh century, Muslim armies operating under different caliphs and different leaders gained control of Egypt and the Byzantine Levant by 645,[32] as well as over all the territories in Mesopotamia and Iran previously controlled by the Sassanid Empire, which ceased to exist by 644.[33] Along with the acquisition of these territories, revenues, and peoples, the newly formed Muslim empire inherited institutional structures, imperial traditions, and establishments that were left in place by the two major late-antiquity empires.[34] Such establishments included churches and temples but also a variety of charitable institutions – including the Byzantine *xenodochia* and leprosaria and the Syriac *xenodochia* – that were attached to different structures of religious or political patronage. The Umayyad Caliphate, which consolidated its rule in 661, moved the capital from Medina to Damascus; doing so signaled a new era, during which Byzantine influences would become more pronounced in many aspects of Umayyad rule.

Under the fifth Umayyad Caliph, ʿAbd al-Malik b. Marwān (r. 685–705), the Umayyads commenced an Arabization of state records,[35] and ʿAbd al-Malik issued orders to mint a coin carrying his own image as the first coin ever minted by the Caliphate (Figure P.2.1).[36] ʿAbd al-Malik also started

[32] In *Maghāzī* literature (Islamic sources describing the battles fought by Muḥammad and his successors), the conquest of the Byzantine Levant started in 629 with the battle of Muʾtah (near Karak in Jordan), where Muslims fought against the Ghassanids (Arab vassals of the Byzantine Empire). The active push in Byzantine territories started five years later under Abū Bakr (the first caliph; r. 632–634) in 634, and then under ʿUmar I (r. 634–644). By 635, most of Palestine, southern Syria, and Jordan were conquered, with Jerusalem surrendering only in 637. Damascus was conquered in 634 after a siege that lasted for only twenty-eight days. Alexandria, the Byzantine capital of Egypt, fell in 641 after a six-month siege.

[33] The conquest of Mesopotamia started under Abū Bakr (r. 632–634) in 633. The Sassanid capital, Ctesiphon (near contemporary Baghdad) fell in 637 under ʿUmar I (r. 634–644). Muslims won the decisive battle of Nahāvand (capital of Hamadan in Eastern Iran) in 641, thus securing their control of Mesopotamia. By 643, they controlled Isfahan and the Tabaristan region around the Caspian Sea and Fars (Southern Persia). The battle of Oxus River in 644 marked their full control of Khurāsān, the largest and easternmost province of the Sassanid empire (including today's northeast Iran, Afghanistan, and parts of Turkmenistan). The last Sassanid emperor Yazdegerd III (b. 624 r. From 632) attempted to instigate rebellions against Umar I and his successor ʿUthmān, until he died in 651 in Merv.

[34] On the Islamization and transformation of Syria, see Khalek, *Damascus after the Muslim Conquest.*

[35] Ibn al-Nadim, *Fihrist*, 339.

[36] Naghawi, "Umayyad Filses Minted at Jerash," 219.

important construction projects in Damascus and in other Levantine cities, the most famous of which is the Dome of the Rock in Jerusalem, completed in 691. ʿAbd al-Malik's son and successor, al-Walīd I (r. 705–715), who ruled over the largest expansion of the Umayyad empire, pursued an aggressive construction program that changed the appearance of Damascus, as well as that of many other important towns and centers in his realm. In Damascus, he seized the Basilica of Saint John and transformed it into the famous Umayyad Mosque in 706; he also completed the construction of al-Aqṣā mosque begun by his father in Jerusalem,[37] and he sponsored major renovations to the prophetic mosque in Medina as well.[38] Both caliphs relied on Byzantine artisans in their constructions and modeled their buildings, whether in Damascus or in Jerusalem, on earlier Byzantine buildings.

Many medieval Arabic sources credit al-Walīd I with building Islam's first bīmāristān in Damascus. For instance, the famous historian Abū Jaʿfar al-Ṭabarī (d. 923) reported two different accounts of al-Walīd's patronage in relation to medicine. The first described his creation of a leprosarium (a place to incarcerate lepers, thus preventing them from begging while at the same time providing for them); the second recounted his creation of a bīmāristān in Damascus.[39] These accounts provide evidence for many modern historians who credit al-Walīd I with sponsoring the first institutions like these under Muslim rule. Dols explains that the establishment sponsored by al-Walīd I was probably unlike the later bīmāristāns of the tenth century and more like a leprosarium, which would have been more consistent with Byzantine practice; as such, it would have paralleled Byzantine leprosaria in other urban centers, like the one originally built by St. Basil in Caeseria.[40] However, these sources on Umayyad institutions

37 Creswell, Gautier-Van Berchem, and Hernández, *Early Muslim Architecture: Umayyads, Early ʿAbbāsids and Ṭūlūnids*.

38 Gibb, "Arab-Byzantine Relations under the Umayyad Caliphate."

39 Al-Ṭabarī, *Taʾrīkh al-Rusul wa al-Mulūk*, 6: 437. Contemporary to al-Ṭabarī, al-Balādhūrī (d. 892) reported al-Walīd's provisions for the lepers, the blind, and the crippled. Also, Al-Ya'qūbī (d. 897) wrote that al-Walīd I built the first bīmāristān in Damascus (Al-Yaʿqūbī, *Tārīkh al-Yaʿqūbī*, 2: 291), and Ibn ʿAbd Rabbih (d. 940) reported the same account in the context of explaining why al-Walīd was one of the best Umayyad caliphs (cited in Conrad, "Did al-Walid I Found the First Islamic Hospital?," 236). Finally, this account was also reported by al-Maqrīzī (d. 1442), who lived his life between Cairo and Damascus and occupied the position of market inspector in Damascus (Al-Maqrīzī, *al-Khiṭaṭ*, 4: 408).

40 Dols, "Origins of the Islamic Hospital," 378. Conrad published an important article on this subject in Aram – "Did al-Walīd Found the First Islamic hospital?" – in which he questioned this narrative of origin, arguing that there is little reason to believe that al-Walīd I did indeed found the first Islamic hospital. Conrad's argument was persuasive to a number of historians, who gradually moved away from the accounts of this Umayyad institution, locating the beginning of the Islamic bīmāristān in Abbasid Iraq (Horden, "The Earliest Hospitals"; Pormann, "Islamic Hospitals").

suffer from the same difficulties found in Umayyad historiography in general. On one hand, there is a serious lack of contemporary narratives that chronicle the Umayyad period.[41] On the other, writings composed under the early Abbasids (who revolted against and then replaced the Umayyads in 750) were generally biased against the Umayyads, especially in relation to institutional developments or their perceived achievements.[42]

Although there is no evidence that the Umayyad institution was similar in any way to the more sophisticated bimāristāns of the eleventh, twelfth, or thirteenth centuries, there is evidence that al-Walīd (or possibly some other Umayyad ruler) established, acquired, or renovated a small facility that provided services to the crippled, blind, and lepers. It is this institution that later sources identified as the first bīmāristān, linking it to their own contemporary and much more sophisticated institution. One small facility, known as al-Bīmāristān al-Ṣaghīr, continued to exist and to serve people in Damascus; it was located adjacent to the Umayyad mosque (where al-Walīd's facility might have existed). This small bīmāristān was identified by Levantine author al-Yūnīnī as the Umayyad Bīmāristān. Similarly, Ibn al-ʿImād in his biographical dictionary *Shadharāt al-Dhahab* wrote:

> Al-Bīmāristān al-Ṣaghīr (the small bīmāristān) in Damascus is older than al-Bīmāristān al-Nūrī. It [is] located opposite the wash basin (*maṭharah*) of the Umayyad mosque. The first to have turned it into a house and ceased the

Pormann did not fully accept that Hārūn al-Rashīd established the first bīmāristān in late eighth-century Baghdad because he found no contemporaneous sources reporting on this event (and rejected later sources as questionable). However, he did not present an alternative narrative, apart from identifying the fact that literature in the second half of the ninth century indicated that the Baghdadi literati were already accustomed to the presence and roles of the bīmāristān. Conrad's source criticism and his meticulous analysis of different accounts are clearly remarkable, but his conclusions merit a closer look. For a detailed discussion of Conrad's proposal, see the Annex.

41 Most historians and scholars writing in the Umayyad period whose work survived focused on collecting materials related to Muhammad's life and conquests (*sīra* and *maghāzī* literature). Many of these also lived in Medina or in Iraq, somewhat removed from Damascus and major centers of Umayyad politics. For instance, ʿUrwa ibn al-Zubayr (d. 712) lived most of his life in Medina and probably wrote a *sīra* of Muḥammad's life but he was said to have destroyed all of his writings before his death (on ʿUrwa, see, for instance, Gorke, "The Historical Tradition about Al-Hudaybiya: A Study of Urwa B. Al-Zubayr's Account.") Abū Bakr al-Zuhrī (d. 742) also lived most of his life in Medina and composed only a *maghāzī*: see al-Zuhrī, *al-Maghāzī al-Nabawīyah*. For al-Zuhrī's biography, see Ibn ʿAsākir, *Tārīkh Madīnat Dimashq: Al-Zuhrī Abū Bakr Muḥammad Ibn Muslim Ibn ʿubayd Allāh Ibn ʿabd Allāh Ibn Shihāb Al-Zuhrī Al-Qarshī*. The most prominent historian of the late eighth century was Ibn Isḥāq (d. 761; active in Medina), who wrote only a biography of Muḥammad that was transmitted by Ibn Hishām (d. 835): see Ibn Hishām, *Al-Sīrah Al-Nabawiyyah*.

42 Robinson, *Islamic Historiography*, 40–42, 52–54. Interestingly, some accounts of Umayyad history were reported in Andalusian historiography, under the Umayyad Caliphate of Cordoba, although most of these accounts are evidently biased against the Abbasids. See Manzano-Moreno, "Oriental 'Topoi.'"

> customs of the bīmāristān (*kharraba rasm al-Bīmāristān*) from it was Abū al-Faḍl al-Ikhnāʾī. Then, it was owned by his brother al-Burhān al-Ikhnāʾī. It is located under the western minaret of the Umayyad mosque towards the west, and is attributed to the constructions of Muʿāwiyah or his son.[43]

This bīmāristān was in fact built by the Seljuk ruler of Damascus, Duqāq b. Tutush (r. 1095–1104),[44] although it is not clear whether this structure or a similar one had existed there before. Ibn al-ʿImād's account indicates that the people of Damascus thought that this institution was indeed the legendary Umayyad one and attributed it to either the founder of the Umayyad dynasty or his son.

"The increasing tendency of the Umayyads to adopt Byzantine usages and to emulate the Greek Emperors is a patent fact."[45] As mentioned before, it was only until the reign of ʿAbd al-Malik b. Marwān (the fifth Umayyad caliph) that a consistent effort to Arabize the state records was undertaken. Also, ʿAbd al-Malik's newly minted coin resembled Byzantine coins, including the fact that he stamped it with his own likeness. "The most striking legacy of the imperial heritage, however, is furnished by the Umayyad policy of erecting imperial religious monuments."[46] This tradition of building religious monuments, particularly mosques, was not adopted by the Abbasids who followed.[47] In this context, al-Walīd's constructions – including the Umayyad mosque and his renovations of the prophetic mosque – were in line with an "imperial ideology"[48] that emulated and attempted to maintain the Byzantine traditions of patronage and monumentality. The Umayyad mosque itself replaced the city's largest Byzantine monument, the Basilica of Saint John the Baptist, which seemed to be a key component of the project. The famous geographer, historian, and Jerusalem native Shams al-Dīn al-Maqdisī (d. 991), explained that

[43] Ibn al-ʿImād, *Shadharāt al-Dhahab*, 3: 407.

[44] Mouton, *Damas et sa Principauté sous les Saljoukides et les Bourides*, 14–15.

[45] Gibb, "Arab-Byzantine Relations," 223.

[46] Ibid., 224.

[47] Ibid. The Abbasids built a number of mosques in Baghdad, such as al-Manṣūr's (r. 754–775) mosque in 762, which was built when Baghdad was built. Also, al-Muktafī bil-llāh (r. 902–908) built the Caliphs' Mosque (*Jamiʿ al-Khulafāʾ*) around 907. There was no attempt, however, to build a mosque as central to its city as the Umayyad Mosque was to Damascus or the Aqṣā Mosque to Jerusalem; furthermore, the previously mentioned Abbasid mosques did not appear to be part of a larger building policy adopted by the Abbasid caliphs. Ibn ʿAsākir reported that when al-Maʾmūn (r. 813–833) visited Damascus and saw the Umayyad mosque, he exclaimed that "it was built like nothing before (*ʿalā ghayr mithāl mutaqaddim*)," even though he had certainly seen al-Manṣūr's mosque and had witnessed the additions and renovations done to it by al-Mahdī (r. 775–785) and al-Rashīd (r. 786–809) See Ibn ʿAsākir, *Tārīkh Madīnat Dimashq*, 1: 304.

[48] Gutas, *Greek Thought, Arabic Culture*. Gutas used the term "Imperial ideology" to refer to the Abbasid willingness to adopt specific practices and views from their Sassanid predecessors.

ʿAbd al-Malik and al-Walīd I built the Dome of the Rock and the Umayyad Mosque for fear that Muslims would be tempted by the magnificence of the Church of the Holy Sepulchre, the Basilica of St. John the Baptist, and other churches in Syria.[49]

Within this context, any establishment that al-Walīd may have built was not a "medical" institution in the sense that the later bīmāristāns of the twelfth and thirteenth centuries would be; rather, it was a charitable one and intended to compete with, replace, and continue the Byzantine practice of building such relief institutions and annexing them to churches or monasteries. When historians like al-Maqrīzī (d. 1440) later traced the genealogy of the bīmāristān to al-Walīd, they were imposing their own experience of the later bīmāristāns like al-Nūrī and al-Manṣūrī and were placing these later bīmāristāns in a broader framework of royal patronage and support for the poor. It was not the medical nature of the institution that animated this genealogy but rather the centrality of royal patronage to the empire's capital. In Egypt, there is no clear evidence of a comparable Umayyd institution in the province's Umayyad capital, thus indicating that the Umayyads may not have built or sponsored similar institutions in the major cities of the provinces.[50] As Horden maintains, Christian institutions of care that existed under the Byzantines in different fashions probably continued to exist in the background, mostly in Egypt, the Levant, and other former Byzantine territories, although they are not necessarily detectable in our Muslim sources.

In the East, in Iraq and Iran, the rise of the bīmāristān in its different forms was not connected to any direct Byzantine influence or motivated by previous pre-Islamic royal patronage traditions. Sassanid charitable initiatives and institutions influenced Abbasid practice in many ways,[51] but, as seen before, Sassanid practice and traditions did not include sites for collective healing or care similar to bīmāristāns or to *xenodochia*. Instead, the *xenodochia* had survived in Syriac Christian forms in the major Syriac centers as Nisbis, Gundisapur, and Ctesiphon, the seat of the Patriarch of

[49] Cited in Gibb, "Arab-Byzantine Relations," 224.

[50] ʿĪsá, *Tārīkh al-Bīmāristānāt fī Al-Islām*, 45. ʿĪsá cited Ibn Duqmāq's (d. 1407) *al-Intiṣār*. ʿAmr ibn al-ʿĀṣ (d. 664) was the commander of the Muslim armies that conquered and annexed Egypt. He supported the rise of the Umayyads, being of the same clan as the Umayyads, and he was appointed the governor of Egypt under the first Umayyad Caliph, Muʿāwiyah (r. 661–680). ʿAmr also built Egypt's first Islamic capital, al-Fusṭāṭ, which would survive as a commercial suburb of Cairo centuries later. He built his mosque in the center of al-Fusṭāṭ, and the mosque has continued to hold symbolic significance in Egypt throughout the medieval and early modern period, up until today.

[51] Gutas, *Greek Thought, Arabic Culture.*

the Eastern Church. Mostly consisting of small infirmaries to support students, monks, and clergy, Syriac *xenodochia* were also sites for medical education and training and were dominated by Galenic physicians who may have been churchmen as well. *Xenodochia* were physicians' projects that Sassanid patrons supported: as such, they were not a sign of the Eastern Church's patronage nor were they a symbol of royal benevolence to the empire's subjects. Rather, these institutions functioned as signs of the royal patronage of particular physicians.[52]

The story of Islamic bīmāristāns in the East (i.e., in Iraq and Iran) is better known and constitutes the major part of the traditional narrative ascribed to the archetypal bīmāristān. Hārūn al-Rashīd (r. 786–809) was credited for asking a famous physician from Gundesapur, Jibrīl ibn Bakhtīshūʿ, to build a bīmāristān in Baghdad.[53] Although there is little contemporary evidence to suggest the veracity of these reports, the mention of the bīmāristān in ninth- and tenth-century literature shows, beyond doubt, that the institution was well-known in Baghdad and that the city's inhabitants had clear ideas of what constituted a bīmāristān's role and mission.[54] Reports place the "first" Baghdadi bīmāristān in the late eighth century or early ninth century, under either al-Rashīd (r. 786–809) or his son al-Maʾmūn (r. 813–833). However, the famous Baghdadi literatus Ibn Ṭayfūr (820–893) wrote a history of Baghdad – of which only the parts describing the reign of al-Maʾmūn survive – and did not mention al-Maʾmūn's having built a bīmāristān; this raises the possibility that it was indeed al-Rashīd who built it, possibly under the influence of his trusted physician Jibrīl ibn Bakhtīshūʿ of Gundisapur.[55] In fact, al-Rashīd's vizir,

[52] On Sassanid patronage and its connection to Zoroastrianism, see Stewart, "The Politics of Zoroastrian Philanthropy."

[53] Dunlop, Colin, and Sehsuvaroglu, "Bīmāristān."

[54] Dols, "The Origins of the Islamic Hospital," Pormann, "Islamic Hospitals in the Time of al-Muqtadir," 354–55.

[55] Ibn Ṭayfūr, *Tārīkh Baghdād.* Ibn Ṭayfūr's history of al-Maʾmūn constructs a largely favorable depiction of the caliph and his achievements. It is, therefore, unlikely that al-Maʾmūn would have established the first Abbasid bīmāristān in Baghdad without it being celebrated by Ibn Ṭayfūr. Peter Pormann rejects the attribution of the bīmāristān to al-Rashīd based only on what he sees as questionable or exaggerated claims about Gundisapur: "As already mentioned, the accounts of Jundaysabūr as a medical academy-cum-hospital in Sassanian and Umayyad times are legendary and thus unreliable. It is therefore not surprising that reports of Harūn al-Rashīd being inspired by Jundaysabilr to set up similar institutions in Baghdad should also be dismissed as fictitious" ("Islamic Hospitals in the Time of Al-Muqtadir," 353–54). As will be explained, and as Pormann correctly identifies, the accounts of Gundisapur's legendary history originated with the patriarchs of the Bakhtīshūʿ family and other physicians who belonged to the town's extended genealogy. What is important to note is that all these accounts did not describe contemporaneous events – that is, conditions in Gundisapur in the eighth or ninth century, to which al-Rashīd and other Baghdadī

Yaḥyā al-Barmakī (d. 806), asked the Indian physician, Mankah, to write a commentary on Indian medicine in the bīmāristān, raising the possibility that the first bīmāristān of Baghdad could have been built by the Barmakids and reacquired by al-Rashīd.[56]

As mentioned earlier, there is evidence that Gundisapur had a Syriac theological school with a *xenodocheion* attached to it and that there was a tradition of medical learning in this *xenodocheion*. It was probably the best of the different Syriac establishments, which would explain why Patriarch Timothy I (r. 780–823) sent one of his students to Gundisapur to learn medicine.[57] The narrative surrounding Gundisapur grew gradually, but consistently, in the hands of the town's sons, especially those of the Bakhtīshū' medical dynasty, who presented Gundisapur as an exemplary site of scholarship and learning and, therefore, as an ideal that Baghdad itself should emulate. Thus, the accounts of Gundisapur, many of which came from the now-lost history of Jibrīl ibn Bakhtīshū' (d. 824) and survived in many other writings – most importantly in the biographical dictionary of 'Alī b. Yūsūf al-Qifṭī (d. 1248)[58] – should not be read as historical accounts of the city. Rather, they should be viewed as idealistic accounts portraying the ideals and aspirations of the new medical elite, a group that arrived in Baghdad in the last decades of the eighth century and came to dominate the medical scene over the following centuries. The bīmāristān of Gundisapur is, therefore, an ideal image, crafted by these physicians and reanimated in the Abbasid bīmāristāns in Baghdad and other cities (and that were supervised by these physicians themselves). The deep commitment of these physicians to this project, the imagined xenodocheion-cum-bīmāristān, reflects previous decades of Sassanid patronage of and connection to the physician and the bīmāristān.

The Lore of the Bakhtīshū's

Accounts of the town of Gundisapur and its medical academy and hospital dominated Arabic writings on medicine and history from the ninth well

elites would have had access – but rather its past glories and lore, many of which exaggerated the size and importance of what probably was a Syriac *xenodocheion* attached to the town's theological school. Although it is not possible for al-Rashīd to have been inspired by something that did not exist, it is possible that he was inspired by the historical (or legendary) narrative of his physician or that his physician attempted to "revive" an establishment that existed only in local legend and lore.

56 Ibn al-Nadīm, *Fihrist*, 421.

57 Macdonald, Twomey, and Reinink, *Learned Antiquity*, 165.

58 al-Qifṭī, *Tārīkh al-Ḥukamā'*.

into the fifteenth century, if not longer. In these accounts, the town was portrayed as a center built by an enlightened sovereign with immense power and wealth for his patronized physicians, philosophers, and other men of knowledge. Gundisapur was also seen as the site of a bīmāristān, an establishment dedicated to the sick and entirely administered by Galenic physicians. Al-Qifṭī wrote:

> The physicians of Gundisapur (*ahl Jundisābūr min al-aṭibbā'*) [have been] skilled and knowledgeable in this art since the time of the Khosraus[59] (*min zaman al-akāsirah*). The reason they reached such [a high] position (*manzila*) is that Shapūr, son of Ardashīr,[60] had made peace with Philip, the Cesar of the Romans,[61] after defeating him in Syria and conquering Antioch. [Shāpūr] asked [Philip] for his daughter in marriage in exchange for something they agreed on, so Cesar agreed. Before she moved to [Shāpūr's], he [Shāpūr] built her a city, which is Gundisapur, in the shape of Constantinople[62] . . . When Cesar's daughter moved to [the city], good physicians (*aṭibbā' afāḍil*) moved with her. When they resided there, they started to teach youngsters (*aḥdāth*)[63] from the town's people. Their . . . science continued to grow stronger (*wa lam yazal amruhum yaqwā fi al-'ilm*), and they improved it and organized the rules of treatment (*yurattibūn qawānīn al-'ilāj*) based on the conditions of their regions [and their] complexions, until they excelled in [all] virtues. Some prefer their treatment and their method to the Greeks and the Indians because they took the best from each faction, increased it with what they extracted on their own, and arranged them in formularies, compendia and books, where they collected all the best.[64]

The excellence of the physicians of Gundisapur, according to al-Qifṭī's account, was rooted in the sources of their medical knowledge and practice: beginning with the best Roman physicians, they integrated their knowledge of the Greeks with that of the Indians, perfecting treatment regimens

[59] Title taken by a number of Sassanid rulers after the mythical ruler Khosrau in the Avesta. In Arabic, the term was used to refer to Sassanid rulers prior to Islam.

[60] Shapur I was the second emperor of the Sassanid empire and ruled from 240 to 270, after Ardashīr I, the founder of the Sassanian empire.

[61] Philip the Arab (Marus Julius Philipus Augustus) ruled from 244 to 249. He was called Philipus Arabus because he was born near Damascus in the Roman province of Arabia.

[62] Syriac accounts describe the building of the city, which was called Bet Lāpāt in Syriac, by captives brought from Antioch after Shapur I's wars (Zacharias Bishop of Mytilene, *The Syriac Chronicle Known as That of Zachariah of Mitylene*). In Middle Persian, the city is called *Veh-Andiyōk-Šābūr*, which literally meant: *Shāpūr [made this city] better than Antioch.* (Wiesehofer, "Gundeshapur"). The connection with Antioch, preserved in the account of the war, was replaced in al-Qifṭī by "Constantinople," probably in an attempt to further the greatness of Gundisapur. Also see Harrak, *Acts of Mār Māri*, 73.

[63] *Aḥdāth* was a term used to describe children before legal majority.

[64] Al-Qifṭī, *Tārīkh al-Ḥukamā'*, 133.

that were based on the conditions of their new region and the "complexions" of the people there. This account highlighted the physicians' training of local youngsters who would then continue to perfect their medical knowledge; in this way, they would maintain the excellent reputation of Gundisapur and its heritage of mixed Sassanid/Persian and Syriac ancestry. Remarkably, the town's Syriac Nestorian legacy and concordant connection with the Church of the East was never referenced, with it instead being presented strictly as a medical center.

For al-Qifṭī, the story of the town of Gundisapur and that of the Bakhtīshūʿ family were intractably, inextricably connected. The Bakhtīshūʿs were not just another medical family in Baghdad: they were the most reputable, well-steeped in medical traditions spanning more than three centuries and multiple generations of physicians. Throughout its time in Baghdad, the family moved from one court to another, serving both rivals and allies;[65] they survived many political upheavals and remained a paragon of excellence in medical practice. For al-Qifṭī, this connection between a family dynasty and Gundisapur itself allowed him to frame the tale of the famed medical school and hospital with another narrative: the biography of the famous patriarch of Banū Bakhtīshūʿ, Jibrīl I ibn Bakhtīshūʿ.

The Bakhtīshūʿs gathered gradually in Baghdad to serve the Abbasid court. First, Jūrjīs I ibn Bakhtīshūʿ, the patriarch living in Gundisapur, was summoned to Baghdad in 765 to treat the Abbasid Caliph al-Manṣūr (r. 754–775). He fared very well and continued to serve the caliph until 769, when he became very sick and was given permission to return to Gundisapur.[66] Jūrjīs's son, Bakhtīshūʿ II (d. 801), who was still in Gundisapur, was then invited to Baghdad by Hārūn al-Rashīd (r. 786–809) in 787.[67] Bakhtīshūʿ II's son, Jibrīl II (d. before 833), served al-Rashīd and eventually served al-Rashīd's two sons, first al-Amīn (r. 809–813) and then al-Maʾmūn (r. 813–833). After the civil war between the two brothers, which ended in the removal and death of al-Amīn, Jibrīl II fell out of favor and was imprisoned by al-Maʾmūn from 813 to 825, when he was released. Ibn Abī Uṣaybiʿah wrote:

[65] For instance, two members of the Bakhtīshūʿ family served Hārūn al-Rashīd (d. 809) and his courtier, Jaʿfar al-Barmakī (d. 803). When Jaʿfar fell eventually out of favor with the Caliph and was executed in what came to be known the "Trial of the Barmakid" in 803, Jibrīl II ibn Bakhtīshūʿ joined the Caliph's service (Ibid., 101–02; Ibn Abī Uṣaybiʿah, *ʿUyūn al-Anbāʾ*, 2: 15–16) before serving his two sons.

[66] Al-Qifṭī, *Tārīkh al-Ḥukamāʾ*, 134–35; Ibn Abī Uṣaybiʿah, *ʿUyūn al-Anbāʾ*, 2: 8–12; Sourdel, "Bukhtīshūʿ."

[67] Ibn Abī Uṣaybiʿah, *ʿUyūn al-Anbāʾ*, 2: 13; al-Qifṭī, *Tārīkh al-Ḥukamāʾ*, 101.

> In the year 210 [825 CE], al-Maʾmūn had a difficult ailment. He was being treated by the best of physician (*wujūh al-aṭibbāʾ*) and he would not improve. He said to Mīkhāʾīl:[68] "the medications you give me increase my ailment. Summon the physicians and consult with them about my condition." [The caliph's brother] told [the caliph]: "O prince of the believers, let us summon Jibrīl. He knows our complexions from our childhood" but [the caliph] ignored what he said ... When al-Maʾmūn was too weak to take medications, they reminded him of Jibrīl so he ordered him summoned. When he arrived, he changed all [the caliph's] medications, so he improved after a day, and was healed in three days.[69]

Ibn Abī Uṣaybiʿah (d. 1269) reported this account on the authority of Qinūn al-Turjumān, a physician and translator of Greek works who was active in Baghdad in the late tenth century. The authenticity of the report cannot be verified by comparing Ibn Abī Uṣaybiʿah to other sources, and it is possible that Jibrīl's heroic come-back to al-Maʾmūn's court was exaggerated by Qinūn, by Ibn Abī Uṣaybiʿah, or by both. However, the real significance of the account lies in its being part of a family lore that was propagated well into the thirteenth century; it was also part of the production of a history of Islamicate medical elites that could be traced back through Baghdad to Gundisapur, through this family and others (as will be explained in depth later). According to this lore, the Bakhtīshūʿs continued to excel on every occasion, thus demonstrating their abilities and their knowledge, and changing the medical landscape of Baghdad.

This lore surrounding the Bakhtīshūʿs consistently emphasized their connection and dedication to the bīmāristān (*xenodocheion*) of Gundisapur from the very beginning of their relationship with the Abbasid elites: when al-Manṣūr (r. 754–775) asked Jurjis I to bring his son Bakhtīshūʿ II to Baghdad, he refused because "Gundisapur is in need of him [his son]. If he leaves, the bīmāristān will fall in ruins."[70] A famous student of Jurjis I, known by the name Ṣahārbakht (fl. 780), was also reported to have refused to leave the bīmāristān at Gundisapur for Baghdad.[71] When Hārūn al-Rashīd funded Jibrīl II (d. 801) for constructing a bīmāristān in Baghdad, the physician sent for his students and aids in Gundisapur to staff the new bīmāristān, further solidifying the connections between the emerging

[68] Mīkhāʾīl ibn Misawayh (d. After 835) was al-Maʾmūn's personal physician. One of his contemporaries reported "He never agreed with any of the physicians on anything more recent than two-hundred years" (Ibn Abī Uṣaybiʿah, *ʿUyūn al-Anbāʾ*, 2: 126). He belonged to the Masawayh family, who were clients of the Bakhtīshūʿs back in Gundisapur, and was also Jibrīl's brother-in-law.

[69] Ibid., 2: 18.

[70] Ibn Abī Uṣaybiʿah and Najjār, *Kitāb ʿuyūn al-Anbāʾ*, 2: 10.

[71] Al-Qifṭī, *Tārīkh al-Ḥukamāʾ*, 247–48.

bīmāristān scene in Baghdad and the old (if often imagined) bīmāristān lore of Gundisapur.[72] Even after the Bakhtīshūʿs had moved almost entirely out of Gundisapur, their direct relations to the old town appear to have continued. For instance, when Jibrīl II b. Bakhtīshūʿ died during the reign of al-Maʾmūn (r. 813–833), his estate included gardens in Gundisapur that his son endowed to a monastery.[73] The bīmāristān in Gundisapur also seems to have survived for decades, even after the gradual departure of many of its elite physicians. For instance, the famous Sābūr b. Sahl (d. 869), who composed the medical formulary "Aqrābādhīn Sābūr," was at the head of the bīmāristān at Gundisapur. The formulary was primarily prepared for the Gundisapur bīmāristān before it became a significant resource for other bīmāristāns in Baghdad and Iraq.[74] Sābūr's son, Sahl b. Sābūr (d. 833), did not continue his father's practice in Gundisapur, but instead traveled to Baghdad where he served al-Maʾmūn and in a number of Baghdad bīmāristāns, alongside his friends and colleagues, Jurjīs II ibn Bakhtīshūʿ and Yūḥanna b. Masawayh.[75]

The Bakhtīshūʿ lore, found in the biographical dictionaries of the thirteenth century, also appears to have relied on reporters and authors from the ninth and tenth centuries. For instance, Ibn Abī Uṣaybiʿah derived the different accounts of the Bakhtīshūʿs from five main sources:[76] Qīnūn al-Turjmān (fl. before 978),[77] Yūsuf b. Ibrāhīm b. al-Dāyah (d. 878),[78] Abū Isḥāq al-Ruhāwī (active in the late tenth century),[79] Thābit b. Sinān (d. 976),[80] and ʿUbayd Allāh b. Jibrīl ibn Bakhtīshūʿ (d. c. 1058).[81] The connections between these five sources and the Bakhtīshūʿs are important for understanding and explaining the

72 Ibid., 383–84. At least one of Jibrīl II's students, Dashtak (fl. 800), was reported to have refused to join the master in Baghdad because he thought that the funds allocated to the new bīmāristān were insufficient. It is unlikely that the bīmāristān in Gundisapur was bigger than the new bīmāristān, which suggests that this account was a later addition to the events surrounding the first bīmāristān in Baghdad. This further highlights the importance of funds and facilities and the Gundisapurians' high standards. It could, on the other hand, be taken as a sign of the high hopes that Dashtak, possibly among other students of the Bakhtīshūʿs, had for the new foundation.

73 Al-Qifṭī, *Tārīkh al-Ḥukamāʾ*, 143.

74 Sābūr Ibn Sahl, *The Small Dispensatory* and *Sabur Ibn Sahl's Dispensatory in the Recension of the Adudi Hospital.*

75 Al-Qifṭī, *Tārīkh al-Ḥukamāʾ*, 196. Sahl b. Sābūr was known by the name Sahl al-Kawsaj.

76 In addition to these five sources, Ibn Abī Uṣaybiʿah relied on three others, reporting one account from each: Maymūn b. Hārūn (fl. 833–842; Ibn Abī Uṣaybiʿah, *ʿUyūn al-Anbāʾ*, 2: 24), Ibrāhīm b. ʿAlī al-Ḥusarī, and Abū Muḥammad Badr b. Abī al-Iṣbaʿ.

77 See ibid., 2: 12.

78 Ibid., 2: 18, 2: 27.

79 Ibid., 2: 20.

80 Ibid., 2: 42.

81 Ibid., 2: 47.

significance and production of this lore. Qīnūn, whom Ibn Abī Uṣaybiʿah cited most often, was a physician in the service of the Buyid emir ʿIzz al-Dawlah Bakhtyār (d. 978). Qīnūn was close to the family and had access to the library of Bakhtīshūʿ III (d. 870), where he found documents belonging to the latter's father, Jibrīl II, related to his service in Hārūn al-Rashīd's court. These outlined his salary and al-Rashīd's food regimens among other things. Although it is not clear whether Qīnūn was, in fact, a client of the Bakhtīshūʿs, his admiration of the family patriarchs and his closeness to their heirs were clear. Ibn Abī Uṣaybiʿah cited Qinūn's opinion of Jūrjis I (fl. 765–769) and of his son, Bakhtīshūʿ II (d. 801):

> Jūrjis and his son were the best of the people of their time for what God bestowed on them of honor (*sharaf*), nobility (*nubl*), [and their] righteousness (*birr*), good-doing (*al-maʿrūf*), and charities (*al-ṣadaqāt*), and [their] treating poor and destitute patients, supporting the fate-stricken (*al-mankūbīn*) and the tired to extents that cannot be described.[82]

The second source, Yūsuf b. Ibrāhīm ibn al-Dāyah (d. 878), was a secretary to the Abbasid heir-apparent Ibrāhīm al-Mahdī (d. 839). After his master's death, he immigrated to Damascus and then to Egypt, where he practiced medicine and astrology. During his sojourn in Baghdad, Ibn al-Dāyah was close to the Bakhtīshūʿs and other members of the medical community in the city.[83] In addition to Qīnūn and Ibn al-Dāyah, Ibn Abī Uṣaybiʿah's other sources included Thābit ibn Sinān (d. 976), who had an illustrious medical career in Baghdad and supervised a number of the city's bīmāristāns; Abū Isḥāq al-Ruhāwī, another physician who is known to us by his famous book "manners of the physician (*adab al-Ṭabīb*); and ʿUbayd Allāh ibn . . . Bakhtīshūʿ (d. c. 1058), who was one of the family's most important and successful biographers and who composed a short history from which Ibn Abī Uṣaybiʿah copied a great deal.

In all these cases, the accounts and stories reported about the famous medical dynasty could be traced to members of the family, their most famous and trusted students and clients, or to other important physicians and medical authors. The lore surrounding the Bakhtīshūʿs and their different exploits should not, therefore, be read as a narration of events or as a chronology of medical elites. Instead, it was a lore that carried significance for the medical elites in Baghdad and elsewhere and that helped to formulate and represent specific ideals of the profession, of

82 Ibid., 2: 32.
83 Ibid., 2: 20.

patronage practices, and of physicians' ideal motives and purposes. In this lore, the bīmāristān figured prominently as part of a physician's relationship to his patrons and to his professional endeavors. At the same time, the lore of the Bakhtīshūʿs was connected to Gundisapur and its bīmāristān, ultimately serving as inspiration for the new bīmāristāns in Baghdad. As explained before, the bīmāristān of Gundisapur, on whose model the Baghdad bīmāristāns were supposedly fashioned, was likely not a real institution that could be visited and emulated by Abbasid elites; instead, it was mainly part of a new and expanding Syriaco-Sassano-Abbasid medical lore that understood the bīmāristān/*xenodocheion* in a specific manner and that intended to bring this understanding to the new bīmāristāns of Baghdad. Finally, in all probability, this model was fictitious or legendary – originating in the Syriac infirmaries – and the new Baghdad bīmāristāns were among the first incarnations of this model.

A Tale of Two Cities and Two Bīmāristāns

One of the earliest documented bīmāristāns in Egypt is al-Bīmāristān al-Ṭūlūnī, which was built by Aḥmad ibn Ṭūlūn (r. 868–884) in 872.[84] Aḥmad ibn Ṭūlūn was an Abbasid emir of Turkic origin who was appointed as the governor of Egypt by the Abbasid Caliph al-Muʿtazz (r. 866–869). He was able to consolidate his power in Egypt, annex the ports of the Levant and Alexandria, and institute a new autonomous state under nominal Abbasid control. In 891, at the peak of the kingdom's expansion, Khumārawayh (r. 884–896), Aḥmad's son and successor, received an edict from the Abbasid caliph granting him and his offspring

[84] Al-Kindī, *al-Wulāh wa al-Quḍāh*, 163. Most of the accounts describing the life, career, and reign of Aḥmad ibn Ṭūlūn and his successors rely on three contemporary (or near-contemporary) sources: *al-Sīrah al-Ṭūlūniyyah* by Ibn al-Dāyah (d. after 904), who wrote a commissioned history for each of the Ṭūlūnid rulers. Ibn al-Dāyah's book did not survive except in a reproduction by ʿAlī ibn Mūsā ibn Saʿīd (d. 1286) in his *Al-Mughrib fī ḥulā al-Maghrib* (Ibn Saʿīd, *Al-Mughrib fī Ḥulā al-Maghrib*), along with other partial reproductions in other works. Another source is *Sīrat Aḥmad ibn Ṭūlūn* (originally named *Sīrat Āl Ṭūlūn,* but the parts dealing with Aḥmad ibn Ṭūlūn's offspring were either lost or never completed, and the book came to be known as *Sīrat Ibn Ṭūlūn*), by ʿAbd Allāh ibn Muḥammad al-Balawī (d. after 933). Al-Balawī consulted Ibn al-Dāyah's work and criticized him for having less details than needed. And yet al-Balawī's history is equally celebratory of Ibn Ṭūlūn and his time. Finally, Muḥammad ibn Yūsuf al-Kindī (d. after 965), to be differentiated from the famous philosopher Yaʿqūb al-Kindī (d. 873), wrote a long chapter on Ibn Ṭūlūn in his book on the rulers and judges of Egypt, *al-Wulāh wa-al-Quḍāh.* Al-Kindī was a well-known genealogist and reporter of prophetic traditions and was well-respected for his accuracy. His history presents the most unflattering image of Ibn Ṭūlūn and includes lengthy quotations of poetry satirizing the emir, none of which is found in Ibn al-Dāyah or al-Balawī.

control over all regions west of the Euphrates as far as Barqah (Cyrenaica, in the east of modern-day Libya) for thirty years. The caliph also married Khumārawyh's daughter, Qaṭr al-Nadā.[85] Although al-Bīmāristān al-Ṭūlūnī was reported to be the first in Egypt by the emir's own biographer, Ibn al-Dāyah, it appears that the term "bīmāristān" was a familiar one to readers in Egypt and the Levant, thus suggesting that it had already made its way to the region.[86]

Ibn Ṭūlūn's bīmāristān was built within a specific political and architectural context. Politically, the emir had succeeded in defeating a number of Abbasid armies that had sought to remove him from power, and he was able to conquer parts of Palestine and Jordan. He also controlled Alexandria, which was a governorship separate from Egypt under the Abbasids.[87] In this year (872) and after returning from Alexandria, where he appointed one of his sons as local governor, Ibn Ṭūlūn ordered the construction of a new mosque close to al-Muqaṭṭam Hill to the west of al-Fusṭāṭ (the original capital of Islamic Egypt and the country's biggest town at the time).[88] The new mosque was to be at the center of a new city built especially for Ibn Ṭūlūn's huge army, which was supposedly so big that people in al-Fusṭāṭ complained to the emir that the old mosque was crowded on Fridays by his soldiers. The new city, termed al-Qaṭāʾiʿ (the quartered city), was divided into quarters, each of which was occupied by a specific ethno-military faction of the emir's army. At the center of the new city, close to the mosque, Ibn Ṭūlūn built a huge palace that overlooked a large hippodrome (*maydān*), which was used for games, processions, and troop inspection and also for the emir to welcome the poor seeking his charities on feast days. His bīmāristān was established nearby, close to the mosque and palace.[89]

The bīmāristān was thus a part of this new royal complex. Along with the mosque and a well providing water to the new city, it was supported by a huge *waqf* that included a number of shops and the entire slave market in al-Fusṭāṭ, thus providing enormous resources for the bīmāristān. The emir

85 Al-Kindī, *Al-Wulāh wa-al-Quḍāh*, 176–78.

86 Both al-Kindī (d. after 964), the author of *al-Wulāh wa-al-Quḍāh*, and Ibn al-Dāyah (d. 951), author of Ibn Ṭūlūn's official history, used the terms "bīmāristān" and "māristān" liberally, with no qualifications or explanations. In the case of Ibn al-Dāyah, his book – which was an official commissioned history – was not expected to be read in Baghdad, but was directed instead toward a local Levantine and Egyptian audience that was probably familiar with the Arabized term.

87 Ibid., 162–63.

88 Ibid., 163.

89 Al-Balawī, *Sīrat Aḥmad Ibn Ṭūlūn*, 54–56. Ibn Ṭūlūn's city was burned and razed after the fall of his dynasty (c. 903). Only the mosque and the bīmāristān survived.

paid special interest to his new institution, visiting it every Friday to inspect the patients and ensure they were receiving good care. According to Ibn Ṭūlūn's chronicler, Ibn al-Dāyah:

> [Ibn Ṭūlūn] mandated (*sharaṭa*) that when a patient is brought, his clothes and his money will be taken [from him] and kept with the bīmāristān's treasurer (*amīn al-māristān*). He is then given clothes, and bedding (*yufrash lahu*), and is visited with medications, food and [by] physicians until he is cured. When he [is able to] eat a chick and a loaf of bread, he will be ordered to leave and be given his money and his clothes.[90]

The emir prohibited soldiers from attending the bīmāristān and receiving treatment there, dedicating it entirely to the poor. It also appears that al-Bīmāristān al-Ṭūlūnī was aimed not at the chronically ill, old, or crippled but rather at those suffering from more acute conditions, the cure of which was indicated by the ability to eat a chick and a whole loaf of bread. The bīmāristān was equipped with two bathhouses, one for men and one for women, both of which served the bīmāristān patients but also accepted other paying customers, with revenues going to the bīmāristān and to the mosque. Al-Balawī explained:

> [Ibn Ṭūlūn's] piety (*al-birr*) was evident with great enthusiasm and proper intentions; [as in his] building the mosque and the bīmāristān, [which] included, in its drug cabinets (*khazā'in*), the most precious (*nafīsah*) and effective drugs, and well-known theriacs, which are only [found] in the drug cabinets of kings and caliphs. His bīmāristān was never missing any of the medications or the major (*ra'īsah*) drugs, such as the musk treatment and others . . . He bought for [the bīmāristān] precious revenues (*mustaghallāt*), [only] some of which would suffice for all the needs [of the bīmāristān], should God protect whoever is administering them.[91]

The emir's piety and charity was a consistent theme when discussing his bīmāristān, which was always linked to the mosque and the charitable well (and well-house) that he constructed, so that the three of them formed a grand, charitable whole. Al-Balawī, in attempting to provide evidence that Ibn Ṭūlūn was rewarded in the afterlife, reported a number of dreams seen by known pious figures. In one of these dreams, Ibn Ṭūlūn told the dreamer that he was received into the afterlife by two pretty women, one representing his jihād against the Byzantines and the other his charities – namely, the well and the bīmāristān. The two women led him away from

[90] Al-Maqrīzī, *al-Khiṭaṭ*.
[91] Al-Balawī, *Sīrat Aḥmad Ibn Ṭūlūn*, 180.

hellfire about to consume him and into paradise.[92] In another dream, he was seen sitting in his mosque as hellfire burned outside. He told his interlocutor that it was the well that had saved him from this hellfire.[93]

Al-Bīmāristān al-Ṭūlūnī was credited by Ibn al-Dāyah, Ibn Ṭūlūn's personal historian, as the first bīmāristān in Egypt, and al-Maqrīzī and others followed this account. Two other bīmāristāns that were not properly dated – Bīmāristān Zuqāq al-Qanādīl and Bīmāristān al-Maʿāfir – might have existed before al-Bīmāristān al-Ṭūlūnī, however. Bīmāristān Zuqāq al-Qanādīl acquired its name from the name of the street close to the oldest mosque in al-Fusṭāṭ, the mosque of ʿAmr ibn al-ʿĀṣ, suggesting that it may have been an Umayyad establishment (since this was the center of the Umayyad capital). Bīmāristān al-Maʿāfir was located in the center of al-ʿAskar, the Abbasid capital built a few miles away from al-Fusṭāṭ, which suggests that it might be traced to early Abbasid rule.[94] Whether or not it was the first in Egypt, however, al-Bīmāristān al-Ṭūlūnī was the biggest and most prosperous institution of its kind to be built in the Egyptian capital region. Both Ibn al-Dāyah and al-Balawī reported that the bīmāristān and its *waqf* cost Ibn Ṭūlūn more than sixty thousand dinars.[95] To put this number in context, the same sources reported that Ibn Ṭūlūn had to pay a total of one hundred thousand dinars a year to the Abbasid court – in taxes and homages – to maintain his and his family's power over Egypt.[96] His son, Khumārawayh, was asked to pay a tribute of three hundred thousand dinars to the Abbasid court in exchange for his appointment and for the appointment of his family as rulers of all regions "from [the] Euphrates to Barqah (Cyrenaica)" for thirty years.[97] The bīmāristān and its rich endowments, therefore, cost the equivalent of one-fifth of the tribute for all of Egypt, the Levant, western Iraq, Arabia, and the southern region of Asia Minor (up to Tarsus). The mosque, however, cost Ibn Ṭūlūn

[92] Ibid., 352–53. The use of dreams and visions seen by known pious figures was a familiar trope, providing evidence for one's fate in the afterlife. In the case of Ibn Ṭūlūn, as with other emirs, rulers, and generals, his violent behavior and his measures against his enemies, as well as the heavy responsibility of ruling, were seen as possible conduits to hellfire unless other acts were done to evade this fate. Ibn Ṭūlūn, appearing in another dream, explained that his actions against spies and against his enemies were enough to have him punished but that his charities saved him. He also added that he was inflicting God's wrath on deserving foes and that he never transgressed against someone who did not deserve such transgression (ibid., 355).

[93] Ibid., 353. This dream stresses the antithetical images of the charitable water (in the well) and the hellfire from which the emir is saved.

[94] ʿĪsá, *Tārīkh al-Bīmāristānāt fī al-Islām*.

[95] Al-Balawī, *Sīrat Aḥmad Ibn Ṭūlūn*, 350.

[96] Ibid.

[97] Al-Kindī, *al-Wulāh wa al-Quḍāh*, 177.

twice as much, with its cost coming to one hundred and twenty thousand dinars; this clearly indicates the relative significance of the bīmāristān's construction within the emir's ambitious building program.[98]

Ibn Ṭūlūn was definitely aware of the bīmāristān tradition that had begun to flourish in Baghdad at the time. He may have also been influenced by Christian charitable institutions especially that he was known to have been in close contact with the Christian communities in Egypt;[99] it is clear, in any case, that al-Bīmāristān al-Ṭūlūnī was not built within a context of the emir's medical patronage. The emir's relations with his physicians – al-Ḥasan ibn Zayrak (d. 884) and Sa'īd ibn Tawfīl (d. 892) – were, in fact, rather strained, and he did not seem to appreciate their advice much.[100] Furthermore, none of the emir's physicians was involved with his bīmāristān or was reported to have practiced there at all. The bīmāristān was instead part of Ibn Ṭūlūn's charitable endeavors, as well as of the building programs that symbolized his consolidation of power in Egypt and the Levant. In this context, the emir's weekly visits to the bīmāristān, where he inspected the wards, visited the patients, and gave instructions to the bīmāristān's attendants, were clear signs of his piety, philanthropy, and dedication to his flock. It appears that the bīmāristān was only able to survive because of the emir's direct care and attention.[101]

In near contemporary Baghdad, we have some detailed information on the career of the famous physician Sinān ibn Thābit (fl. 908–932, d. 942), whose life and career were deeply connected to the bīmāristāns of Baghdad.[102] Around 920, Sinān ibn Thābit was reportedly managing all

[98] Al-Balawī, *Sīrat Aḥmad Ibn Ṭūlūn*, 350. It is, of course, possible that these numbers were exaggerated by al-Balawī and Ibn al-Dāyah. However, the huge size of the bīmāristān probably made this exaggeration seem legitimate to these authors' readers and contemporaries.

[99] Ibn Ṭūlūn was known to have frequented a Coptic monastery in the desert, south of al-Fusṭāṭ, known as al-Qaṣīr. He used to stay alone in one of the monks' cells to think. His son, Khamārawayh ibn Ṭūlūn, built a room for himself inside the monastery, which he – like his father – used to visit (Al-Balawī, *Sīrat Aḥmad Ibn Ṭūlūn*, 118). Ibn Ṭūlūn also used a Christian architect, Sa'īd ibn Kātib, to supervise his building projects, including the Nilometer, the mosque, and possibly the bīmāristān (ibid., 181).

[100] Ibn Abī Uṣaybi'ah, *'Uyūn al-Anbā'*, 3: 345–53; Al-Balawī, *Sīrat Aḥmad Ibn Ṭūlūn*, 312–16.

[101] Al-Maqrīzī, *al-Khiṭaṭ*. The interruption to Ibn Ṭūlūn's visits was explained by a particular incident: the emir visited the bīmāristān one Friday to inspect the mad. One of the chained madmen, who looked more composed and well-dressed than the rest, told him that he had been wrongly locked up in the bīmāristān because of his enemies' conspiracies. The emir believed him and ordered him released, giving him a pomegranate at the inmate's request. The inmate then threw the pomegranate at the emir, soiling his clothes (or injuring him). After this event, Ibn Ṭūlūn hardly visited the bīmāristān again.

[102] Ibn Abī Uṣaybi'ah, *'Uyūn al-Anbā'*, 2: 208–14. Ibn Abī Uṣaybi'ah copied most of his accounts of the life of Sinān ibn Thābit from the history written by his son, Thābit II ibn Sinān, also a physician

the bīmāristāns in Baghdad and elsewhere.[103] Sinān was close to the Abbasid Caliph al-Muqtadir (r. 908–932) and to his mother Shaghab (d. after 932) – an influential figure herself in the Abbasid court since the reign of her consort, al-Muʿtadid (r. 892–902) and one that played a significant role in her son's accession to the throne. Sinān motivated both his patrons to build two different bīmāristāns in Baghdad, which he supervised and arranged:

> Thābit ibn Sinān said: On the first of Muḥarram of the year 306 AH [June, 918 CE], my father inaugurated (*fataḥa*) Bīmāristān al-Sayyidah (the Lady's Bīmāristān; in reference to Shaghab), which he established (*ittakhadha*) for her in Sūq Yaḥya (a neighborhood in Baghdad). He sat there, arranged the physicians [in shifts] (*rattaba al-mutaṭibbīn*), and admitted (*qabala*) patients. He built it overlooking the Tigris, and its expenditure was six hundred dinars a month. In this year as well [306 AH/918–919 CE], my father [Sinān ibn Thābit] advised (*ashāra*) al-Muqtadir ... to build a bīmāristān that [would] carry his [name], so he [al-Muqtadir] ordered him [Sinān] to establish it (*amarahu bi-itikhādhihi*). [Sinān] established it at the Gate of the Levant and named it al-Bīmāristān al-Muqtadirī, and spent on it [from the Caliph's] money two hundred dinars a month.[104]

These two bīmāristāns were not the only bīmāristāns in the city for we are told that Sinān had already been presiding over other bīmāristāns for roughly a decade before these two were built. Sinān continued to instigate his patrons to build yet more bimāristāns in different parts of the capital and in other Iraqī cities. After the death of the Caliph al-Rāḍī (r. 934–940), whom Sinān served, the physician was called to the service of Bajkam al-Makānī (d. 941), commander of the Abbasid armies and the effective ruler of the capital. Bajkam trusted Sinān deeply and took him on as a physician, courtier, and also a teacher of manners. Sinān advised Bajkam to build another bīmāristān in Baghdad to support the sick poor.[105] Sinān was also concerned with protecting the funds and the resources of the capital's different bīmāristāns, such as Bīmāristān Badr – built by and named after the Abbasid general and courtier Badr al-Muʿtaḍidī (d. 901). The bīmāristān shared the revenues of a *waqf* with the Abbasid royal family. It appears that, at one time, the revenues reaching Bīmāristān Badr had

in the Abbasid court. Peter Pormann has compared a number of accounts from Ibn Abī Uṣaybiʿah's biography of Sinān with other contemporary sources, concluding that the biography provided accurate reproductions of Thābit II's history ("Islamic Hospitals").

103 Ibid., 360. Ibn Abī Uṣaybiʿah, *ʿUyūn al-Anbāʾ*, 2: 208.

104 Ibid., 2: 210.

105 Ibid., 2: 213.

been delayed for some months; Sinān sought the intervention of the vizir ʿAlī ibn al-Jarrāḥ (fl. 908–934, d. 941) to ensure that these funds were delivered in time. Sinān was successful, and the vizir intervened, rebuking the *waqf* supervisor and ordering him to give the bīmāristān precedence over the royal family.[106]

These various accounts present a completely different image from the one observed in Egypt. In Baghdad, the chief physician of the city and of its bīmāristāns was responsible not only for managing the bīmāristāns and for supervising medical practice there, but he was also personally invested in these projects. For Sinān, the construction of bīmāristāns (and stimulating his patrons to build even more of them) was, as he saw it, a significant part of his own career and role; this was reported and described by his son, another important physician, who inherited his father's roles and positions. The bīmāristāns of Baghdad were not part of larger building programs intended to immortalize the patron's name and symbolize his greatness and wealth; they were instead integral to the patronage of medicine and physicians and were directly influenced by the chief physician's medical career and agenda.

The controversy surrounding the finances of Bīmāristān Badr is particularly instructive. On one hand, Sinān perceived himself as the defender of the bīmāristāns under his supervision, going to great lengths to provide sufficient funds – using both his clout and his relationship with the vizir, Ibn al-Jarrāḥ to force an arrangement favorable to the bīmāristān. On another level, the story of this particular bīmāristān reveals details not only about itself, but also about the environment in the Abbasid capital. The bīmāristān was built by Badr al-Muʿtaḍidī (d. 901), a famous courtier and general under al-Muʿtaḍid (r. 892–901), who fell out of favor rapidly and dramatically after his patron's death and was eventually assassinated. Badr did not have many friends in the capital in the first decades of the tenth century, and yet his bīmāristān survived even though it carried his name, protected by the chief physician and the vizir.[107] The *waqf* in question was said to have been established by the royal mother and consort, Sijāḥ, who was the mother of al-Mutawakkil (r. 847–861) and who most likely died before the establishment of Badr's bīmāristān. It was therefore impossible for the bīmāristān to have been an original beneficiary of the *waqf*, which would

[106] Ibid., 2: 210.
[107] Al-Dhahabī, *Al-Tārīkh al-Kabīr*.

have given Sinān more arguments in support of his claims. What is more plausible is that the Bīmāristān Badr was not necessarily a new bīmāristān, but rather a renovation of an older institution that benefitted from the *waqf* at hand. Renovating and renaming institutions was not an unusual practice. In fact, al-Bīmāristān al-ʿAḍudī (built in 981), which was one of the largest and most celebrated in Baghdad, was an old institution renovated and expanded by ʿAḍud al-Dawlah (d. 983), who named the renovated bīmāristān after himself.

The intervention and dedication of the medical elites made possible the survival of different institutions in the names of out-of-favor courtiers and statesmen, along with the expanding tradition of renovating various functional bīmāristāns, which were certainly sites of pride for their patrons and namesakes. However, none of the bīmāristāns sponsored by Sinān carried the same political significance, centrality, or comparative charitable impact as Ibn Ṭūlūn's bīmāristān. Al-Bīmāristān al-Ṭūlūnī was the only functioning institution of its type and size located at the center of governance and under the direct supervision and care of the founder, whereas Bīmāristān al-Sayyidah or al-Bīmāristān al-Muqtadirī were additions to a larger network (made up mostly of smaller pieces) that were generally acts of medical patronage directed to the individual physician's professional self. Here, it is instructive to note Ibn Ṭūlūn's weekly visits to his bīmāristān after Friday prayers and his personal inspection of the bīmāristān and its patients. Ibn Ṭūlūn's visits were central to the functioning of the bīmāristān. Soon after the emir stopped his visits, the bīmāristān's conditions started deteriorating. By contrast, it was Sinān who inaugurated the Bīmāristān al-Sayyidah and al-Bīmāristān al-Muqtadirī, not the patrons themselves. Nor were the latter interested in the institutions' affairs.

Conclusion

When al-Manṣūr Qalāwūn was planning his bīmāristān, the concept and the institution that it stood for were not a novelty. The Mamluk sultan, aiming to consolidate his rule and that of his dynasty, was maintaining the tradition of previous kings and sovereigns who had invested in similar projects. Bīmāristāns were also a notably physical, material presence in the Middle East: they occupied the centers of many towns and cities, punctuated pilgrimage routes and travel itineraries, and provided needed care for the many sick and poor. Qalāwūn's bīmāristān, much like those bīmāristāns built before and after it, was embedded in this rich history, relying on available sets of developing meanings and changing significances in order to construct its own meaning.

The bīmāristān – both as a physical entity marking the urban landscape and as a metaphorical presence in collective history – developed via a rich tradition, the most relevant episodes of which began with the Byzantine institutions that symbolized the care of Church and sovereign for the poor. In this way, the bīmāristān, in its care for the poor, was not alone; it was instead part of a complex system of institutions that defined the Byzantine philanthropic landscape. Institutions of this nature morphed gradually into monuments for emperors, bishops, and devout donors who spent large funds to establish loci of care in city centers throughout the Eastern Mediterranean, defining both urban spaces and local identities. It was this model that persisted in Egypt and the Levant, where bīmāristāns were built under the auspices of political authorities and rich patrons, while physicians played a limited role in the management and maintenance of these institutions. Regardless of their degree of medicalization (which increased with time), these bīmāristāns continued to be markedly charitable projects, built as part of a sovereign's urban and charitable plan.

In the East, the Byzantine tradition had filtered through the Nestorian Schism and moved with the immigrating Syriac Nestorian Christians to the Sassanid empire. In the new institutions of learning and scholarship, the church, academy, and *xenodocheion* were three major components of the new Syriac urban centers: Nisbis and Gundeshapur, among others. The Sassanid royal patronage of these immigrant Christians enabled them to build new institutions that sustained Byzantine philanthropic tradition. However, these institutions were necessarily limited in scope; they were infirmaries, dedicated to students, clerical communities, and members of the Nestorian Church in the small Syriac communities surrounding Church centers and had little impact on Sassanid society as a whole.[108] Instead of being symbols of greatness and power, Syriac *xenodocheia* were intracommunal relief institutions, sites for medical care and medical education for students. When the Abbasids inherited the Sassanid tradition in the early eighth century, the xenodocheion-cum-bīmāristān continued to prosper as a sign of royal favor to specific physicians who now served the new caliphate. The new Abbasid bīmāristān was, then, a hybrid of the politico-charitable institutions of the Eastern Mediterranean: it came to

108 Ibid.

play a charitable role in the urban centers while still cloaked in the garb of the Syriaco-Sassanid function of serving physicians and their careers. The bīmāristān of Gundeshapur, which had prospered under the Abbasids, was a prime example of Abbasid patronage of their Syriac physicians, as well as the original Syriac centers that were slowly fading from view.

PART I

Building a Bīmāristān

Bīmāristāns in the Politico-Architectural Landscape

CHAPTER 1

From Jerusalem to Damascus: The Monumental Bīmāristāns of the Levant

The Bīmāristān as a Monument

Al-Bīmāristān al-Manṣūrī, like other large architectural projects, was a monument: it was intended to create a lasting memory of the patron, to symbolize his good works. It also served to insert Qalāwūn into the architectural fabric of the capital in a striking manner by changing the directions of people's movement, modifying the city's landscape, and erasing memories that had been embodied in previous buildings.[1] As well as being charitable and medical institutions, this and other bīmāristāns were also architectural projects built with a specific intent and providing significant meaning beyond their functions.[2] An urban "monument" was an artifact of historical interactions. As such, it was a physical structure of a magnitude intended to be "memorable," to be woven into the fabric of discursive and embodied "memory." It was designed to invoke acts of "remembrance" that were often ritualized.[3] In creating a memorable structure, the creator engaged in acts of "violence" against a specific physical order that involved both physical structures (including distinctive shapes of buildings, design of streets) and the performances of these structures (in their orientation of transit, their functions as shopping locations, ritual sites, etc.). In all these cases, a monument etched its memorability into the preexisting urban structures and the relations that it modified. At the same time, that monument itself evoked degrees of familiarity and was presented as a continuation of, or modification to, preexisting objects of knowledge and experience. In building a bīmāristān, a mosque, or another site of service, one attempted to recreate previously existing objects in an act that violated the structural integrity of the proposed location or site. The

1 See al-Harithy, "Space in Mamluk Architecture."
2 See al-Harithy, "Urban Form and Meaning"; Humphreys, "Expressive Intent."
3 On monuments and monumentality, see Williams, "Urbanization and Monument Construction"; O'Kane, "Monumentality in Mamluk and Mongol Art and Architecture."

monument thus invoked, while breaking with, the genealogy of imageries and metaphors attached to these types of structures, acquiring much of its meaning through these associations. Finally, the monument occasioned sets of ritualized acts of remembrance – from Quran recitals to requested prayers to even the ceremonial writing of appointment decrees that recalled the act of founding and the intentions of the founder.

Take, for instance, a previous example. Aḥmad ibn Ṭūlūn's (d. 884) bīmāristān was part of a larger architectural and urban project of building an entirely new capital. In the center of this capital, the major and unifying establishments of the new city were built: the governor's famous mosque (the only surviving monument of the city), a hippodrome for training and games, the governor's palace, and the bīmāristān.[4] The different components of the city's center played important roles in symbolizing the governor's power and control and also in uniting his army behind the ideal of a stable new polity in the making. The mosque and the palace reflected the central components of Islamic urban design of the time, reflecting the emir's piety and power. The military and celebratory buildings like the hippodrome – used for games, expositions, and the training of elite troops – emphasized the emir's military might. The bīmāristān played a similar role by showing the emir's care for his people, his desire to rule them under nominal Abbasid control but in his own name, and his intent to establish a dynasty from the new capital al-Qaṭṭāʾiʿ.

In Damascus, Nūr al-Dīn Zankī (d. 1174) built his bīmāristān as a symbol of his dominance and control over the Levantine capital and also as the crown jewel of the urban reorganization program with which he intended to refashion the city as the Zangid capital.[5] He chose to build the bīmāristān in the center of the city, close to the already large Umayyad monument; in so doing, he linked the city's past to its present and future. Along with his bīmāristāns, both in Damascus and in Aleppo, Nūr al-Dīn's patronage extended to important madrasas and Sufi monasteries, all of which played significant roles in emphasizing both his Sunni agenda against the Shiite population (as in Aleppo), as well as his jihad against the Crusaders. Similarly, Ṣalāḥ al-Dīn al-Ayyūbī (d. 1193) was also building a new state as he put an end to the Fatimid Caliphate, restoring Egypt to the nominal power of the Abbasid Caliphate and thereby enabling his emerging dynasty to control the region. Ṣalāḥ al-Dīn's built patronage,

[4] Swelim, *The Mosque of Ibn Ṭūlūn*; Fattal, *Ibn Tulun's Mosque*; Corbet, "Life and Works of Aḥmad Ibn Ṭūlūn."

[5] On Nūr al-Dīn's architectural patronage in Aleppo before moving his capital to Damascus, see Tabba, *Constructions of Power*; Tabba, "The Architectural Patronage of Nur Al-Din, 1146–1174."

which, like Nūr al-Dīn's, included madrasas, Sufi monasteries, and bīmāristāns, signaled his intent to transform the landscape of his new empire from a Shiite-dominated to a Sunni polity, all while building a castle and restructuring the Fatimid capital in Egypt.[6] He also aimed to challenge existing Crusader structures in Jerusalem and other Levantine cities and to build a new Muslim population in these regions.[7]

Al-Bīmāristān al-Manṣūrī (c. 1285) in Cairo shows even more profoundly the political significance of location. Al-Bīmāristān al-Manṣūrī was established as part of a large sultanic complex that included the sultan's tomb and a madrasa. However, the bīmāristān was not only the largest of the complex's three components – which were all essentially under one roof, separated by small hallways – but was also the most prominent and most famous of the three; indeed, the entire complex, including the shrine and the madrasa, was referred to as the bīmāristān. The complex was built in the center of Cairo, facing the shrine of the last Ayyubid Sultan, al-Malik al-Ṣāliḥ Ayyūb, and the madrasa of the famous Mamluk Sultan, al-Ẓāhir Baybars, while at the same time replacing a large Fatimid palace, al-Dār al-Quṭbīyyah. The location was chosen in relation to the tomb and madrasa of al-Ṣāliḥ Ayyūb, who was the most prominent figure for the Mamluk elite at that time, as he was for al-Manṣūr Qalāwūn himself, and whose complex had been the site for taking oaths of allegiance since the Mamluk reign had begun three decades earlier. The bīmāristān was therefore a part of an older, deeper architectural patronage, one extending to the beginning of the Mamluk reign, that merits closer examination.

In various accounts of the construction of al-Bīmāristān al-Manṣūrī, Qalāwūn was reported to have been deeply influenced and inspired by al-Bīmāristān al-Nūrī, which was built by the Nūr al-Dīn Zankī (ca. 1154), in Damascus. A number of these accounts repeat the same narrative: al-Manṣūr Qalāwūn – still an emir under al-Ẓāhir Baybars (d. 1277) – was leading a campaign against Crusaders in the Levant when he fell ill, close to Damascus. As he camped there, medications were brought to him from al-Bīmāristān al-Nūrī. During this episode of sickness or after his recovery, Qalāwūn pledged to build a bīmāristān should God grant him the throne of Egypt. When Qalāwūn finally came to the throne and was able to consolidate his power, he built the bīmāristān he had promised.[8] None

[6] Rabbat, *The Citadel of Cairo*; Mackenzie, *Ayyubid Cairo*.
[7] See Frenkel, "Islamic Religious Endowments."
[8] Al-Maqrīzī, *al-Khiṭaṭ*, 4: 409.

of these writings provide an accurate account of his sickness, nor do they clearly identify the aforementioned campaign; nevertheless, they betray the fact that Qalāwūn and his entourage were indeed impressed by (and wished to emulate) Nūr al-Dīn's bīmāristān.

The link between al-Bīmāristān al-Manṣūrī and its founder Qalāwūn, on the one hand, and al-Bīmāristān al-Nūrī and its founder Nūr al-Dīn, on the other, was also emphasized by Qalāwūn's controversial emir and trusted aide Sanjur al-Shujāʿī (as cited by al-Maqrīzī), who supervised the construction of the complex. After the construction was completed, a number of scholars accused the sultan and his emir of extracting land by force and coercion and of using forced labor and stolen materials in building the bīmāristān; these actions rendered the waqf illegitimate, in their view, and prompted them to issue fatwas prohibiting prayers in the complex. Al-Manṣūr Qalāwūn dispatched his emir – who was already directly supervising the construction – to plead with these concerned scholars and attempt to both mitigate their anger and establish the complex's legitimacy. In al-Maqrīzī's account, Al-Shujāʿī pleaded to the chief judge that the sultan had only wanted to "follow the example of the martyr Nūr al-Dīn, but he received only blame while [Nūr al-Dīn] received praise."[9] This connection proposed by al-Shujāʿī located the institution within a specific pious, philanthropic tradition and linked the Mamluk Sultan to the celebrated Zangid sovereign. Qalāwūn showed his appreciation of al-Bīmāristān al-Nūrī, too, by renovating it and adding more to its waqfs after becoming sultan, even though he did not have any other major building projects in Damascus. Similarly, Qalāwūn was also influenced by the bīmāristāns of Jerusalem and other Levantine cities, including the structures built by the Crusaders (some of which continued to function under his reign), as well as the bīmāristān built by Ṣalāḥ al-Dīn in Jerusalem after he annexed the city. In fact, one of Qalāwūn's earlier construction projects was a bīmāristān in Hebron, which was regarded as part of the regular visitation to Jerusalem (as will be seen later) and which was deeply influenced by the two bīmāristāns dominating the Holy City: the Crusaders' and Ṣalāḥ al-Dīn's. This chapter will visit the Levantine scene and trace the role and place of the Bīmāristān in Nūr al-Dīn's architectural patronage, as well as the precedents established by the Hospitallers and Ṣalāḥ al-Dīn in the Levant.

[9] Al-Maqrīzī, *al-Khiṭaṭ*, 4: 409.

Nūr al-Dīn Zankī and His Bīmāristāns

Nūr al-Dīn's Architectural Program

The life and history of Nūr al-Dīn Maḥmūd Zankī (1118–74) was a source of inspiration for the Ayyubid and Mamluk dynasties following the short-lived Zangid dynasty. His successful career culminated in his control of most of the Levant and his emergence as one of the more significant political actors in the Middle East for most of the twelfth century. Nūr al-Dīn's most important achievements were his consolidation of power over a quasi-united Levant – ruled first from Aleppo and later Damascus – and his efforts to extend to Egypt the protracted Sunni revivalism project that had begun under the Seljuks, who had been the Zangids' masters. In Egypt, his endeavor came to fruition under his protégé-turned-rival, Ṣalāḥ al-Dīn, who was finally able to put an end to the Shiite Caliphate of Cairo, unite Egypt and the Levant with the East of Islamdom under Abbasid tutelage, and mount serious challenges against the Crusaders. Nūr al-Dīn's military and political projects were mirrored in his urban development and constructions in a number of cities in the Levant, especially in Aleppo and Damascus, from where he presided over his realm. In both cities, Nūr al-Dīn established three major types of institutions that are particularly relevant to this discussion: the madrasa, the dār al-ʿadl (lit. house of justice), and the bīmāristān.[10]

Aleppo was Nūr al-Dīn's capital from 1146 to 1154, until he was able to conquer Damascus and move his capital there. Aleppo had a large Shiite community, and Nūr al-Dīn's father, ʿImād al-Dīn Zankī, had maintained a policy of general tolerance of the Shiite population. Nūr al-Dīn's first "monument" was, in fact, a renovation of an older Shiite shrine – Mashhad al-Imām al-Muḥsin – a move that perpetuated his father's policies. Nūr al-Dīn commissioned a hall of ablution and a cistern in the Mashhad and spent a small fortune renovating it.[11] His second monument, however, was not an attempt to appease the local Shiite population; rather, it marked the beginning of his program of Sunni revival, which was spearheaded by the building of madrasas teaching Sunni law. Establishing madrasas was a consistently employed strategy of the Sunni revivalist project, which had been growing in the Abbasid Caliphate's urban centers since the late tenth

[10] Nūr al-Dīn's mausoleum was located in his madrasa in Damascus. For more information on Nūr al-Dīn and his works, see Talmon-Heller, *Islamic Piety in Medieval Syria*; Mourad and Lindsay, *Intensification and Reorientation*.

[11] Tabba, "The Architectural Patronage of Nur Al-Din, 1146–1174," 47.

century, partially in response to the rise of Shiism that had culminated in the consolidation of the Fatimid Caliphate in Cairo and then the Buyids in Iraq and Iran. Under the Seljuks, the madrasa institution reached its apogee as a site for regularizing and spreading Sunni Islamic law,[12] and, in 1149, Nūr al-Dīn commissioned his first madrasa in Aleppo, al-Madrasa al-Ḥallāwiyyah.

Al-Madrasa al-Ḥallāwiyyah was built after the Second Crusade (ca. 1145–1149), during which a number of important victories had begun to provide Nūr al-Dīn with sufficient political capital to commence a more ambitious Sunni revivalist program in Aleppo.[13] Choice of site, as in earlier examples, played a significant role in constructing the meaning and significance of the structure. The madrasa was built near the Congregational Mosque of Aleppo – dominated by the Shiite majority – and faced the famous Mashhad al-Imām al-Muḥsin, which was the largest Shiite monument in the town and the same mashhad Nūr al-Dīn himself had renovated more than a year earlier. Like any new structure built in an already well-established urban settlement, al-Madrasa al-Ḥallāwiyyah was not built in an empty space; instead, it had to efface its predecessors in order to assert its own monumental existence. The madrasa usurped the remains of the Byzantine Cathedral of St. Helena, which was the largest church in the town, an important center of the Byzantine Church, and a symbol of Byzantine Empire's control of the city.[14] It survived until 1124, when Judge Ibn al-Khashshāb – "the caretaker" of Aleppo during prolonged periods of instability – converted it into a mosque in response to Frankish attacks on the city.[15] However, Ibn al-Khashshāb's conversion was an impromptu act and did not transform the outer or the inner structures of the church. It was Nūr al-Dīn who presided over the ambitious project of permanently effacing the cathedral, replacing it with a huge structure that would symbolize his victories over the Crusaders, his new status in the city and in the Levant, and his new policies toward the Shiite population. Nūr al-Dīn's inscriptions in the new madrasa showed that he perceived this monument to be a sign of his new-founded rule: he deleted the title "Atābik" – which his family had borne for decades as deputies and

[12] Makdisi, "Muslim Institutions of Learning"; Makdisi, "Scholastic Method in Medieval Education."
[13] Ibn al-Shiḥnah and al-Batrūnī, *Tārīkh Ḥalab*, 109.
[14] Tabba, "The Architectural Patronage of Nur Al-Din, 1146–1174," 51.
[15] Ibn al-Shiḥnah and al-Batrūnī, *Tārīkh Ḥalab*, 110. Ibn al-Shiḥnah was familiar with this school's history and *waqf* because his father had taught in it. He explained that Ibn al-Khashshāb's conversion of the cathedral was in retaliation to the Franks having dug up and burned Muslim graves during their 1124 siege of Aleppo.

generals of Seljuk suzerains – thereby severing his connections with the Seljuk sultan and pronouncing himself independent from his suzerainty. He then added the title "Mujāhid" (warrior of the holy war) to his epithets for the first time, thus inaugurating his career of warring against the Crusaders, the Shiites, and other Levantine powers alike.[16]

Months later, in 1150, Nūr al-Dīn built another madrasa whose location proved, yet again, his and his entourage's awareness of the significance of place. Facing the Antioch gate, he built al-Madrasa al-Shuʿaybiyyah and its magnificent *qasṭal* (fountain) at a site believed to be that of the city's first mosque. The mosque bore the name of the second caliph, ʿUmar I, and had been built hurriedly after Muslims seized the city, at the place where they first "laid their weapons" after entering from the Gate of Antioch.[17] The mosque gradually decreased in significance after the Umayyads built the city's big congregational mosque, which was renovated by the notable Shiite Abū al-Ḥasan al-Ghaḍāʾirī and controlled by the town's Shiite elite ever since.[18] By building a madrasa and a fountain as a monument of his victory with inscriptions that recalled ʿUmar I's legacies – linking Nūr al-Dīn to the Guided Caliph revered by the Sunnis but disliked by Shiites – Nūr al-Dīn reclaimed the Islamic history of the city while attempting to efface both its pre-Islamic past and its Shiite present.

Al-Bīmāristān al-Nūrī

Nūr al-Dīn's last large monument in Aleppo and first monument in his new, much-coveted capital of Damascus were his two bīmāristāns. Both bore the title al-Bīmāristān al-Nūrī, but only the Damascene institution survived and received many deserved accolades. The bīmāristān of Aleppo was located in Jallūm al-Suflā, the urban sector in which Nūr al-Dīn was also establishing a large intramural water project. The bīmāristān in Damascus was located near the Umayyad congregational mosque; Nūr al-Dīn annexed his other major monument in Damascus, Dār al-ʿAdl (House of Justice), to the Umayyad mosque as well. Together, these two monuments encircled the Great Mosque, which stood as the major architectural monument of Damascus and a reminder of the city's glorious past as the capital of the Umayyad Caliphate. By choosing this location, Nūr

[16] Tabba, "The Architectural Patronage of Nur Al-Din, 1146–1174," 262–65.
[17] Ibid., 53. Ibn Al-Shiḥnah and al-Batrūnī, *Tārīkh Ḥalab*, 107. The madrasa was reportedly built for an Andalusian *faqih*, Shuʿayb ibn Abī al-Ḥasan, after whom it was named.
[18] Tabba, "The Architectural Patronage of Nur Al-Din, 1146–1174," 266.

al-Dīn attached himself to the city's past and thus consolidated his position as a major figure in the history of Damascus. Furthermore, al-Bīmāristān al-Nūrī's presence there made Nūr al-Dīn's complex a central part of Damascus for centuries to come and required that reigning authorities under the Ayyubids, the Mamluks, and the Ottomans support the bīmāristān as a central landmark of the city's architectural heritage.

Nūr al-Dīn's bīmāristāns in Aleppo and Damascus were not the first in either city. Both cities had previously enjoyed bīmāristāns built during the Abbasid and Seljuk periods. At the time that Nūr al-Dīn was planning his construction of the Damascene bīmāristān in 1154 – the first year of his reign in Damascus – another small bīmāristān was close by, on the west side of the Umayyad mosque, according to Ibn Jubayr's account of his 1184 visit to Damascus.[19] Ibn al-ʿImād (d. 1679) wrote that the people of Damascus claimed that this smaller bīmāristān dated as far back as the Umayyad times and was indeed built by the first Umayyad caliph, Muʿāwīyah (r. 661–680).[20] Although there is no evidence that Muʿawīyah was involved in any constructions of this sort, the local Damascene story reported by Ibn al-ʿImād was probably superimposing the story of an Umayyad institution (likely built by al-Walīd I) on this bīmāristān due to its proximity to the Umayyad mosque. Although al-Walīd's establishment may have been built beside, or annexed to, the mosque, this particular institution was built by the Seljuk ruler Duqāq ibn Tatash, who also renovated the Umayyad mosque.[21] Al-Bīmāristān al-Nūrī eclipsed the older bīmāristān, which was henceforth called al-Bīmāristān al-Ṣaghīr or the small bīmāristān.

Nūr al-Dīn "revived" not only the institution of the bīmāristān – and the Umayyad legacy of which the Damascus bīmāristāns were then perceived to be a part – but also another important Umayyad institution: Kashf al-Maẓālim. With his construction of the Dār al-ʿAdl, Nūr al-Dīn recreated an old Umayyad institution designed to allow people to complain to the caliph or governor as a final appeal. This renewed institution was given a new building close to the Umayyad mosque, possibly near the original building of Kashf al-Maẓālim. Nūr al-Dīn sat there once or twice a week to listen to complaints. The survival of the Umayyad form was not limited to the existence of these institutions. In his study of Nūr al-Dīn's architectural patronage, Yasser al-Tabba explains that the Umayyad style of

19 Ibn Jubayr, *Riḥlat Ibn Jubayr*, 272.
20 Ibn Al-ʿImād, *Shadharāt al-Dhahab*.
21 Mouton, *Damas et sa Principauté sous les Saljoukides et les Bourides*, 14–15.

ornamentation was produced in the Levant into the eleventh and twelfth centuries and was apparent in Nūr al-Dīn's own edifices surrounding the Umayyad mosque. He explains that this

> may be a rare document of the survival of Umayyad-style ornament long after its disappearance in other parts of the Muslim world, with the possible exception of Spain. Or it could in fact be an example of deliberate revival of Umayyad ornament, much in the tradition of the Umayyad-style mosaics of the Aqsa mosque in Jerusalem, done under the Fatimid Caliph al-Ẓāhir in 1035. Of course even a deliberate revival implies in part survival, namely the existence of craftsmen who could still faithfully render ornament which preceded them by more than three centuries.[22]

In his visit to Damascus, Ibn Jubayr was quite impressed with al-Bīmāristān al-Nūrī:

> Its daily expenses are about fifteen dinars. It has attendants that have records that contain the names of patients, the expenses that they need for medications and nourishment. Physicians go there early every morning, inspect the patients, and order the preparation of what is good for [each of them] of medications and nourishment. [. . .] The incarcerated mad also [receive] a form of treatment while they are chained. May God protect us from plight and bad fate.[23]

A foundational myth wove al-Bīmāristān al-Nūrī in Damascus into the fabric of Nūr al-Dīn's work and career. Most anecdotes explained how Nūr al-Dīn captured a Crusader lord and that his emirs disagreed on what to do with him; they could not decide whether to execute him or hold him for ransom. Nūr al-Dīn decided on the ransom and later used this money to build the bīmāristān.[24] The bīmāristān, therefore, was a charitable institution that exemplified Nūr al-Dīn's piety and care in its own right, while remaining linked to his jihad and his war against the Crusaders.

The bīmāristān has a cruciform floor plan with four rooms (*īwāns*), each covered by barrel vaults and opening onto a courtyard that probably had a garden or water fountain in its center (see Figure 1.1). In addition to the four open *īwāns*, four other large rooms would open to the courtyard, two from the east and two from the west, each lying alongside its respective barrel-vaulted *īwān*. Four more rooms, smaller than the others,

22 Tabba, "The Architectural Patronage of Nur Al-Din, 1146–1174," 89–90.
23 Ibn Jubayr, *Riḥlat Ibn Jubayr*, 272.
24 Al-Maqrīzī, *al-Khiṭaṭ*, 4: 408.

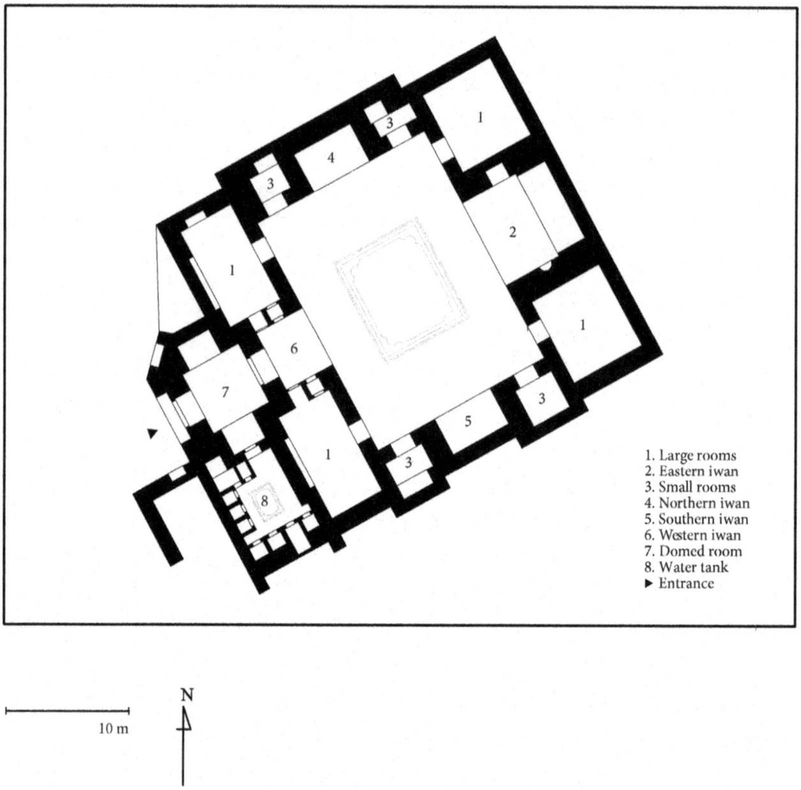

Figure 1.1. Floor plan of al-Bīmāristān al-Nuri

open onto the courtyard alongside the northern and southern vaulted *īwāns*, two on each side. The entryway of the western *īwān* leads into the bīmāristān, practically creating a gateway to the main court from the street. "The main entrance on the street has a most unusual vault over a bay whose depth is only one-quarter of its width, the vault itself being a semidome with its depth reduced to half its radius."[25] The semidome creates a gradation in the entryway, increasing the size of the door while simultaneously luring the gaze inward. This then leads to a small corridor, which opens onto a room whose huge domed ceiling rises over two semi-domes on the north and south walls. This domed room leads into

[25] Herzfeld, "Damascus: Studies in Architecture I," 7.

another corridor, where a second door provides access to the west *īwān* of the main court. On the southwestern side of the building, a smaller court with a water tank in it, surrounded by baths and lavatories, probably served as the bīmāristān's bathhouse. It opens to the domed room in the entryway.[26]

Herzfeld recorded three main inscriptions in the bīmāristān, which provide important information on the bīmāristān's history, as well as on the usage of its massive structure. In the eastern *īwān*, on the southern wall (located to the right of a person entering the *īwān*), the dedicatory inscription appears on a plate of white marble and reads as follows:

> This [bīmāristān] which completion (*tamām*) was ordered; not for [the purpose of] immortality (*al-khulūd*) but for [the purpose of] respite (*al-baqā'*) for the duration of one's reckoned fate (*al-ajal al-muḥṣā*), and pre-ordained and predestined life (*al-ʿumr al-muqaddar al-maqḍī*), by the needy to God in his bountiful mercy, our lord, the just, the scholar (*al-ʿālim*), the knower (*al-ʿārif*), the ascetic (*al-zāhid*), the holy warrior (*al-mujāhid*); Nūr al-Dīn, the pillar of Islam and Muslims; Abū al-Qāsim Maḥmūd ibn Zankī ibn Āqsunqur; the helper of the Commander of the Faithful, in the year 549 [AH, 1154 CE].[27]

The dedicatory text echoed a pietistic formulation of medicine, and it presented the role of the bīmāristān as a site where medical practice was not intended to bestow immortality. Rather, its purpose was to provide an abode for the period of one's predestined life, which would end when God ordained, regardless of the illness or its treatment. This understanding of medical practice as the conduit of a predestined fate – and not as an attempt to defy God's will by seeking immortality or escaping death – could, at that time, be found in many religious texts addressing questions of medicine. Most notable among these are writings on prophetic medicine, a genre that had existed since the ninth century but flourished in the thirteenth and fourteenth centuries. The introductory chapters of these texts discussed the legitimacy of medical practice and used this explanation

[26] Ibid., 2–11.

[27] Tabba, "The Architectural Patronage of Nur Al-Din, 1146–1174," 229–30; Herzfeld, "Damascus: Studies in Architecture I," 3. Tabba corrected Herzfeld's Arabic text to read as follows: "basmalah . . . hadhā mā 'amar bi-tmām ("bi-itmām" in Herzfeld) ʿimāratih al-ʿAbd al-faqīr ilā Allāh fī siʿat raḥmatih lā lil-khulūd ("lil-tajāwud" in Herzfeld) fīh bal lil-muqām bih muddat al-ajal al-muḥṣā wa-l-ʿumr al-muqaddar al-maqḍī wa dhalik fī sanat tisʿ wa arbaʿīn wa khams mā'ah, mawlānā al-malik al-ʿādil al-ʿālim al-ʿārif al-zāhid al-mujāhid Nūr al-Dīn rukn al-islām wa-l-muslimīn abū al-qāsim Maḥmūd ibn Zankī ibn Āqsunqur nāṣir amīr al-mu'minīn." This translation relies on Tabba's text and corrections, but not his translation.

of the purpose of medicine to argue for its legitimacy alongside a tradition (sometimes attributed to the Prophet and other times to a number of companions) that stated: "God created a cure for every illness."[28] The dedication included a long series of honorific titles, as well, which recalled important components of Nūr al-Dīn's political persona: warrior (*mujāhid*), ascetic (*zāhid*), knower (*ʿārif*, in reference to esoteric knowledge of the divine), and the supporter and helper of the Abbasid caliph (in reference to his war against Shiites).

The second inscription was also located in the eastern *īwān*, on a dado around the *īwān*'s left and right walls – in the case of the right, under the dedicatory inscription – where a number of Quranic verses concerning health and treatment were written.

> Right wall: "O mankind! There hath come unto you an exhortation from your Lord, a balm for that which is in the breasts (Q10: 57). There cometh forth from the bellies [of the bees] a drink divers of hues, wherein is healing for mankind (Q16: 69)."
>
> Left wall: "[He] who created me, and He doth guide me; And Who feedeth me and watereth me; And when I sicken, then He healeth me; And Who causeth me to die, then giveth me life (again); And Who, I ardently hope, will forgive me my sin on the Day of Judgment (Q26: 78–82)."[29]

The verses on both walls speak of treatment and healing, but they do not all emphasize healing the body. On the right, the first verse does not speak of physical healing but rather of healing (*shifāʾ*) hearts through belief. The second addresses the healing of bodily ills: in this case, explaining the "miraculous" nature of honey as a treatment for many ills. By juxtaposing these verses about different types of "healing" (*shifāʾ*), the inscription highlights their similarity. This linguistic connection emphasizes God's ability to heal every illness, spiritual or physical. The bīmāristān was to be a space where such comprehensive healing can occur. At the same time, the pious ruler's role is to seek God's reward by ensuring that these spaces for healing are built and maintained; the patron's support of such institutions is itself a demonstration of his piety.

[28] Examples of these writings include Ibn Qayyim al-Jawzīyah, *Al-Ṭibb al-Nabawī*; Ibn Ṭūlūn, *Al-Manhal al-Rawī fī al-Ṭibb Al-Nabawī*; al-Dhahabī, *Al-Ṭibb al-Nabawī*; al-Aṣbahānī, "Al-Ṭibb al-Nabawī"; al-Suyūṭī, *Al-Raḥmah fī al-Ṭibb wa-al-Ḥikmah*. See also Pehro, *The Prophet's Medicine*.

[29] Tabba, "The Architectural Patronage of Nur Al-Din, 1146–1174," 228; Herzfeld, "Damascus: Studies in Architecture I," 5. The translations of these verses come from Marmaduke Pickthall's translation of the Quran.

On the left wall, five verses describe God as the grantor of guidance, of life and sustenance, of healing and death. Their rhythm – staccato, strong – blatantly underscores the message found on the right wall: the power to heal is, ultimately, God's. Why these particular verses were selected, or whether they held any special significance beyond their apparent meaning and reference to healing, is unclear. However, it is clear that the room that these verses (and dedicatory inscription) adorn, the eastern *īwān*, was – functionally – the heart of the entire building, serving as the site of the bīmāristān's most official activities. The Quranic verses lining this space, therefore, literally encircled the bīmāristān's material functions with an acknowledgment of the institution's sacred purpose.

Ibn Abī Uṣaybiʿah (d. 1269) learned and worked within al-Bīmāristān al-Nūrī for a number of years. His descriptions of the bīmāristān, found in a number of biographies of physicians who worked in al-Nūrī, name three main areas of the bīmāristān: halls for patients, where patients had beds and were examined by physicians;[30] a place where physicians sat to examine the patients who came to them;[31] and a space where physicians could read and teach their students.[32] The patients' halls were probably the eight rooms (with the four large rooms opening onto the eastern and western walls and the four small rooms opening onto the northern and southern walls) described previously in this chapter. Both Ibn Abī Uṣaybiʿah and Ibn Jubayr also cited specific places for those whom Ibn Abī Uṣaybiʿah called "melancholic" (*mamrūrīn*) or whom Ibn Jubayr called "the mad" (*majānīn*). According to Ibn Abī Uṣaybiʿah, these inmates were kept in halls where they received treatment; Ibn Jubayr wrote, however, that they were chained. The hall where the mad were kept may have been one of the eight rooms, or it may have been the southwest annex (which opened onto the domed entry room). It is likely, as well, that men and women were kept in separate halls. Elsewhere, it was written that the bīmāristān's library and the weekly or daily lessons were held in a large *īwān*; this was most likely the eastern *īwān*, which was the largest and, with its verses and inscriptions, would have been well-suited for such purposes.[33] Physicians probably examined patients in the northern and southern *īwāns*, which lend themselves most easily Ibn Abī Uṣaybiʿah's description of the place where a

[30] See, for instance (in the context of the biography of Muhdhdhab al-Dīn ibn ʿAbd al-Raḥīm, who will be discussed in more detail later), Ibn Abī Uṣaybiʿah, *ʿUyūn al-Anbāʾ*, 4: 327.

[31] For more reading on Muhdhdhab al-Dīn ibn ʿAbd al-Raḥīm, see Ibn Abī Usaybiʿah's *ʿUyūn al-Anbāʾ*, 4: 325–26.

[32] Ibid., 4: 328.

[33] Tabba, "The Architectural Patronage of Nur Al-Din, 1146–1174," 228.

physician sat on a bench and examined the patients who had come to see him. Patients were probably examined in the eastern *īwān* as well. Herzfeld suggests that some additional buildings were attached to the bīmāristān, which may have included cells for the mad, along with rooms for preparing drugs and medications, and the like.

The third inscription Herzfeld describes foregrounds the connection between al-Manṣūr Qalāwūn and Nūr al-Dīn Zankī. In the entryway, just before the second door, another dedicatory plate was inserted to commemorate the renovations and additions that al-Manṣūr Qalāwūn ordered in al-Bīmāristān al-Nūrī. The plate reads: "What was out of repair [in] its building and *waqf* was replaced by the Sultan Qalāwūn in 682 [1283 CE]."[34] The placement of the plate is curious: it is the first text encountered upon entering the bīmāristān, thereby dominating the institution and reattributing it to Qalāwūn. It was not attached to any specific site Qalāwūn had added, and it also mentioned repairing the *waqf*, which financed the entire institution. At the same time, the inscription is strikingly short and blunt, with no honorific titles attributed to Qalāwūn – not even his regal title al-Manṣūr – and makes no specific mention of any of Qalāwūn's renovations. The deliberate prominence of the plate's location, noticeable to anyone entering the bīmāristān's court and most official space, belies its simplicity and modesty. Moreover, the plate was likely installed at the end of the aforementioned renovations in 1283, just two years before al-Bīmāristān al-Manṣūrī was built in Cairo, and, as such, demands further investigation into the relationships between these two rulers and their places of healing.

Qalāwūn's choice to renovate al-Bīmāristān al-Nūrī and to replace some of its (probably no longer profitable) *waqfs* illustrates the depth of Qalāwūn's inspiration by the Damascene bīmāristān. If the anecdote recounting his treatment by medications from al-Bīmāristān al-Nūrī is accurate, it could very well explain his interest in the renovation. In either case, the renovation – just two years before the construction of his own bīmāristān – reveals that the connection between the two bīmāristāns was not arbitrary, nor was it contrived by Qalāwūn's historians or emirs after the construction of al-Bīmāristān al-Manṣūrī. Instead, it was rather more deliberate and had deeper roots into Qalāwūn's ten-year rule. This makes Qalāwūn's modest plate and the lack of any glorifying terms or titles, or even descriptions of his piety (all of which could be found on other buildings he established), particularly interesting. Although the inscription recognizes the act of renovation – reattributing the building to Qalāwūn at

[34] Herzfeld, "Damascus: Studies in Architecture I," 5.

its very entrance and linking the Mamluk sultan to the history of the bīmāristān – it does so with a modesty that suggests a genuine reverence for Nūr al-Dīn. If this, Qalāwūn's personal admiration for Nūr al-Dīn, is what it seems, then the plate's inscription marks his renovation as a simple act of restoring the building and its *waqfs* to their original status in memory of Nūr al-Dīn.

Crusader Hospitals: Friendship, Animosity, and Competition

In August 2013, the Israel Antiquities Authority concluded their excavation of what appears to be the ruins of the famous Crusader hospital in Jerusalem, parts of which date to 1099 or even earlier. The excavation, which was performed in what was a vegetable market, revealed a structure stretching out over fifteen dunams (or 15,000 square meters). This huge space was not all dedicated to the Crusaders' famous hospital, but was most likely the entire complex of the Order of the Hospital, which included a chapel, residences, animal stables, and possibly even barracks.[35] Parts of the large Crusader edifice were converted by Ṣalāḥ al-Dīn into a bīmāristān bearing his name: al-Bīmāristān al-Ṣalāḥī, eventually giving that neighborhood in Jerusalem its current name, "al-māristān." Ṣalāḥ al-Dīn gave a number of Hospitaller friars permission to stay and continue caring for Christian patients, and, throughout the Mamluk period, al-Bīmāristān al-Ṣalāḥī continued to function and to serve as the second-largest bīmāristān in the Levant (after al-Bīmāristān al-Nūrī), alongside a smaller Crusader hospital. This model for establishing these institutions – transforming a Hospitaller House into a bīmāristān – was not limited to Jerusalem, but was repeated in other Levantine towns as Ṣalāḥ al-Dīn conquered them, the most famous of which was the Hospitaller House turned bīmāristān in Acre. Crusader-cum-Ayyubid bīmāristāns had a significant influence on the establishment of bīmāristāns in the Levant and Egypt throughout the twelfth century, and they were a substantial part of the environment that eventually produced al-Bīmāristān al-Manṣūrī and similar institutions in that region.

The origins of the earliest Crusader/Latin hospital date to the early ninth century, when Charlemagne reportedly asked for Hārūn al-Rashīd's

35 Israel Antiquities Authority, "Enormous 1,000 Year Old Hospital Building" (August 2013). Animal bones, including those from horses and camels, were found, along with large quantities of metals, likely used for shoeing horses and making weapons.

permission to build and renovate a number of establishments in Jerusalem – including a hospital.[36] There is no local contemporary evidence that the request for, or the actual building of, the hospital ever took place, making it likely that it was attributed to Charlemagne at a later date. Pope Gregory I had built a Latin *xenodocheion* in 632, which may have been renovated by Charlemagne. This *xenodocheion* was dedicated to the service of Latin pilgrims coming to the holy town, but it was either destroyed or seized by the Fatimid Caliph al-Ḥākim bi-Amr Allah (d. 1021), who was known for his severe measures against Christians. In the writings of William of Tyre, the destruction of the hospital under al-Ḥākim was evidence of the deterioration of the conditions of Christians under his reign; the fortunes of the hospital were linked to the fortunes of Christians, and the survival of the hospital – as well as other sites of pilgrimage support and care – symbolized the success of the Latin endeavor in the East: to protect and serve pilgrims and to liberate the Christians from the Muslim yoke.[37] Its destruction symbolized the opposite:

> Earlier sources confirm the outlines of William's account and add further details. The South Italian chronicler Amato of Montecassino recorded the establishment of hospitals in Jerusalem and Antioch at the initiative of a rich Amalfitan called Mauro of Pantaleone, whose family had a close relationship with the abbey of Montecassino; he joined Amato as a monk there shortly before his death. An Amalfitan chronicle described how Archbishop John of Amalfi (c. 1071–1081/82) made a pilgrimage to Jerusalem and was received there by his countrymen, who, a few years before, had built two hospitals, one for men, which must be the Hospital of St John, and one for women.[38]

The Amalfitan patronage of the pilgrims did not stop at Jerusalem; the Benedictine monastery of Sancta Maria was built in Constantinople by 1060 and still existed in 1256. "The Hospitallers conceivably took over some such Latin foundation at an early date, in much the same way that elsewhere they secured possessions and churches originally destined for the Holy Sepulchre."[39]

By the twelfth century, the pilgrimage land route that passed through Eastern Europe and Constantinople was marked by the Order's hospitals, including its house in Constantinople itself. However, the death of the Byzantine Emperor Manuel I, in 1180, and the collapse of Byzantine control over Serbia and Hungary rendered land routes less safe and reliable,

[36] William of Tyre, *Deeds Done beyond the Sea*, 64–65.
[37] Ibid., 64–68.
[38] Riley-Smith, *The Knights Hospitaller*, 17.
[39] Luttrell, "The Hospitallers," 227–28.

and most travel shifted to the direct sea route through the Adriatic. This coincided with the building of a number of Hospitaller houses "along the roads to the Adriatic in Friuli, Carinthia, Carniola, Istria, Styria and Croatia as well as in western Hungary."[40] Anthony Luttrell links the change of travel patterns – as well as the subsequent change in the distribution of hospitals and of the Order's activities – to the changing political circumstances in the Byzantine empire and the increasing hostility toward Latins in the last decades of the twelfth century:

> In the twelfth century, the Hospital had founded or acquired pilgrim hospices in the Levant as well as in western Europe. These included the hospice on the overland route from central Europe to Syria which passed through Constantinople, where the Hospitallers, along with other Latins, often enjoyed good relations with the Greeks. After 1182, however, pilgrims and other westerners increasingly travelled by sea rather than overland through Constantinople, where political conditions had in any case become unfavourable to Latin communities.[41]

The charitable function of the Order, its role in serving pilgrims, and its connection to the hospital of Jerusalem were further regularized in the Papal Bull that officially initiated the Order in 1113:

> Paschal the Bishop, servant of the servants of God, to his venerable son Gerard, founder and Provost *(prepositus)* of the *Xenodochium* ... of Jerusalem, and to his lawful successors forever. A pious request and desire should meet with satisfaction and fulfillment. For as much as of thine affection thou hast requested that the *Xenodochium,* which thou hast founded in the City of Jerusalem, near to the Church of the Blessed John the Baptist, should be supported by the Apostolic See, and fostered by the patronage of the Blessed Apostle Peter. We therefore, being much pleased with the piety and earnestness of thine hospital work [*hospitalitas*], do receive thy petition with paternal kindness, and we ordain by virtue of the present decree that the House of God the *Xenodochium* shall always be under the guardianship of the Apostolic See and the protection of Blessed Peter.[42]

The Papal Bull not only established the connection between the Order and the hospital of Jerusalem but also reiterated the hospital's origins asserting that it was founded by Frere Gerard, who was also the founder of the Order. The hospital soon occupied a central position in Crusader Jerusalem, attracting the attention and comments of many pilgrims who visited the city. In addition to its size and its central location, the hospital

[40] Ibid., 228.
[41] Ibid., 232.
[42] Qtd. in Hume, *Medical Work of the Knights Hospitallers*, 424.

was a crucial site for pilgrims, both for practical and symbolic purposes. In his enthusiastic report on the "medical works of the Knights Hospitallers of St. John of Jerusalem," Edgar E. Hume quotes a number of accounts from visitors and pilgrims. Among them, John of Wurzburg wrote in 1160:

> Over against the Church of the Holy Sepulchre, on the opposite side of the way towards the south, is a beautiful church built in honor of John the Baptist, annexed to which is a hospital, wherein in various rooms is collected together an enormous multitude of sick people, both men and women, who are tended and restored to health daily at every great expense. When I was there I learned that the whole number of these sick people amounted to two thousand, of whom sometimes in the course of one day and night more than fifty are carried out dead, while many other fresh ones keep continually arriving.[43]

Theodorich, in 1187, echoed John of Wurzburg's observations on the size of the hospital and the number of patients while also describing how the hospital was, in fact, part of his and his company's pilgrim route: "Indeed, we passed through this palace, and were unable by any means to discover the number of sick people lying there; but we saw that the beds numbered more than one thousand."[44] While discussing its enormous expenses, Theodorich also made reference to the grand possessions of both the Hospitallers and the Templars (who likewise were responsible for flourishing charity institutions and hospitals): "It is not everyone even of the most powerful kings and despots who could maintain as many people as that house does every day; and no wonder, for, in addition to its possessions in other countries . . ., the Hospitallers and the Templars have conquered almost all the cities and villages which once belonged to Judaea, and which were destroyed by Vespasian and Titus, together with all their lands and vineyards."[45]

Shortly before Theodorich's visit, in 1163, Rabbi Benjamin of Tudela in Navarre visited the city and wrote about two hospitals run by the Hospitallers and the Templars: "There are in Jerusalem two hospitals, which support four hundred knights and afford shelter to the sick; these are provided with everything they may want, both during life and death; the second is called the hospital of Solomon, being the place originally built by King Solomon."[46] The mention of the Templars' hospital and other institutions reveals the importance of the charitable framework that

[43] Ibid., 412–13.
[44] Ibid., 413–14.
[45] Ibid., 414.
[46] Ibid., 413.

served the pilgrims and established the legitimacy of the Orders in the Holy Land.

The hospital in Jerusalem and the other houses of the Hospitaller Order attracted the attention of many European sovereigns and noblemen, who often bestowed gifts and endowments on these institutions. With the first capture of Jerusalem and the coronation of Godfrey de Bouillon as Godfrey I of Jerusalem in 1099, the new king gave the knights and their newly acquired hospital two bakeries and the Casal Hessilia[47] – and this even before the Order was formally recognized in 1113. Similarly, other European noblemen and sovereigns donated to the Order in the form of either monetary donations or the granting of fiefs. King Bela III of Hungary (d. 1196), who was the heir to Manuel I's Byzantine imperial throne, donated generously to the Order's hospitals in Hungary, which served the land route to Jerusalem.[48] Bela's younger son, King Andrew II the Jerosolimitan (d. 1235) – who was one of the heirs to the Latin Imperial throne of Constantinople – continued his father's amicable relations with the Order and was affiliated to the Order as Confrater. He bestowed upon the Order

> the customs duties of the port of Bobeth at Soprony (Oldenburg), together with the land between the Drave and the Csurgo, and extensive privileges in the Magyar realm. . . . The King a little later granted the Order the sum of 500 marks of silver (a mark weighed eight ounces) each year, secured upon the royal salt-works at Szalacs. When the King visited the Knights' castles of Margat and Le Crac, he made a further donation, likewise secured upon the saltworks of Szalacs, of 100 marks of silver a year to each fortress, to be used in strengthening the defenses.[49]

Similarly, the first Latin emperor of Constantinople Baldwin I (formerly Baldwin IX of Flanders; d. 1205) supported the Order by granting it fiefs in the newly Latin territories in Asia Minor, such as in the principality of Morea, and in Pergamon, although this region never came under Latin control and the gift never materialized.[50]

In spite of the significance of the various hospitals scattered along the pilgrimage routes, the hospital of Jerusalem continued to be the most important of the Order's possessions; other houses and prioris were required to send supplies to Jerusalem every year. For instance, the Chapter-General

[47] Ibid., 404–05.
[48] Luttrell, "The Hospitallers," 228.
[49] Hume, *Medical Work of the Knights Hospitallers*, 418–19.
[50] Luttrell, "The Hospitallers," 230–31.

of 1181 under Grand Master Roger des Moulins, Master of the Hospital, adopted a number of statutes to regulate the yearly supplies sent to the Jerusalem hospital from other priories around Europe. In these statutes:

> The Prior of the Hospital of France should send each year to Jerusalem one hundred sheets of dyed cotton, . . . the Prior of Italy each year should send to Jerusalem for our lords the sick[51] two thousand ells of fustian . . . of divers colors, . . . and the Prior of Pisa should send likewise the like number of fustians. And the Prior of Venice likewise, and all should be reckoned in their *Responsions.*

Neither were establishments in the Levant exempt from sending supplies to Jerusalem:

> The Bailiff of Antioch should send to Jerusalem two thousand ells of cotton cloth . . . for the coverlets of the sick. The Prior of Mont Pelerin [i.e., Tripolis] should send to Jerusalem two quintals [i.e., 200 pounds] of sugar for the syrups, and the medicines and the electuaries. . . . For this same service the Bailiff of Tabarie [Tiberias] should send there the same quantity. The Prior of Constantinople should send for the sick two hundred felts.[52]

However, the Crusaders' changes in fortune – including their defeats by the Ayyubids and, ultimately, the fall of Jerusalem to Ṣalāḥ al-Dīn in 1163 – forced the Hospitallers to abandon the hospital of Jerusalem; they moved first to Acre, then to Rhodes and, eventually, to Malta, following successive military defeats. The hospital at Acre was equally famous and impressive as that of Jerusalem, attracting the admiration of many travelers and visitors. In one (likely apocryphal) account, Ṣalāḥ al-Dīn himself was one of these visitors. He masqueraded as a patient demanding to be treated only by eating the Grand Master's horse; the freres were terrified by the request, but the Master complied and ordered his horse slaughtered for the unknown patient. Fortunately for the horse, Ṣalāḥ al-Dīn revealed himself to the Master and commended his dedication to the service of patients. He wrote to the Master upon his return: "Let all men know that I, Saladin, Soldan [sic] of Babylon, give and bequeath to the Hospital of Acre a

[51] To this day, the Order refers to the sick poor as the "Poor of Christ" or the "Poor of Our Lord." The Order's rule explains that "they belong to our Lord Jesus Christ and they are to be treated like the Lord himself (cf. chapter 16 of the Rule). They are called 'the Blessed, our Lords, the sick.' The members of the Order made the promise 'to be servants and slaves to our Lords, the sick.' The brothers, on the one hand and the sick on the other hand, are mutually representing Christ, making life in the community of the hospital a mutual encounter with the Lord and therefore an event of salvation." (See for instance, the Order of Malta official webpage: http://smom-za.org/spirituality.htm. Last accessed on December 18, 2014)

[52] Hume, *Medical Work of the Knights Hospitallers*, 428.

thousand besants of gold, to be paid every year in peace or war, unto the Grand Master be he who he may, in gratitude for the wonderful charity of himself and his order."[53] In Jerusalem, Ṣalāḥ al-Dīn maintained parts of the Latin hospital while converting the rest to the service of Muslims.

In his analysis of the Hospitallers' activities, Hume furnishes us with extensive citations from various Hospitallers' statutes describing the manner in which they envisioned their institutions' models of care. The statutes clearly identify the sick received by the hospital as Latin Catholics who would "partake of the Holy Sacrament, first having confessed his sins to the priest" before being taken to bed.[54] Another rule issued at the Chapter-General in 1176 under Frere Jobert, the Master of the Hospital, insisted that white bread was to be provided to the patients in line with Raymod du Puy's rule, which stipulated that they would be "refreshed with the best of food."[55] Another statute from 1181 specified that "for three days in the week the sick are accustomed to have fresh meat, either pork or mutton, and those who are unable to eat it have chicken."[56]

The Chapter-General of 1181 was even more specific, discussing bedding and covers, with every patient receiving a cloak of sheepskin, boots, and caps of wool. The statute affirmed that every bed should have its own sheet and every patient his own cover.[57] The statute also discussed pilgrim women, especially those who gave birth during their pilgrimage, and stipulated that the newborn should lie in a little cradle to sleep separately "in no danger from the restlessness of its mother."[58] The statute also indicates the type of medical practice required in these hospitals and of those who practiced there: "And secondly, it is decreed with the assent of the brethren, that for the sick in the Hospital of Jerusalem there should be engaged four wise doctors, who are qualified to examine urine, and to diagnose different diseases, and are able to administer appropriate medicines."[59] This description, with its emphasis on examining urine, recalled one of the most famous acts of Galenic physicians in Latin lore, which would have been clear to the authors of the statute. The physicians were probably not members of the Order because they were not described as freres or confereres; this suggests that the Order hired these physicians to

[53] Ibid., 420. The story is consistent with the favorable views that many Crusaders and Crusade chroniclers held toward Ṣalāḥ al-Dīn as an honorable warrior, pious sovereign, and worthy rival.
[54] "The Rule of the Blessed Raymond du Puy" (c. 1150), qtd. in ibid., 426.
[55] Ibid.
[56] Ibid., 428.
[57] Ibid., 426.
[58] Ibid., 427.
[59] Ibid., 426.

provide medical service inside the hospital, but also that their roles were likely limited to administering medical care. The management of the hospital, on the other hand, was clearly the prerogative of the freres, as it was in similar institutions in the region.

The number of physicians – four – is very small compared to the number of patients, described in the hundreds or even thousands by the travelers. Although it is likely that the reported number of patients was exaggerated, it is also possible that the hospital received and served such huge numbers on specific occasions on the Latin religious calendar and that the number of physicians did not correspond to the number of patients at times like these. The strong focus of the statutes on matters related to patients' housing, bedding, food, and the like reveal that the hospital was not only a site for medical practice; rather, it was also primarily a site of charity toward pilgrims that included but was not limited to medical care. The form of care the statute presents as vital was not as centered on treating illness as it was on providing proper food and proper living conditions, which the pilgrims did not have. In fact, the same statute of 1181 listed a number of other functions that the hospital performed: "Every year the House of the Hospital is accustomed to give to the poor one thousand cloaks of thick lamb skins. And all the children abandoned by their fathers and mothers, the Hospital is accustomed to receive and to nourish. To a man and woman who desire to enter into matrimony, and who possess nothing with which to celebrate the marriage, the House of the Hospital is accustomed to give two bowls or the ration of two brethren."[60] The hospital's role extended, then, to meeting many needs of the poor in Jerusalem; it was a site of charitable giving that was rooted in the image of "Our Lord the Sick" but that embraced children, the poor, and the needy as well.[61]

The hospital in Jerusalem and the other hospitals and houses on Latin Europe's pilgrimage routes were not a completely isolated phenomenon; they were part of a larger, longer history of similar institutions in Europe, which inspired, influenced, and were influenced by the institutions of the East. As far back as the sixth century, the Merovingian King Childebert I (d. 558) established a hospice for the pilgrims in Laon. Other hospitals were scattered throughout Merovingian Gaul, including one built by Bishop St. Praeiectus of Auvergne (d. ca 674) in Claremont, which housed only twenty patients. Similarly, Saint Adalard of Corbie

[60] Ibid., 428.
[61] Riley-Smith, *The Knights Hospitaller*, 17–18.

(d. 827) built a *xenodocheion* for pilgrims before his cousin, Charlemagne, presumably built his famous hospital in Jerusalem, thus marking the beginning of a long line of Carolingian hospitals throughout Latin Europe.[62] Many of these were annexed to monasteries and functioned as a service for monks; the Abbey of Saint Gall (built ca. 719), for example, included a hospital dedicated to serve its monks.[63] It appears that the hospital in Jerusalem – although dedicated to the service of pilgrims – also paid close attention to the freres, housing them separately and instituting severe punishments against any lack of care or attention by their comrades or superiors; this is explained in detail in the statute issued in the Chapter-General of 1304.[64] The Hospitallers built more hospitals throughout Europe, like the hospital of the Holy Sepulchre and Saint John in Pisa (1113) and the Holy Spirit in Montpelier (1145). Other orders, such as the Order of Teutonic Knights, built a number of hospitals in Germany in the last decades of the twelfth century, and the Order of the Knights of the Temple annexed the hospital of the Holy Sepulchre in Florence in 1205 only to have it inherited by the Knights of the Hospital in 1213.[65]

This hospital tradition, whether in Latin Europe or in the Latin East, was connected to the older Byzantine tradition and to the Islamic traditions of the East. In fact, Latin sources, including the Papal Bull establishing the Order of the Hospital, used the Greek term *xenodochium* to refer to the institution, echoing the older Byzantine usage, which had been dropped in favor of *nosokomion*. Henri Pirenne argues that the spread of hospitals in Merovingian Gaul was connected to the migration of Syrians, Greeks, and Jews from Byzantine territories to Gaul at the wake of the Arab expansion and that they brought the heritage of hospitals with them. Saint Praeiectus of Auvergne was said to have been influenced by the Oriental traditions in establishing the hospital of Clermont; similarly, other cities and regions in close contact with "Eastern" traditions maintained important hospitals and similar institutions, such as the hospital founded by Bishop Masona of Merida (d. 606) in Visigothic Spain and other hospitals in Rome. "At Merida many of the bishops were Greeks and trade with Byzantium was brisk; at Rome men from the eastern Mediterranean were often elected to the papacy, and Greek monasteries were numerous."[66]

[62] Miller, "Knights of Saint John," 710.
[63] Ibid., 711.
[64] Hume, *Medical Work of the Knights Hospitallers*, 430.
[65] Ibid., 409.
[66] Miller, "Knights of Saint John," 711.

The Crusader Hospital was, clearly, a significant part of the larger hospital tradition in the Middle East and exerted a strong influence on the Levant, Egypt, and Asia Minor where contact with the Crusaders was greatest. Firmly tied to religious institutions, the Crusader Hospital accentuated the connection between the Byzantine Xenon and the Byzantine Church, holding forth a model of religious philanthropy that was also dominant in nearby Islamic territories. In this region, it appeared that "the hospital" – whether in its Byzantine, Islamic, or Crusader iterations – played a crucial role in symbolizing religious and sovereign care for the poor and needy, effectively establishing these categories as representations of the Self in opposition to the Other.

Ṣalāḥ al-Dīn and Inheriting the Hospitaller Heritage

Ṣalāḥ al-Dīn's relations with the Order of the Hospital can be traced to their encounters on the battlefield during Ṣalāḥ al-Dīn's wars in the Levant. The Hospitallers controlled a number of important forts, such as Ṣafad,[67] Crec de Chevalliers,[68] and Sion,[69] which had to be conquered in order for Ṣalāḥ al-Dīn's plans to bear fruit. Ibn Shaddād (1145–1234), a judge and bureaucrat working closely with Ṣalāḥ al-Dīn and his brother al-ʿĀdil I, described many of these battlefield encounters in his biography of Ṣalāḥ al-Dīn. After the decisive battle of Ḥaṭṭīn in 1187, which all but sealed Ṣalāḥ al-Dīn's control over the Levant, Ṣalāḥ al-Dīn decided to execute all the prisoners belonging to the Orders of the Hospital and the Temple, although he released a number of other prisoners and dignitaries.[70] Ṣalāḥ al-Dīn's aggression toward the Hospitallers was probably motivated by their growing military strength over the twelfth and thirteenth centuries. But this aggression mingled with an appreciation of their role in the Crusader politics of the time; Ṣalāḥ al-Dīn had to allow the Master of the Hospital to act as the mediator between him and Richard Coeur Lion during their negotiations.[71]

At the same time, the Hospitallers' presence in the Levant was not limited to their forts or political prowess, but could also be seen in their different Houses, which anchored the pilgrimage routes and functioned as important sites for the support of Latin (and possibly local)

67 Ibn Shaddād, *The Life of Saladin*, 31.
68 Ibid., 125.
69 Ibid., 130.
70 Ibid., 114.
71 Ibid., 263.

Christians.[72] As mentioned before, the largest house of the Order was the Hospital of Saint John in Jerusalem, which included an infirmary and a hospice, housing sick pilgrims but also the tired, destitute, and disabled, as confirmed by William of Tyre. This nature and role of the Crusader Hospital raises questions about the reciprocal influences between this *xenodocheion* and neighboring Islamic bimāristāns, which evidence suggests were more medicalized and more or less restricted to housing patients.[73] When the Amalfitan community first established its hospitalia in Jerusalem, another bīmāristān had stood there for decades, as is evident in the writings of Nāṣir-i Khusraw (d. 1088), who visited Jerusalem in 1047 and who described a well-endowed bīmāristān staffed with physicians and where various drugs were available to patients.[74]

Although the exact date of the first Amalfitan institutions is not clear – nor is it clear whether there were indeed earlier Carolingian institutions or what shape they took – there is little doubt that these Latin institutions were influenced by the pre-Crusade bīmāristān in Jerusalem, if not also by the other bīmāristāns in surrounding Levantine cities. It is important to remember, however, that the bīmāristān described by Khosraw was, as with bīmāristāns in other cities, part of a larger network of charity that included many religious and political institutions ranging from mosques, hostels, sabīls, and public kitchens to charities endowed by political authorities. The Amalfitan institution (followed by that of the Hospitaller), on the other hand, may have been the major site for many of these functions, making it more inclusive in its charitable role than neighboring Muslim institutions. This would explain the huge size of the Hospitaller complex, which appears to have been much more than an infirmary.

Sources contemporary to Ṣalāḥ al-Dīn's conquest of Jerusalem described his effort to alter the city, undermine its Crusader nature, and highlight its new Sunni Muslim character. ʿImād al-Dīn al-Isfahānī (d. 1200), a bureaucrat in Ṣalāḥ al-Dīn's service who accompanied him in Jerusalem, described the process of the islamization of the city in some detail. One of Ṣalāḥ al-Dīn's first steps was to clean and reopen the Aqṣā mosque and the Dome of the Rock. The Aqṣā mosque was supposedly used as a residence for the Templars; its prayer niche had been blocked by

[72] On local Christians in Crusader Levant, see Macevitt, *Crusades and the Christian World*, 50–73, 136–49.

[73] See William of Tyre, *Deeds Done beyond the Sea*, 1: 244.

[74] Kedar, "A Note on Jerusalem's Bīmāristān," 7. As Kedar explains, Khusraw's travelogue, edited by Thackston, does not have any details on the hospital save for mentioning its existence on the eastern side of the city (Khusraw, *Book of Travels*, 23.)

improvised wooden walls, and many of its inscriptions had been covered. Ṣalāḥ al-Dīn ordered the wall taken down. The walls and prayer space were cleaned, the inscriptions revealed. As for the Dome of the Rock, al-Isfahānī claimed that it had been turned into a church and that Ṣalāḥ al-Dīn ordered it to be restored to its original shape and function. The sultan also appointed preachers and teachers at both sites and ordered the renovation of all mosques in the town.[75] Al-Iṣfahānī spoke of a potential change in the town's demography after almost a century of Latin rule:[76] while all Latins were asked to leave the town or enter slavery, local Christians were not part of this agreement. They were not required to leave the town, and only some of them left. Al-Iṣfahānī appears to have expected them to leave town and follow the Franks, but, to his surprise, they refused to leave and asked instead to return to the *dhimma* status that Christians held in other contemporary Islamic polities. Al-Isfahānī's evaluation of the situation appeared to be colored by his and his bureaucrat contemporaries' dismay at the appointment of Christians to state offices: he mentioned that the remaining local Christians had been appointed to the town's administration under Ṣalāḥ al-Dīn. This statement contradicted his assertion that their stay was unwelcome and that it involved severe humiliation.[77] This also casts doubts on whether all Latin Christians did, indeed, leave or were enslaved as al-Isfahānī described.

Following these reclamation projects aimed at the restoration of pre-Crusader Islamic buildings, Ṣalāḥ al-Dīn proceeded with new constructions that fell within the preexisting categories of built patronage he had sponsored in Cairo and in other cities: namely, the madrasa and the Sufi khānaqāh, both of which were also favorite forms for Nūr al-Dīn Zankī's architectural patronage. Ṣalāḥ al-Dīn confiscated the church of Sancta Anna and converted it to a madrasa for Shāfiʿī scholars and then converted the Episcopal palace into a Sufi monastery (*ribāṭ*).[78] The two establishments were located close to the Church of the Holy Sepulchre, which Ṣalāḥ

[75] Al-Iṣfahānī, *Al-Fatḥ al-Qussī fi-l-Fatḥ al-Qudsī*, 76–81.

[76] In his visit in 1047 (about half a century before Crusader control), Nāṣir-i Khusraw mentioned that the city had 20,000 people and that many Muslims in the Levant would visit it for pilgrimage if they could not visit Mecca. Although there is no evidence that the reported population of 20,000 was accurate, Jerusalem was certainly an important pilgrimage site for many Levantine Muslims, and itself may have had a large population of Muslims, who appeared to have left during the Crusader period.

[77] Ibid., 76. At several incidents, al-Isfahānī's writings betray the fact that he expected Ṣalāḥ al-Dīn to impose more retribution on Latin Christians and to prevent them from taking Church possessions with them.

[78] Ibid., 82. Frenkel dates the seizure of Sancta Anna and the establishment of the madrasa in 1189 without explaining the sources for this dating. However, al-Iṣfahānī's narration indicates that these

al-Dīn may have contemplated demolishing, confiscating, or at least closing; but, according to al-Isfahānī, he was dissuaded by his entourage from doing so. Choosing to build a madrasa and a Sufi monastery was consistent with Ṣalāḥ al-Dīn's Sunni building patronage and was also consistent with his desire to attract more Muslim settlers to the city. Before he left the town to continue his battles, Ṣalāḥ al-Dīn was reported to have distributed charities to the poor and fiefs to his commanders and officers.[79] However – up until he left – there was no mention of his intentions to build a bīmāristān in Jerusalem or to effectively alter or adapt the Hospitallers' infirmary. "Of course, we know that directly after the re-conquest Saladin allowed ten Hospitaller brothers to remain in the Hospital for a year to tend the sick there."[80] However, the huge size of the Hospitaller complex would have allowed Ṣalāḥ al-Dīn to establish a bīmāristān while allowing the Hospitaller brothers to keep their infirmary. The reason may have been that Ṣalāḥ al-Dīn was not prioritizing ridding the city of all Christian influences, so the brothers' presence did not register as an impediment to refashioning the city as Islamic. Ten Hospitallers, caring for some patients or the disabled, likely did not present as a serious threat to the city's new Islamic character.

Ṣalāḥ al-Dīn revisited Jerusalem in 1192, at the conclusion of his battles with Richard Coeur Lion during the Third Crusade, as peace was being promulgated between the two sovereigns. Although his visit involved supervising the renovation of the city's fortifications, there was no imminent danger – except perhaps that the negotiations might fall through – and his efforts were directed not only at renovating the city but also at emphasizing his victory and dominance. It was then that he decided to build his bīmāristān. Again, ʿImād al-Dīn al-Isfahānī provides us with the most detailed account, which was copied afterward by other historians:

> [Ṣalāḥ al-Dīn] asked the Sufis about their conditions, and followed his question by answering their demands and requests. He had endowed the Patriarch's Palace near [the Church of the Holy] Sepulchre a monastery for them, and had instituted a [public] meal every day, so he increased the *waqf* [of the monastery] and invested them with [the authority to] spend [from the *waqf*] in charity. He had also [ordered] the church of Sancta Anna near the Gate of the Lions [transformed into] a madrasa for the Shāfiʿī scholars, and returned it [to its pre-Crusade state] as a building built on piety, so he

acts were promulgated shortly after the conquest of 1187. See Frenkel, "Islamic Religious Endowments," 5.

79 Al-Iṣfahānī, *Al-Fatḥ al-Qussī fi-l-Fatḥ al-Qudsī*, 84.

80 Richards, "Saladin's Hospital," 72.

> increased its *waqfs*, and provided for its various expenses. He ordered that the church close to the House of the Hospitallers near the Sepulchre be made a bīmāristān for the sick. He created in it [the church] places for those with different ailments to satisfy their needs. He endowed estates for it, and ordered rare medications and drugs to be taken to it, and appointed al-Qāḍī Bahā' al-Dīn [ibn Shaddād] as the judge [of Jerusalem] and to oversee [all] these waqfs.[81]

Ibn Shaddād himself confirmed that he was ordered to supervise the construction of the bīmāristān in 1192, although he did not go into details in the same florid manner as al-Isfahānī's narrative.[82] In al-Isfahānī's account, building the bīmāristān was connected to inspecting the two major establishments built in 1187: the new additions to the 1187 buildings show that they were built quite hastily, without sufficient *waqfs* to support them. In a way, the new projects of 1192 were continuations of earlier projects, only with the addition of the bīmāristān. Two questions can be asked about the new bīmāristān: why choose a church rather than use the Hospitallers' infirmary? And why now? Because the Hospitallers were mediating the negotiations between Ṣalāḥ al-Dīn and Richard the Lionheart, it is plausible that he decided against confiscating their properties especially if their infirmary (or parts of their House) had existed before the Crusades and could have been legitimately granted to the Amalfitan community. Parts of the Hospitaller complex had already been taken back when Jerusalem was conquered in 1187, such as the palatium, which became a place to house visitors to the city and even the city's governor. A year later, one of Ṣalāḥ al-Dīn's sons seized part of the complex and transformed it into a mosque.[83] Yet, the core of the establishment, which may have dated back to the middle of the eleventh century, continued to serve Latin pilgrims well into the fourteenth century.[84]

The Hospitallers and their establishments appear to have played a significant role in housing Latin pilgrims even after the conquest of Jerusalem in 1187. For instance, when these pilgrims were allowed to visit holy sites after the conquest – presumably after Ṣalāḥ al-Dīn disregarded the idea of demolishing or closing the Sepulchre – they were "lodged by the Moslem authorities outside the city in what were during the Crusader period the stables (asinerie) of the Order of St. John [the Hospitaller Order]."[85]

[81] Al-Iṣfahānī, *Al-Fatḥ al-Qussī fi al-Fatḥ al-Qudsī*, 319.
[82] Ibn Shaddād, *The Life of Saladin*, 394.
[83] Richards, "Saladin's Hospital," 72.
[84] Ibid.
[85] Schein, "Latin Hospices," 82.

Although lodging the pilgrims in the stables may have been a move serving to both protect against spies and to humiliate Latin visitors (as Schein suggests), it is instructive that the chosen site belonged to the Order of the Hospital at the same time that the Order kept a small infirmary inside Jerusalem. This infirmary and the Hospitaller palatium would return to the Order during the brief period of Latin control between 1229 and 1244.[86] A century later, in the 1330s, the hospice inside the city was a site where Latin pilgrims could reside during their visits to the city, and it continued as such during the Mamluk period and well into the fifteenth century.[87] Although it is not clear when the infirmary inside the Hospitaller complex was made available to Latin pilgrims, it is plausible that the Hospitaller's infirmary was visited by pilgrims even though they were residing outside the city walls. With no evidence that the infirmary was closed or that visitors were prevented from frequenting it, it is not unlikely that it continued to function modestly and was visited by Latin pilgrims in need of charitable care and support.

If this was indeed the case, we may be able to find an explanation of Ṣalāḥ al-Dīn's decision to build his bīmāristān in 1192 in the accounts given by al-Isfahānī. According to our chronicler, Ṣalāḥ al-Dīn, during his negotiations with Richard Coeur Lion in 1192, purposefully encouraged Latin pilgrims to visit Jerusalem so that they would understand that they could get to the holy sites in peace (thus diminishing their resolve to fight for control of those sites). Richard may have caught on to this plan because he requested that Ṣalāḥ al-Dīn prohibit all Latin pilgrims except those carrying Richard's personal permissions, but Ṣalāḥ al-Dīn refused to comply.[88] The increasing number of pilgrims visiting the city, and possibly visiting the Hospitaller's infirmary, likely motivated Ṣalāḥ al-Dīn not only to ensure that the previously built foundations were better endowed – and thus able to attract more students and Sufis – but also to build a bīmāristān that would be a larger and more elaborate establishment than the then-impoverished Hospitaller's infirmary. Nonetheless, as with a number of his other sites of architectural patronage, Ṣalāḥ al-Dīn decided not to build a new structure but instead to utilize an existing one. In the bīmāristān, patient halls were adapted from rooms within the existing church he restructured as a bīmāristān. Because the Hospitaller infirmary continued to function, however, it is unlikely that Ṣalāḥ al-Dīn's new bīmāristān

86 Ibid., 83.
87 Ibid., 84.
88 Al-Iṣfahānī, *Al-Fatḥ al-Qussī fi-l-Fatḥ al-Qudsī*, 318–19.

would have been smaller or less remarkable than the Hospitallers' institution. It is more likely that the new arrangement converted much of the Hospitallers' property to serve other functions – including a guesthouse, a Sufi monastery, and a madrasa, along with a bīmāristān – while setting aside a small space for the Crusader institution to continue to function.

Conclusion

The overwhelming presence of al-Bīmāristān al-Nūrī cannot be overlooked in any attempt to understand the history of bīmāristāns in the Levant and Egypt. This is particularly true regarding the history of al-Bīmāristān al-Manṣūrī, which was explicitly linked to al-Bīmāristān al-Nūrī and its founder. The life and history of Nūr al-Dīn Maḥmūd Zankī (1118–1174) were sources of inspiration for the Ayyubid and Mamluk dynasties that followed the short-lived Zangid dynasty; his successful career culminated in his control of most of the Levant and in his emergence as one of the more significant political actors throughout most of the twelfth-century Middle East. His architectural projects served as templates for Ṣalāḥ al-Dīn and, later, for al-Manṣūr Qalāwūn as well. Qalāwūn was inspired by Nūr al-Dīn, by his accomplishments both as a builder and patron of charitable foundations and as a warrior and dominant king. He renovated Nūr al-Dīn's bīmāristān and added to its *waqfs* ensuring its flourishing but chose to mark his deeds with the humility owed to a figure like Nūr al-Dīn. The latter's bīmāristān, which figured prominently in the making of Qalāwūn's bīmāristān was a significant source of inspiration – both in how Qalāwūn envisioned his project in the framework of his patronage and in how al-Bīmāristān al-Manṣūrī itself was built to mirror the patterns of al-Bīmāristān al-Nūrī.

At the same time, the presence of the Crusader states, their legacies, and their enduring impact on the architectural landscape of the region were equally influential on the architectural projects of al-Manṣūr Qalāwūn – at the heart of which lay al-Bīmāristān al-Manṣūrī. The Crusader Hospital of Jerusalem continued to function under Qalāwūn's reign to serve pilgrims to the Christian holy sites, and it continued to attract donations and gifts from European nobility. The role played by this hospital motivated Ṣalāḥ al-Dīn to build his own bīmāristān in Jerusalem once Christian pilgrimage was allowed and pilgrims started to fill the city streets. Ṣalāḥ al-Dīn may have wanted to build a structure that was bigger and more impressive than the Hospitallers' House. He may also have wanted to provide services for Muslims visitors and pilgrims, as well as to students and Sufis, whom he wanted to attract to the city. The focus on the pilgrims and serving them through bīmāristāns was manifested in Ṣalāḥ al-Dīn's other bīmāristān in Alexandria, as will be discussed in Chapter 2. More importantly, this interest was undoubtedly influenced by the role played by Hospitaller Houses in the Levant in the preceding century. Qalāwūn, a warrior against Crusaders in his own right, appeared to have been also interested in patronizing Jerusalem and the Muslim visitation and pilgrimage sites there. He built a bīmāristān in Hebron, which was part of the regular visits to the sites in Jerusalem. His projects in Hebron were aimed at facilitating visitations and pilgrimages in the same way that the Hospitaller Houses and al-Bīmāristān al-Ṣalāḥī in Jerusalem did.

CHAPTER 2

Reclaiming the Past: The (New) Bimāristāns of Egypt

Ṣalāḥ al-Dīn's New Capital: The Making of Cairo Cityscape

Before Cairo: The Making of the Capital Region

In 1285, al-Manṣūr Qalāwūn built his complex in the center of Cairo – a relatively young city, a little more than three centuries old that was undergoing a series of modifications illustrating its diverse history. Although the capital region at the south of the Nile Delta had been and would continue to be an important center for the Nile Valley and for the Egyptian province for a longer period of time, Cairo was built under the Fatimids in 909 as the new caliphal capital of the emerging empire. The capital region was the site of the Byzantine city of Babylon, which was one of the more important centers in Byzantine Egypt after the capital Alexandria.[1] After the Islamic conquest of Egypt (639–642, with Babylon falling in 640) ʿAmr ibn al-ʿĀṣ (d. 664), the commander of Muslim armies, ordered the construction of a new town named al-Fusṭāṭ alongside Babylon on the eastern bank of the Nile, possibly in 643.[2] A number of reports linked the origin of the name to ʿAmr ibn al-ʿĀṣ's tent (*fusṭāṭ*), as the town was said to have been built in the same location of the conqueror's original encampment:

> When the Muslims conquered the fort [Babylon] ʿAmr [ibn al-ʿĀṣ] determined to march on Alexandria. So he [started the] campaign in Rabīʿ al-Awwal of the year twenty [March 641], and ordered his tent (*fusṭāṭ*) to be taken down, but a dove was found to have had laid eggs on top of it. So

[1] On cities in Byzantine Egypt, see Alston, *The City in Roman and Byzantine Egypt*; Bagnall, *Egypt in the Byzantine World, 300–700*; Ruffini, *Social Networks in Byzantine Egypt*. On the transformation of Byzantine cities after Islamic conquest, see Cotton, *From Hellenism to Islam*. Also see Sheehan, *Babylon of Egypt*.

[2] Jomier, "Al-Fusṭāṭ."

> [ʿAmr] said, "It sought refuge in our vicinity. Leave the tent until [the eggs] hatch and her chicks fly." So they left the tent, and it was ordered that the dove not be disturbed until its chicks became independent. This is why [the town] was called al-Fusṭāṭ.[3]

The first and most significant building in the new center was the congregational mosque (*al-masjid al-Jāmiʿ*),[4] which served as a site for prayers but also for government. In the following years and decades, new buildings were erected, and the new town drew significant migration from neighboring Babylon.[5] Al-Fusṭāṭ remained the major center for the new Islamic province throughout the Rāshidūn period (c. 632–661) and during the Umayyad rule (c. 662–750) as well. Different Umayyad rulers continued to improve, expand, and renovate the city's major structures including the mosque, which was renovated by ʿAbd al-ʿAzīz ibn Marwān (d. 705) in 696, while he was the governor of Egypt. At the same time, the capital region continued to expand:

> Plague hit Egypt in 689, ʿAbd al-ʿAzīz [ibn Marwān] left [al-Fusṭāṭ] heading to al-Sharqīyah and [camped] in Ḥulwān and liked it. So he took it [as a center], [and] settled the guards, aides, and police in it. ... [There], ʿAbd al-ʿAzīz built houses, mosques, and other [buildings] and planted its vines and its palm trees.[6]

ʿAbd al-ʿAzīz ibn Marwān, one of the most important Umayyad governors of the province, was the heir apparent to the Umayyad throne that was occupied by his brother, the celebrated ʿAbd al-Malik ibn Marwān (r. 685–705). ʿAbd al-ʿAzīz's building projects in al-Fusṭāṭ may have been linked to the larger Umayyad projects undertaken by his brother at the same time, and they may also have been related to the plague and resulting devastation experienced by the city seven years earlier. As explained by al-Kindī, it was the plague that motivated the governor to build a new suburb closer to the desert in the southeast of al-Fusṭāṭ for himself and his armies. However, ʿAbd al-ʿAzīz's suburb, Ḥulwān, did not play a significant role in

[3] Al-Kindī, *Al-Wulāh wa al-Quḍāh*, 10.

[4] The mosque was the first to be built in Egypt, and it remained the major congregational mosque in al-Fusṭāṭ (and possibly in all of Egypt) until the end of the Umayyad empire. It appears that the mosque continued to be called the Congregational mosque well into the middle of the tenth century, as is evident in the writings of al-Kindī (d. 964). In Ibn Duqmāq's (d. 1407) and al-Maqrīzī's (d. 1442) writings, the mosque is often referred to as the Old Congregational [mosque] (*al-Jāmiʿ al-ʿAtīq*). See Denoix, al-Maqrīzī, and Ibn Duqmāq, *Décrire le Caire Fusṭāṭ-Miṣr d'après Ibn Duqmāq et Maqrīzī*. Currently, the mosque is referred to by the name of its founder, as the mosque of ʿAmr ibn al-ʿĀṣ.

[5] Jomier, "Al-Fusṭāṭ"; see also Bareket, *Fustat on the Nile;* Sayyid, *La Capitale de L'Egypte*.

[6] Al-Kindī, *al-Wulāh wa al-Quḍāh*, 39–40.

the capital region, and al-Fusṭāṭ remained the effective seat of government for the remainder of the Umayyad period.[7]

Under the first Abbasid governor of Egypt, Ṣāliḥ ibn ʿAlī al-ʿAbbāsī (d. 768), the major functions of the administration moved gradually to the new Abbasid capital of al-ʿAskar (the city of the soldiers), which Ṣāliḥ ibn ʿAlī built before 753 to the northeast of al-Fusṭāṭ. The new center was mainly a series of garrisons for the Abbasid armies that served as a starting point for Abbasid invasions of North Africa.[8] Al-ʿAskar did not entirely replace al-Fusṭāṭ, which continued to grow in size and importance and continued to play important roles in the administration of the region. In fact, Ṣāliḥ ibn ʿAlī himself expanded the old mosque in al-Fusṭāṭ in 750, and the mosque remained the main congregational mosque of the capital region. Soon, the two cities became twin centers, each of which required its own police chief (*sharṭah*) and its own market inspector (*muḥtasib*).[9]

This model continued until the reign of Aḥmad ibn Ṭūlūn (r. 868–884), who built his new capital al-Qaṭāʾiʿ to rule over his own autonomous realm, which he was establishing under Abbasid banners. Similar to al-Fusṭāṭ, Ibn Ṭūlūn's city was also centered around a mosque, which is now the only surviving monument of the city. Facing the mosque, the emir built a huge palace that included a hippodrome (*maydān*), which was used for games, ceremonies, and processions at different occasions, and for the emir's distribution of fiefs and honors to his commanders, as well as charities to the poor. The hippodrome was so large and significant to the new city that the entire palace was called *al-maydān* (the hippodrome). Close by, Ibn Ṭūlūn built his famous bīmāristān, which was seen by some as the earliest bīmāristān built in Egypt. More significantly, the construction of al-Qaṭṭāʾiʿ seems to have dislodged al-Fusṭāṭ from its original position as the central town in the capital region in part by moving the

[7] Jere L. Bacharach questions the notion of "the capital" in the Umayyad context, including Damascus as the imperial capital, and argues that the major Umayyad cities such as Damascus and Jerusalem played important roles as seats of special government functions but that there was no reason to argue for the concept of "capital" in this period. Bacharach admits that most government offices, the mint (newly established by ʿAbd al-Malik ibn Marwān), and major Umayyad palaces were built in Damascus, giving it the function (and appearance) of a capital, but he explains that not all caliphs resided there for extended periods of time and that not all caliphal architectural patronage was directed to the city. Although Bacharach's arguments do not question the notion of the capital sufficiently before issuing such judgment about Damascus, it is useful for thinking about the function of al-Fusṭāṭ as a center for administration in relation to other settlements, such as Ḥulwān, where Umayyad governors resided at times. See Bacharach, "Marwanid Umayyad Building Activities."

[8] Al-Kindī, *al-Wulāh wa al-Quḍāh*, 74–79.

[9] Ibid., 77; Stilt, "The Muḥtasib, Law and Society."

congregational prayer to the new Ṭūlūnid mosque. After the fall of the Tulunids, the new Abbasid rulers would settle in al-ʿAskar, which became the real center of the province. In 935, when another Abbasid governor, Muḥammad ibn Tughj al-Ikhshīd, started his own autonomous hereditary rule over Egypt (which lasted through five sovereigns until 969), he also ruled from al-ʿAskar. In fact, the Ikhshidids played a significant role in expanding al-ʿAskar while adding a bīmāristān to the old capital of al-Fusṭāṭ.[10] Throughout this period (from 640 to 970), al-Fusṭāṭ continued to grow in size and in population, and settlements extended to bridge the distance between al-Fusṭāṭ and al-ʿAskar. However, after the Umayyad period, and except for modest renovations in the al-Fusṭāṭ congregational mosque by Ṣāliḥ ibn ʿAlī in the wake of the Abbasid control of the province, there is no evidence of any major Abbasid construction projects in the old city. This leaves the small bīmāristān of al-Fusṭāṭ, known as bīmāristān zuqāq al-qanādīl, as a project without a clear owner or any known patron, and it strengthens the possibility that this small, old bīmāristān was indeed built under the Umayyads.

The last in this series of neighboring capitals is al-Qāhirah (Cairo), which was built by the Fatimids after their armies took control of Egypt in 969. The foundations for the new city were laid by the Fatimid commander Jawhar al-Ṣiqillī, who led the Fatimid invasion of Egypt, wrestling the province from the Ikhshidids. The new city was to the northeast of the al-Fusṭāṭ-ʿAskar urban area and, similar to al-ʿAskar's original design, was designed as an abode for the Fatimid elites and the caliphal family. Along with the walls that Jawhar built, almost none of which survives today, the new capital's major buildings were al-Azhar mosque and the Fatimid palace complex in the center of the new city.[11] Both al-Azhar and the caliphal palace complex were located along the major avenue (*qaṣabah*) of the new city, Bayn al-Qaṣrayn (lit. between the two palaces), which acquired its name because of the eastern and western Fatimid palaces on either side of it.[12] Al-Azhar became the new congregational mosque of the capital when the first prayer was held there in 972, and it was located at the far east of the city, a short distance from Bayn

[10] Al-Maqrīzī, *al-Khiṭaṭ*, 4: 406.

[11] Behrens-Abouseif, *Islamic Architecture in Cairo*, 58. For more information on Fatimid architecture, see Pruitt, *Fatimid Architectural Patronage*; Khemir, "The Palace of Sitt Al-Mulk." On al-Azhar and other Fatimid institutions of learning, see Walker, "Fatimid Institutions of Learning."

[12] Rizq, *Aṭlas al-ʿImārah al-Islāmīyah wa-al-Qibṭīyah*; Williams, "Urbanization and Monument Construction," 34.

al-Qaṣrayn avenue.[13] But it was the palatial complex that dominated the architectural layout of the new city and imposed its character as a caliphal capital. The complex was not only a palace and a residence for the caliph and imam, but it was also the "residence" of the dead imams because it included the cemeteries of the Fatimid caliphs.[14] Cairo, which became the new caliphal capital, continued to grow and develop over time. For instance, al-Azhar was transformed into a college in 989, and a new congregational mosque, the mosque of al-Ḥākim, was built under the Caliph al-Ḥākim bi-Amr Allāh (r. 996–1021) at the other end of the city in 1002, opening directly on Bayn al-Qaṣrayn.[15] The famous vizier and commander Badr al-Jamālī (d. 1094 at about eighty years of age) completed important building projects in the city, including a new wall and the city's famous gates, in addition to new mosques and tombs.[16] Al-Jamālī's works were among the most significant Fatimid contributions to the city since its foundation.

In all these incidences, the new capital signaled the beginning of a new order and the control of a new sovereign. Each of these cities was centered around certain significant structures that played an important role in the urban life of the new center, such as the congregational mosque in

13 Behrens-Abouseif, *Islamic Architecture in Cairo*, 58. Al-Azhar continued to be one of the city's most important mosques and colleges even after the Fatimids (with its importance declining during the Ayyubid period in particular). The mosque's importance motivated significant additions and renovations through its long history that changed the nature of the original building and dramatically increased its size. For a discussion of these developments, see Rabbat, "Al-Azhar Mosque."

14 Funerary complexes in the Fatimid period continue to be a topic of extreme importance. Jonathan Bloom argues that the Fatimids (and Shiites) played a significant role in the making of funerary complexes and the development of the cult of the dead in Egypt (Bloom, "The Mosque of the Qarafa"). The same theory was propagated by Caroline Williams "Fatimid Monuments of Cairo, Part I: The Mosque of al-Aqmar" and "Fatimid Monuments of Cairo Part II: The Mausolea." Williams argues that the Fatimids promoted a public cult of the saints centered physically in the Eastern Cemetery (al-Qarāfah), which became all the more important as the authority and legitimacy of the Fatimid imams were being contested in the later decades of the empire. At the same time, they sponsored a private cult around the dead caliphs, which was centered (physically) in *turbat al-zaʿfarān*, the caliphal tombs in the palace complex. This argument is questioned by Ragib, who argues for a much older and more diverse cult of the saints centered in the Eastern Cemetery, to which the Fatimids contributed (see Ragib, "Les Premiers Monuments Funèraires de L'Islam"; also see "Al-Sayyida Nafīsa," "Les Mausolées Fatimides," and "Les Pierres De Souvenir"). More recently, Christopher Taylor argues along Ragib's lines for a more comprehensive view of the cult of the dead and for the rise of funerary complexes in Egypt and in other parts of the Islamicate world: see Taylor, "Development of Monumental Islamic Funerary Architecture," "Social Construction of Moral Imagination in Egypt," and *In the Vicinity of the Righteous*. For more on Fatimid architecture and funerary complexes, see Ragib, "Deux Monuments Fatimides" and "Un Oratoire Fatimide"; Khemir, "The Palace of Sitt Al-Mulk"; Behrens-Abouseif, "The Façade of the Aqmar Mosque"; and Uthmān, *Al-Jāmiʿ al-Aqmar*.

15 Behrens-Abouseif, *Islamic Architecture in Cairo*, 63; Bloom, "The Mosque of al-Ḥākim." Work on the mosque started under al-Ḥākim's father; al-ʿAzīz (r. 975–996) in 990 but was not completed until 1002.

16 Becker, "Badr al-Djamālī"; Behrens-Abouseif, *Islamic Architecture in Cairo*, 67–72.

al-Fusṭāṭ; the Abbasid palace and garrisons in al-ʿAskar; the *maydān* (hippodrome), mosque, and hospital in al-Qaṭṭāʾiʿ; and the caliphal palaces and mosques in Cairo. The connection between new political orders and trajectories and new physical and architectural realities is evident throughout these periods and the Ayyubid and Mamluk periods afterward. At the same time, the population mass that occupied the capital region was changing with these new architectural additions. These changes coincided with political and social events and sometimes epidemics, all while a more stable population core was consistently centered around the old town of Babylon as it gradually became part of the populous al-Fusṭāṭ.[17] The new architectural programs and the new cities that housed them represented important changes in the movement patterns and circulation lines of people, especially when these architectural programs included structures intended to serve large numbers of people (such as a bīmāristān or a mosque) or to be visited and frequented by people (such as tombs, shrines, etc.). In these instances, the choice of location for these establishments was probably part of an implicit understanding of where people should and would go and who the intended audiences of these institutions were.[18] At the same time, it is important to remember that these previous instances of city-building were also reclamation projects

[17] It could be argued that the arrival of thousands of troops at specific instances contributed to a change in the population mass of this region. For instance, ʿAmr ibn al-ʿĀṣ was reported to have arrived with 3,500 troops and later reinforced with 12,000 more under the command of al-Zubayr ibn al-ʿAwwām (al-Kindī, *al-Wulāh wa al-Quḍāh*, 10). These thousands of troops probably required significant structures that rendered their encampments equivalent to new cities. For instance, when ʿAmr laid the foundations for al-Fusṭāṭ, he ordered his troops stationed in Jīzah (on the west bank of the Nile opposite al-Fusṭāṭ, where they were stationed to protect the bridge head to the west of the Nile) to cross to al-Fusṭāṭ. The troops reportedly refused, arguing that they had been in Jīzah for months and that it would be difficult for them to move. The conflict between ʿAmr and his commanders on the west bank was so intense that it required the intervention of caliph ʿUmar I in Medina, who authorized the troops to stay but demanded that they build a fortress in Jīzah. The incident shows that the troops had erected important structures and invested time and effort during their garrison so that it was difficult for them to move. Significantly, these structures apparently did not include a fortress, hence ʿUmar I's request (Guest, "Foundation of Fustat"). Similarly, Aḥmad ibn Ṭūlūn's motivation for building his new mosque was reported by his biographer as related to the complaints of the people of Fusṭāṭ that his armies crowded the congregational mosque on Fridays. He, therefore, decided to build a new city with a new mosque for the troops (Al-Balawī, *Sīrat Aḥmad Ibn Ṭūlūn*). However, in all these cases, the consistent growth of al-Fusṭāṭ provided a significant population center that continued to animate the socioeconomic life of the city and of the entire capital region.

[18] Guides describing important sites for visitations (*ziyārah*), as part of the cult of the dead, were popular throughout the tenth and eleventh centuries. These books were important representations of a prestylized movement that guided and depicted the possibilities (and obligations) of visitors and pilgrims. See al-Harawī and Meri, *Wayfarer's Guide to Pilgrimage*; and Taylor, "Saints, Ziyāra, Qiṣṣa" and *In the Vicinity of the Righteous*. On a different level, travel patterns were equally predictable and well-known, impacting geographical knowledge and travel habits alike, see Touati, *Islam et Voyage*. More recently and more pertinent to this discussion, see Antrim, *Routes*

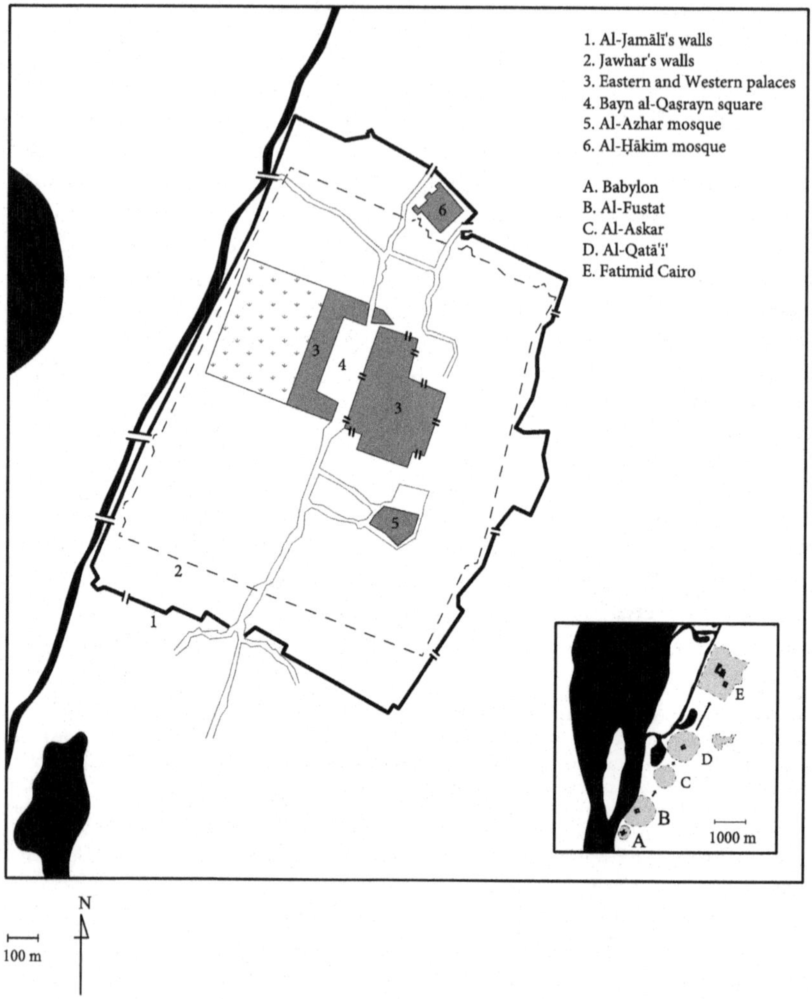

Figure 2.1: Map of Fatimid Cairo

that ended up incorporating uninhabited regions into the capital region and its urban mass. Al-Fusṭāṭ, al-ʿAskar, al-Qaṭāʾiʿ, and Fatimid Cairo were all built on the outskirts of existing urban colonies, and they relied on these colonies for their own support (at least in the beginning). In this

and Realms. All these instances appear to suggest the existence of awareness of movement patterns at the level of the city of the realm(s).

process, city-building did not necessarily include concerted efforts at demolishing or effacing.[19]

Ayyubid Cairo: Building on Ruins

The Ayyubid city constructed by Ṣalāḥ al-Dīn al-Ayyūbī (r. 1174–1193) after he took control of the Egyptian region in 1174 and ended the Fatimid Caliphate was not as ambitious a project as were previous ones. His was not a new city with new centers and major architectural programs resembling the Fatimids' Cairo or even Ibn Ṭūlūn's al-Qaṭāʾiʿ. Rather, it was a more systematic process of effacing the main characters of the Fatimid city by enlarging it to include all the other cities in the capital region, opening it (more) to the public by strengthening its connection to al-Fusṭāṭ, and desecrating, erasing, and rebuilding the core of the city in an attempt to replace the major characters of Fatimid Shiite usage with new Sunni establishments. The first task undertaken was the building of new walls that surrounded the "new" city-conglomerate and provided important visual and material proof of Ṣalāḥ al-Dīn's commitment to the war against the Crusaders.[20] The northern and southern portions of the new wall were united by a large castle complex, the Mount Citadel (*Qalʿat al-Jabal*), in reference to Mount al-Muqaṭṭam, which overlooked Cairo from the east.[21] Although the citadel would have a limited role in defending the city against the Crusaders (they never did arrive at the city walls), it became the seat of power for some of the Ayyubid sovereigns and for all the Mamluk sovereigns after that.[22] Moving the seat of power from the intracity palatial complexes to the citadel further signified the sources of legitimacy for both the Ayyubids (particularly Ṣalāḥ al-Dīn) and the Mamluks after them, and it connected this legitimacy directly and unmistakably to jihad.[23]

[19] When Abbasid forces regained control of Egypt after the fall of the Tulunids, they razed al-Qaṭṭāʾiʿ almost entirely except for the mosque. This act, however, was not intended to provide space for new buildings but rather to erase the Tulunid capital and all it stood for.

[20] The last Crusader attack on Egypt managed to threaten Fatimid rule sufficiently. Many parts of al-Fusṭāṭ were burned to protect it from a potential Crusader take-over, except for the port on the Nile and the older settlements close to the old congregational mosque.

[21] Rabbat, *The Citadel of Cairo*.

[22] Behrens-Abouseif, *Citadel of Cairo*.

[23] The central role of jihad in legitimizing Mamluk rulers could be seen in many writings of the early Mamluk period. Most significant among these writings is a book composed by Muḥammad ibn Ibrāhīm ibn Jamāʿah (d. 1333 at about ninety years of age), who was the chief Shāfiʿī judge and was very close to the Mamluk Sultan al-Manṣūr Qalāwūn (r. 1279–1290) and his sons, including al-Nāṣir Muḥammad (r. 1293–1341; with two interruptions). Ibn Jamāʿah's book, *Taḥrīr al-Aḥkām fī Tadbīr Ahl al-Islām*, presents an interesting look at the perception of political power and sources of political legitimacy for the Sultan (as opposed to the caliph) as seen by those closest to the circles of power. In

Inside the city, Ṣalāḥ al-Dīn's program was intended to modify the Fatimid city center and change its major characters. This project is evident in a number of Ṣalāḥ al-Dīn's major constructions inside the Fatimid city and the capital complex: three madrasas (al-madrasa al-Nāṣirīyyah, al-madrasa al-Qamḥīyyah, and al-madrasa al-Sayfīyyah), a Sufi monastery (Khānaqāt Sa'īd al-Su'dā'), and a bīmāristān (al-Bīmāristān al-Nāṣirī). Ṣalāḥ al-Dīn established his first madrasa for Shāfi'ī scholars, known as al-madrasa al-Nāṣirīyyah, in al-Fusṭāṭ in September 1170, on the site of the former Fatimid police quarters in al-Fusṭāṭ. His second, al-madrasa al-Qamḥīyyah, was also built in al-Fusṭāṭ for the Maliki scholars only few days later. In 1175, he ordered his vizier al-Qāḍī al-Fāḍil to convert the house of the Fatimid vizier al-Ma'mūn al-Baṭā'iḥī, which was adjacent to the huge (Shiite) mausoleum of al-Ḥusayn, into a madrasa for Hanafi scholars known as al-madrasa al-Sayfīyyah.[24] The khānaqāh was the first of its kind built in Egypt, and it introduced an important new element to the city: the Sufi orders. Sufis and Sufi monasteries would soon become part of the charitable and religious map of the city in its new Sunni garb, and their role would increase with time. Ṣalāḥ al-Dīn's khānaqāh was one of the biggest and richest for more than a century, and its *shaykh* occupied an important position in the hierarchy of religious scholars under the Ayyubids and Mamluks. More interestingly for the purposes of our discussion, the khānaqāh, consecrated for poor Sufis, was built in the palace of a Fatimid eunuch and vizier, Sa'īd al-Su'adā', replacing one of the most beautiful and luxurious Fatimid palaces (aside from the caliphal palaces).[25] The *khanāqāh* was a more common establishment in the Seljuk East, from which Ṣalāḥ al-Dīn and his mentor and master Nūr al-Dīn drew their inspiration for spreading Sunnism in Egypt and the Levant.[26]

Ṣalāḥ al-Dīn's bīmāristān, built in 1171, was even more significant in the process of opening the Fatimid city to the poor and ending the exclusive nature of the Fatimid capital. Ṣalāḥ al-Dīn divided the Fatimid palace complex, which dominated the center of the Fatimid capital, among

the book, Ibn Jamā'ah highlighted the importance of jihad as the major duty of the sultan and the real reason why a sultan should undertake the earthly affairs belonging in origin to the authority of the caliph (Ibn Jamā'ah, *Taḥrīr al-Aḥkām*). Similar themes can be seen in some correspondences belonging to Mamluk Sultans with their deputies; see Fernandes, "On Conducting the Affairs of the State." On similar themes about the perception of Mamluks and the legitimacy of their rule, see Haarmann, "Rather the Injustice of the Turks."

[24] Frenkel, "Islamic Religious Endowments," 3.

[25] Fernandes, "Foundation of Baybars al-Jashankir," 21.

[26] As explained earlier, after conquering Jerusalem, Ṣalāḥ al-Dīn commissioned the conversion of the palace of the Jerusalem patriarch into a khānaqāh, as well: Richards, "Saladin's Hospital," 71.

his generals and emirs as he moved his own seat of power to the newly established citadel. He then took one of the pavilions of the larger Eastern Palace, which was built by the Fatimid Caliph al-ʿAzīz (r. 975–996) in 994 and transformed it into a bīmāristān. The narratives surrounding the establishment of this bīmāristān explain that the hall turned into a bīmāristān was known to have had a particular talisman that protected it from ants (and possibly other insects); it was when Ṣalāḥ al-Dīn heard about this that he ordered it turned into a bīmāristān.[27] As explained before, this was not the first bīmāristān in the capital region, and it was not even a departure from the earlier Fatimid custom. In fact, the Fatimids had at least three different bīmāristāns operating at different times, with one of them surviving until the reign of Ṣalāḥ al-Dīn.[28] At least two bīmāristāns are possibly dated to the Fatimid period, one of which was built outside the southern gate of Zuwaylah (Bāb Zuwaylah) in the al-Saqṭiyyīn area between Cairo and al-Fusṭāṭ,[29] and the other, known as Bīmāristān al-Qashshāshīn (after a neighborhood of the same name), was located inside the walls, also to the south of the city and facing al-Azhar mosque, close to the mint house built by the Fatimid vizier al-Maʾmūn al-Baṭāʾiḥī for the Caliph al-Āmir (r. 1101–1130).[30] Whereas Bīmāristān al-Saqṭiyyīn was located outside the city walls closer to al-Fusṭāṭ, where the majority of the bīmāristān's clientele would reside, Bīmāristān al-Qashshāshīn was inside the walls but close to al-Azhar, in an area frequented by students, scholars, and other commoners. The inner quarters of the city and its northern parts dominated by the caliphal palace were quite far from the two bīmāristāns. As such, Ṣalāḥ al-Dīn's act of transforming al-ʿAzīz pavilion into a bīmāristān was significant in terms of desecrating the Fatimid center of power (and the tombs of the Fatimid caliphs inside the palace complex as well) and bringing commoners, patients, and the poor seeking care into the center of the old Fatimid city, inside the caliph's palace.

Ibn Jubayr provides us with some interesting descriptions of the bīmāristāns and other establishments built by Ṣalāḥ al-Dīn, a sovereign who Ibn Jubayr greatly admired. The first bīmāristān described in his travelogue was, in fact, in Alexandria, and it apparently paid special

[27] Al-Maqrīzī, *al-Khiṭaṭ*, 2: 407.

[28] Ibn Jubayr, *Riḥlat Ibn Jubayr*, 21. Al-Maqrīzī, reporting from Ibn ʿAbd al-Ẓāhir, explained that Ṣalāḥ al-Dīn also renovated the old bīmāristān in al-Fusṭaṭ, although it is not clear which bīmāristān he was referring to. See al-Maqrīzī, *al-Khiṭaṭ*, 2: 407.

[29] ʿĪsá, Tārīkh al-Bīmāristānāt fī al-Islām, 51.

[30] Al-Maqrīzī, *al-Khiṭaṭ*, 3: 40.

attention to strangers and visitors, whom Ibn Jubayr cared more about, being a traveler himself:

> The sultan's care of these visiting strangers was so expansive that he ordered bathhouses to be assigned to them to bathe in when they need to. He erected for them a bīmāristān to treat whoever falls ill among them, and appointed physicians to inspect their conditions, with servants working [for these physicians] whom [the physicians] order to take care [of the strangers'] affairs in relation to treatment and nourishment. He also appointed people designated to visit the patients, who refrain from attending the bīmāristān [on account of its being debasing to them], especially [patients who are] strangers [to the town], and recount their conditions to the physicians so that they take care of their treatment.[31]

There is little information about these establishments in Alexandria, and it is hard to find other sources corroborating Ibn Jubayr's accounts. However, the nature of his travelogue as a detailed description of his pilgrimage and his deep interest in explaining and asking about amenities available to travelers, especially *maghribīs* (visitors from the Maghreb and al-Andalus), lend more credibility to his accounts, which could have served as guides for future travelers from the Maghreb. This bias to information useful for travelers might explain why the description of these facilities appears to have been directed more toward visitors and strangers. That being said, Alexandria's role as one of the major ports on the Mediterranean and the first point of encounter in Egypt for land travel across northern Africa, could have led to the bīmāristān's being used mostly by travelers and visitors. At this level, the bīmāristān of Alexandria seemed reminiscent of Crusaders' Hospitals destined to serve pilgrims en route to Jerusalem. Apart from this, the Alexandria bīmāristān described here does not appear to have been much different from other bīmāristāns; it had physicians who attended to patients, and they were aided by attendants and servants who helped take care of patients and executed the physicians' instructions. Moreover, the bīmāristān extended its care to people outside its walls by sending treatment to those who refrained from attending the bīmāristān, which was a common practice as evidenced in the more detailed accounts about al-Bīmāristān al-Manṣūrī, which will be discussed later. Ibn Jubayr also explains that the "messengers" sent from the bīmāristān not only intended to provide medications but also to ask about patients' conditions and report back to physicians, which is a relatively unique practice not found in other accounts about al-Bīmāristān al-Manṣūrī, for instance.

[31] Ibn Jubayr, *Riḥlat Ibn Jubayr*, 10.

In the case of al-Manṣūrī, the bīmāristān's supervisor (*nāẓir*) was instructed to send medications to the homes of patients who were sick and poor.[32] The process probably entailed family members' visiting the bīmāristān, explaining the patient's condition to the physician, and taking out medications (whether in person or having them delivered by the bīmāristān's pharmacists). This is reminiscent of accounts by physicians such as al-Rāzī, who mentioned how he was informed of some patients' conditions by a family member, especially in cases of sick children or women who did not come to the bīmāristān.[33] It is conceivable that a family member might have sought consultation at the bīmāristān for a sick relative who did not need to attend the bīmāristān in person by virtue of having family members able to take care of him or her. Ibn Jubayr's description is different in two respects: the patients he described refrained from attending the bīmāristān because they found it debasing or shameful, but they also needed its provisions because they were strangers. At the socioeconomic level, they may have been much better off than those who normally would have attended the bīmāristān. However, as travelers and strangers, they were in need of the bīmāristān's help because they had little to no social support. For this same reason, they may have needed attendants to report their complaints to physicians, who would then prescribe treatments for them. That being said, it is likely that this practice was limited because it would have extended the bīmāristān's funding and staff to unimaginable lengths.

Ibn Jubayr also describes Ṣalāḥ al-Dīn's more famous bīmāristān in Cairo. His account indicates that the palace pavilion may have been transformed into a bīmāristān without much change in its structure. He wrote:

> One of the prides of this sultan [Ṣalāḥ al-Dīn] is the bīmāristān that is in the city of Cairo. [The bīmāristān] is such a remarkable palace in its beauty and its size, which he [Ṣalāḥ al-Dīn] designated for this virtue [being a bīmāristān] seeking [divine] reward. . . . In the stalls of the palace, beds with full bedding were laid for patients. . . . Alongside this space, another space was separated for women patients, and they too have someone who takes care of them. Beside these two spaces, another space with a wide courtyard, which had stalls with iron windows, which were made cells for the mad. They too have someone who checks their conditions every day.[34]

As opposed to the cruciform structure of al-Bīmāristān al-Nūrī, al-Bīmāristān al-Nāṣirī seems to have relied on the palace structure, which

[32] Ibn Ḥabīb, *Tadhkirat al-Nabīh*, 1, line 292.
[33] Meyerhof, "Clinical Observations by Rhazes." On women patients and this style of consultation, see Pormann, "Female Patients and Practitioners."
[34] Ibn Jubayr, *Riḥlat Ibn Jubayr*, 21.

probably had a number of parallel bays separated by columns with stalls overlooking the central bay. The term "stall" (*maqṣūrah*), which Ibn Jubayr used, was commonly used to describe a small enclosure, sometimes slightly raised, where dignitaries prayed close to the *qibla* niche.[35] The palace's stalls (*maqāṣīr*) may have been originally used by emirs and state dignitaries to overlook the procession of delegates in the central bay, and these stalls were then converted into patient halls simply by laying beds in them. The women's hall appears to have been separated in an improvised manner; hence, Ibn Jubayr's term *uqṭutiʿa*, which indicates its being separated from the original structure rather than being built separately. It is unclear how Ibn Jubayr arrived at this conclusion and whether he was told about the palace or that the separation of the women's hall was clearly impromptu or made of different materials (like wood, for instance). The cells of the mad appear to have originally been separate, overlooking what might have been a court. Although the palace court might have had a garden or a pool, similar to other contemporary courts, this one is described simply as courtyard (*fināʾ*). Considering how Ibn Jubayr was impressed by Ṣalāḥ al-Dīn, it is likely that he would have mentioned a garden should there have been one.

As opposed to Nūr al-Dīn (and later to Qalāwūn), and as explained previously, Ṣalāḥ al-Dīn's building program did not rely on acquiring and replacing existing structures. Instead, he focused on transforming their functions and usage. Yet, Ṣalāḥ al-Dīn was not only establishing new, important institutions; he was also erasing significant Fatimid (and – in the case of Jerusalem – Crusader) monuments, which was a political as well as a material necessity of building in a crowded city. The Fatimid palaces and houses of government were not only sites without owners (or with owners who lost power and influence), but they were also important sources for building materials or *spolia*, which played a significant role in underwriting the building projects by the Ayyubids and the Mamluks.[36] Although every

[35] See, for instance, Kuban, *Muslim Religious Architecture*.

[36] Despoliation was one of the more common consequences of invasion or of serious changes in political rule, and spolia were commonly reused in new structures. On the use of spolia in Mamluk architecture, see Mathews, "Mamluks and Crusaders." See also Flood, "The Medieval Trophy" for a discussion of the utilization of Coptic and Byzantine artifacts in Islamic architecture. In the context of Nūr al-Dīn Zankī's buildings, see Raby, "Nur Al-Din, Qastal al-Shuʿaybīyah, and 'Classical Revival.'" A prominent example is al-Nāṣir Muḥammad b. Qalāwūn's use of a Crusader gate acquired by his brother al-Ashraf Khalīl in the former's *madrasa*, which is located beside his father's complex. Al-Ashraf Khalīl (d. 1293) was assassinated before using the gate that he acquired in his battles in Acre. The gate, which fell to his brother, was first used by al-ʿĀdil Kitbughā (d. 1297), then re-despoiled by al-Nāṣir Muḥammad as he retook his throne from Kitbughā. (See al-Harithy,

building or structure patronized by Ṣalāḥ al-Dīn had its own unique purpose and its specific audience, be it the citadel, the khānaqāh, the madrasas, or the bīmāristān, the pattern through which these institutions were chosen and built reveal Ṣalāḥ al-Dīn's program to modify the city and reappropriate it as a new Sunni capital of his empire in a manner reminiscent of his master's, Nūr al-Dīn's, program of built patronage. This program was also carried out in Jerusalem, where Ṣalāḥ al-Dīn also attempted to erase and rebuild the city's identity after about a century under Crusader rule.

Al-Manṣūr Qalāwūn's Architectural Patronage

Before al-Bīmāristān: Trends and Tendencies

Al-Manṣūr Qalāwūn, who inaugurated al-Bīmāristān al-Manṣūrī in 1285, was the seventh Mamluk sultan after the Mamluk emirs wrestled the throne from the Ayyubids of Cairo and took control of the largest component of the Ayyubid empire. When Qalāwūn came to the throne in 1279, he was evidently the strongest emir in the empire. He had been the guardian of the young sultan who preceded him, the son of al-Ẓāhir Baybars, Qalāwūn's comrade-in-arms and previous sultan. Over the first five years of his reign, Qalāwūn faced a number of political challenges from some of his old comrades who occupied important positions in the army and empire. The most important of these was Sunqur al-Ashqar, the viceroy of the Levant, who rebelled against Qalāwūn and declared himself a sultan in Damascus (ca. 1280). The imperial armies from Cairo defeated him with difficulty,[37] and even after a truce was signed with the sultan, Sunqur managed to retain his army, acquire a title, and remain one of the most important generals in the empire. However, when he rebelled again in 1286, Qalāwūn was in a much more powerful position and was able to defeat the Levantine insurrection handily. This time around, Sunqur was stripped of all his titles and fiefdoms and was kept in the court at Cairo with no official position. When Qalāwūn's son al-Ashraf Khalīl took the throne after his father's death in 1290, Sunqur was executed as punishment for his past sins.[38]

Qalāwūn started his building and architectural patronage very early in his tenure, and his early buildings were all located in holy cities such as Medina and Jerusalem. In 1279, he began his architectural patronage by

"Space in Mamluk Architecture"; Ḥāmid and Ismāʿīl, *Al-Nāṣir Muḥammad Ibn Qalāwūn*; Al-Shujāʿī, *Tārīkh al-Malik al-Nāṣir*.)

[37] Baybars Al-Mansuri, *Zubdat al-Fikrah*, 183–93.

[38] Ibid., 285–86. For details on Qalāwūn's life and career, see Northrup, *From Slave to Sultan*.

building a dome on the prophet's tomb in Medina,[39] which still remains the most distinctive feature of the prophetic mosque (although it has been renovated several times, of course). The last renovations of the Prophetic mosque before Qalāwūn's had been those sponsored by Baybars I (r. 1260–1277) in 1261, shortly after his own ascension to the throne. Qalāwūn appeared to be following in the footsteps of Baybars I in beginning his tenure by patronizing the prophet's tomb. The massive dome was made of wood and covered with lead, square-shaped at its base and fully surrounding the tomb at ground level before rising to form an octagon that supported the massive domed structure.

A year later, Qalāwūn started a construction project around another holy tomb, this time that of Abraham, in Hebron. When Ṣalāḥ al-Dīn took control of the town in 1187, he converted the Latin church of St. Abraham, which was built near the tomb, into a mosque that was (and continues to be) known as *al-Ḥaram al-Ibrāhīmī* (the Abrahamic Sanctuary)[40] and that remained a site of patronage during the Ayyubid and early Mamluk period. Before Qalāwūn's patronage, Baybars I had ordered the renovation of this mosque, increased its *waqfs*, and prohibited Christians from visiting it. During their Islamic history, Hebron and Jerusalem were seen as twin towns; their histories were told together, and patronage acts in one were seen as connected to the other, but Jerusalem continued to enjoy most of the built patronage as the larger and more significant of the pair.[41] Also following in Baybars's footsteps, Qalāwūn directed his attention to Hebron and sponsored a number of building projects intended to make the small town well-equipped as a pilgrimage site. In addition to adding a huge gate to the Abrahamic Sanctuary, Qalāwūn built a Sufi monastery in 1280, which provided hospitality to Sufis but also provided meals to other visitors and pilgrims. In 1281, he built a bīmāristān in Hebron, also known as al-Bīmāristān al-Manṣūrī and also designed to serve visitors and pilgrims.[42] Al-Bīmāristān al-Manṣūrī in Hebron was not large or exceptionally rich, at

[39] Ibid., 85.

[40] The term "*ḥaram*" is the same used to describe the holy mosque of Mecca, the prophet's mosque in Medina, and the al-Aqṣā mosque in Jerusalem.

[41] For instance, the major source for the history of this region links Jerusalem and Hebron as one entity; see Al-ʿUlaymī, *Al-Uns al-Jalīl bi-Tārīkh al-Quds wa al-Khalīl*. Similarly, al-Maqrīzī, al-ʿAsqalānī, and others continued to group the two towns together in their narratives. Also, Ibn Jubayr's (d. 1217) itinerary shows that the two towns were normally part of the same journey. Mujīr al-Dīn used the term "the two sanctuaries (*al-ḥaramayn*)," which originally referred to the mosques of Mecca and Medina to refer to those of Jerusalem and Hebron, which further indicates how the connection between the former and latter pair of cities was seen as similar. Even before the Crusades, Nāṣir-i Khusraw visited Hebron right after visiting Jerusalem; see Khusraw, *Book of Travels*, 35.

[42] Al-ʿUlaymī, Al-Uns al-Jalīl bi-Tārikh al-Quds wa al-Khalīl, 434.

least in comparison to its counterpart (al-Bīmāristān al-Ṣalāḥī) in Jerusalem. However, it might have been the first in the town because Ibn Jubayr, who paid special attention throughout his travelogue to facilities available to visitors and pilgrims, did not mention any similar structure in Hebron. The building of this bīmāristān clearly reveals Qalāwūn's interest in this institution from early on in his career, and it constituted a significant step in making Hebron a site of pilgrimage equipped with tools to receive and care for visitors.

In the four years following, Qalāwūn did not sponsor any major building projects as he struggled to solidify his rule and control the affairs of the state against a number of internal and external challenges. By 1284, Linda Northrup explains, he was in a much better state because "a number of events, over which he had no control, were to occur which would render the Mamluk position among the powers of the Mediterranean Basin less vulnerable."[43] The first major construction that he commissioned was a mausoleum for Fāṭimah Khātūn, his wife of twenty years and the mother of his favorite son and heir apparent, al-Ṣāliḥ; she died in 1283 or 1284. The construction was supervised by Qalāwūn's trusted emir and favorite construction manager (*shādd al-ʿamāʾir*), ʿAlam al-Dīn Sanjar al-Shujāʿī, who would also supervise the construction of Qalāwūn's bīmāristān complex in the following year. Qalāwūn's heir apparent al-Ṣāliḥ would die in 1288 during his father's life and be buried in his mother's mausoleum, which would be known as both *al-Qubba al-Ṣāliḥiyyah* (the Ṣāliḥī mausoleum) and *Qubbat Fātimah Khātūn Umm al-Ṣāliḥ* (mausoleum of Fatimah Khātūn, mother of al-Sāliḥ).

The choice of a site for this mausoleum was significant, especially when considered with the site chosen for Qalāwūn's complex and mausoleum, the construction of which was started a few months later and may have been in the planning stage at the time. Fāṭimah Khātūn's mausoleum was located opposite the mausoleum of Shajar al-Durr (d. 1257), who was the strong wife of the last Ayyubid ruler al-Ṣāliḥ Ayyūb (Qalāwūn's master) and who built al-Sālīḥ Ayyūb's mausoleum and her own when she ruled Egypt independently for about a year in 1250. Similar to Shajar al-Durr's mausoleum, which contained a madrasa along with her tomb, Fāṭimah Khātūn's mausoleum contained a madrasa as well and was probably as big as its older predecessor. Whereas the building of a mausoleum for the sultan's wife was a unique act and was only done for a wife of twenty years who witnessed the all the ups and downs of her husband's career, placing

[43] Northrup, *From Slave to Sultan*, 112.

this mausoleum opposite that of Egypt's most famous woman ruler, who could be considered the true founder of Mamluk rule in the realm, brought the two women together and linked their two husbands, the last Ayyubid ruler al-Ṣāliḥ Ayyūb and Qalāwūn. Even in the name of the new mausoleum, which was formally named "Qubbat Umm al-Ṣāliḥ," the name of the Ayyubid master was recalled in the title of Qalāwūn's son and heir, a title Qalāwūn no doubt chose for his son to match that of his master. Yet, the new mausoleum was not only a neighbor to Shajar al-Durr's but also to a number of other important tombs, *mashhads*, and mausoleums located in this area of Cairo.

In 1250, Shajar al-Durr commissioned the construction of two mausoleums, one for her dead husband al-Ṣāliḥ Ayyūb and one for herself.[44] Her husband's was to be attached to his madrasa, which he had built in the center of Cairo on parts of the old Eastern Fatimid Palace, and set back to back with Ṣalāḥ al-Dīn's aforementioned bīmāristān. This location was one of the most valuable in the capital and lay at the center of its major avenue. Attached to the madrasa, this mausoleum, the first built inside the city walls, dominated the cityscape and secured the dead king's legacy as the effective end of the Ayyubid line and the beginning of the Mamluk one. For her own mausoleum, Shajar al-Durr did not attempt to find a spot inside the city walls. Instead, she chose a spot in the cemetery close to the shrines of a number of women saints, built during the Fatimid period, in order to commemorate women belonging to Muḥammad's lineage.[45] Across the street from Shajar al-Durr's mausoleum (and then beside Fāṭimah Khātūn's) was the *mashhad* of al-Sayyidah Ruqayyah,[46] Muḥammad's great-granddaughter. Close by one can find the mausoleums and the *mashhads* of al-Sayyidah Nafīsa, al-Sayyidah ʾĀtika, and al-Sayyidah Sukaynah, most of which were sites built during the Fatimid period and celebrated the women saints of the Cairo pilgrimage scene.[47]

Although these sites and mosques of women saints lay very close to one another, they were not necessarily seen as part of a woman-saintly

[44] Behrens-Abouseif, *Islamic Architecture in Cairo*, 92.

[45] Ibid., 93.

[46] Al-Sayyidah Ruqayyah was the daughter of al-Ḥusayn, Muḥammad's grandson and claimant to the caliphate. In Shiite lore, she was four or five years old when her father died in the battle of Karbala in 680, and she, among other women and children, was brought to the Umayyad court of Yazīd I. When Yazīd heard her loud weeping, he ordered that her father's head be brought to her. She burst into violent weeping and perished on the spot. Ruqayyah never visited Egypt, so her mosque is not a mausoleum or tomb but rather a *mashhad ruʾyah*, or a mosque commemorating her at a site that would invite her saintly apparition in visions and dreams.

[47] See al-Maqrīzī, *al-Khiṭāṭ*, 4: 436–43.

sanctuary but rather as part of a group of other sanctuaries and mausoleums of descendants of Muḥammad, such as the mausoleums and mashhads of Zayn al-ʿĀbidīn, al-Jaʿfarī, and Ibn Sīrīn on the lane known as "The Lane of [Muḥammad's] Family" and, nearby, the *mashhads* of al-Qāsim al-Ṭayyib, Kulthūm bt. al-Qāsim, Fāṭimah al-Nabawīyyah, Yaḥyā al-Shabīh, ʿĀʾisha bt. Jaʿfar al-Ṣādiq, and, of course, that of al-Ḥusayn himself, among others.[48] The tombs of the Ayyubid sultans and the Ayyubid ruling family were not close by but lay rather at the other end of the cemetery close to the tomb of al-Shāfiʿī. Shajar al-Durr, who departed from the Ayyubid custom when she built her husband's mausoleum inside the city, did not place her own tomb close to those of other Ayyubids, but rather chose a part of the Lane of the Family where the tombs of a number of women saints congregated. Her own mausoleum interrupted the continuity of the tombs of the Family and effectively created a niche of women saints in this area. Fāṭimah Khātūn's mausoleum followed Shajar al-Durr's tradition and further emphasized the nature of this niche carved in the middle of the city's cemetery. More significantly, Fātimah Khātūn's mausoleum further emphasized the connection between her husband, al-Manṣūr Qalāwūn, and Shajar al-Durr's, al-Ṣāliḥ Ayyūb.

Building al-Bīmāristān al-Manṣūrī

A Founding Account for a Bīmāristān

It appears that the model for building a tomb across from another one, the techniques used to relate one building to another, and the overall building style used in Fāṭimah Khātūn's mausoleum formed the basis of Qalāwūn's most famous built patronage, his bīmāristān-madrasa-mausoleum complex, which was planned and supervised by Sanjar al-Shujāʿī as well. Although Qalāwūn's complex was made up of the mausoleum, the bīmāristān, and a madrasa, the spatial arrangement of these structures lent more emphasis to the bīmāristān and highlighted its importance. The portal to the complex faced the complex of al-Ṣāliḥ Ayyūb, creating a feeling of symmetry with the monument across the street while jeopardizing the symmetry of the Qalawunid complex itself because the portal was situated closer to the southern end of the complex rather than its middle. The mausoleum, which was on the right/north and the madrasa on

[48] Today, these mausoleums are located along and close to one lane called the Lane of the Family of the House [of Muḥammad].

the left/south upon walking through the portal, had windows that opened to the corridor, whose floor was lower than that of either structure. This had the effect of recreating the corridor in the image of the outside street leading up to the bīmāristān, which stood out as the center of the complex. The portal is "set back in three layers. . . . The treatment of the portal as a succession of three layers achieves two effects. First, it breaks down the scale of the portal as it rises to the height of the building; second, it is an inviting gesture, generating inward visual movement and strengthening the continuity between the street and the great corridor."[49]

The construction of al-Manṣūr Qalāwūn's complex in the center of Cairo was a significant architectural and urban event: it modified the center of the city, restructured spaces and movements, and had significant political implications as well.[50] Different historians and chroniclers explained the construction process by narrating specific anecdotes in order to make sense of this immense project. Although these accounts were not generally intended to defend the complex or the project – since they were composed at times when the complex was perceived positively[51] – they represent important sources for our understanding of the perception of the project and its place in the sultan's life, career, and patronage. Whether these accounts were written by Qalāwūn's commissioned historians, his close aides and emirs, or near contemporaries who had no direct connection to the sultan, their different perspectives afford us important vantage points from which to observe the sultan's complex within his architectural patronage and political career.

When al-Maqrīzī (d. 1442) described the construction of al-Bīmāristān al-Manṣūrī, he narrated a story that linked the project to an illness suffered by al-Manṣūr Qalāwūn. While he was still an emir under al-Ẓāhir Baybars, al-Manṣūr Qalāwūn was leading a campaign against the Rūm in 1276 when he fell ill close to Damascus. As he camped there, physicians and medications were brought to him from al-Bīmāristān al-Nūrī in Damascus. Either during this episode of sickness or sometime after his recovery, Qalāwūn pledged to build a bīmāristān should God grant him the throne of Egypt. When Qalāwūn finally came to the throne and was able to consolidate his power, he built the bīmāristān as pledged. The Mamluk historian and

49 Al-Harithy, "Space in Mamluk Architecture," 81.

50 Ibid.

51 It appears that the bīmāristān was universally perceived favorably but that the *madrasa* may have generated some opposition and created some backlash that may have extended to the entire complex: see Northrup, *From Slave to Sultan*, 122–24. However, and as will be seen later, these objections soon disappeared, and the complex became very well accepted and appreciated.

bureaucrat Shāfiʿ b. ʿAlī, who worked for al-Manṣūr Qalāwūn (1252–1330) and was the nephew of the famous bureaucrat and author Muḥyī al-Dīn ibn ʿAbd al-Ẓāhir (1223–1292)[52], composed a history of al-Manṣūr Qalāwūn that may have been one of his commissioned biographies. In this biography, he hinted at the same story later narrated by al-Maqrīzī as he explained that Qalāwūn, after his authority was consolidated and his power established, recalled that he had made a vow to God to build a bīmāristān.[53] Shāfiʿ did not explain this vow, but he may well have been referring to the vow later described by al-Maqrīzī, although the latter's sources are not clear. Muḥyī al-Dīn ibn ʿAbd al-Ẓāhir's regnal biography did not mention this account, and instead linked the construction of the bīmāristān to the sultan's charitable impulses when he inaugurated the mausoleum and madrasa of his deceased wife. There, "he aspired to do good and to establish charity" and decided to build a bīmāristān for the people.[54] Whereas al-Maqrīzī's account is likely apocryphal, it portrayed a perceived connection between al-Manṣūr Qalāwūn and his bīmāristān, on one hand, and Nūr al-Dīn Zankī and his bīmāristān, on the other.[55] This connection is evident through other projects undertaken at the time, including Qalāwūn's aforementioned renovation of Nūr al-Dīn's bīmāristān. Similarly, Ibn ʿAbd al-Ẓāhir's account clearly links the bīmāristān to a desire to do good on the part of his patron, but without ever really explaining his motives.

In both cases, the details of these accounts are significant on many levels. Summarizing the complex in the bīmāristān, these accounts reduced the entire complex, including the sultan's mausoleum – the first mausoleum built by its own owner inside the capital[56] – to the bīmāristān and its

[52] Ibn ʿAbd al-Ẓāhir was a renowned secretary and esteemed bureaucrat under al-Ẓāhir Baybars and wrote his commissioned biography, "Al-Rawḍ al-Zāhir fī Sirat al-Malik al-Ẓāhir." Ibn ʿAbd al-Ẓāhir remained in al-Manṣūr Qalāwūn's trusted entourage and composed what appears to be Qalāwūn's commissioned biography "Tashrīf al-Ayyām wa-l-ʿUṣūr fī Sirat al-Malik al-Manṣūr." See Ibid., 25.

[53] Ibn ʿAlī, and Lewicka, *Biography of Qalāwūn*, 405.

[54] Ibn ʿAbd al-Ẓāhir, *Tashrīf al-Ayyām*, 55–56.

[55] Sabra, *Poverty and Charity in Medieval Islam*, 76. Ibn Iyās (d. 1522) mentioned another account in which Qalāwūn ordered his mamluks to slaughter the commoners after they had stoned them. The slaughter lasted for three days before the sultan was convinced to stop the massacre. In repentance, he decided to build the bīmāristān. However, there is no evidence for this story before the sixteenth century.

[56] Al-Harithy, "Space in Mamluk Architecture." Ayyubids built their mausolea in the cemetery outside Cairo alongside the tomb of al-Imām al-Shāfiʿī, which was built by Ṣalāḥ al-Dīn. As mentioned before, only the last Ayyubid sovereign, al-Ṣāliḥ Ayyūb (d. 1249), was buried inside the city in the mausoleum that faced Qalāwūn's complex, but the mausoleum was built by al-Ṣāliḥ Ayyūb's consort, Shajar al-Durr (d. 1257), in 1250 after his death. See ʿUthmān, *Madāfin Ḥukkām Miṣr al-Islāmīyah bi-Madīnat Al-Qāhirah*.

charitable value, relegating the other components of the complex to the status of accessories or embellishments. In the writings of these authors, two of whom were writing Qalāwūn's regnal history, the mausoleum did not appear at the discursive center of the complex, but rather was presented as a shrine commemorating the founder of the bīmāristān, a view consistent with the fact that many authors and historians used the word bīmāristān to describe the entire complex.[57]

Another founding account was reported by Shihāb al-Dīn al-Nuwayrī (d. 1333) in his *Nihāyat al-ʿArab fī Funūn al-Adab*.[58] Al-Nuwayrī supervised the bīmāristān as the deputy of the famous vizier Ibn ʿIbādah and was given absolute authority to manage the entire complex and its *waqf* and even to report directly to the sultan, thus surpassing his supervisor.[59] Al-Nuwayrī explains:

> When the Sultan considered (*raʾā*) the mausoleum of al-Sāliḥ Ayyūb (*al-turbah al-ṣāliḥiyyah*), he ordered the building of a mausoleum (*turbah*), a *madrasa*, a bīmāristān and a charitable *maktab* (*maktab sabīl*). So al-Dār al-Quṭbīyah and its environs were bought [using] the sultan's own money, and its inhabitants were compensated with the palace known as Qaṣr al-Zumurrud. The emir ʿAlam al-Dīn al-Shujāʿī was appointed a supervisor on the construction (*mashaddan ʿalā al-ʿimārah*), so he showed unheard-of interest and care, and it was completed in the shortest of periods. If one sees this great edifice (*al-ʿimārah al-ʿaẓīmah*) and hears that it was completed in such short period, he may [not believe].[60]

Al-Nuwayrī did not explain the construction through any specific anecdotes but rather as part of a well-designed plan in which the mausoleum of al-Ṣāliḥ Ayyūb was the main source of inspiration for the complex. The account narratively restructured the space by bringing the mausoleum to the forefront as the centerpiece of the complex and pushing the bīmāristān, madrasa, and *maktab* to the background.[61] The finances of

[57] The complex would continue to be designated as al-Bīmāristān, when referring to its three different components, in the writings of many historians such as al-Maqrīzī, Ibn Duqmāq, and al-ʿAynī, among others.

[58] Al-Nuwayrī, *Nihāyat al-ʾArab*, 31: 105–06. Al-Nuwayrī occupied several positions in the state of al-Nāṣir Muḥammad b. Qalāwūn (r. 1293–1341, with two interruptions totaling five years), albeit not at the highest end of the bureaucratic hierarchy.

[59] On al-Nuwayrī, see Chapoutot-Remadi, "Al-Nuwayrī."

[60] Ibid., 31: 105–06. Al-Nuwayrī's account starts with "He said" in reference to his source, which he did not identify. Al-Nuwayrī borrowed from many sources, but the most significant for the Mamluk period were in fact Ibn ʿAbd al-Ẓāhir and Baybars al-Manṣūrī. The account was copied verbatim in Ibn al-Furāt (d. 1405): see Ibn al-Furāt, *Tārīkh Ibn al-Furāt*.

[61] This particular arrangement is similar to how Huwayda al-Harithy read the architectural intent of the complex: Al-Harithy, "Space in Mamluk Architecture."

the complex, in al-Nuwayrī's account, reflected a slightly different picture from the discursive and intention-based design of the complex:

> When the construction (*al-ʿimārah*) was completed, the sultan endowed [the bīmāristān] with *Qayāṣir*, hotels, shops, bathhouses, trade monopolies among other things such as real estate in the Levant; all of this fetched a huge sum every month. He dedicated most of this to the bīmāristān, then (*thumma*) the mausoleum (*al-Qubbah*). He [also] arranged the *madrasa*'s *waqf* but it falls short of its needs, and he arranged for the *maktab* a sufficient *waqf* in the Levant.[62]

Although the bīmāristān collected the majority of the revenues, the mausoleum had sufficient waqfs as well. But the madrasa's *waqfs* appeared to be lacking in the eyes of al-Nuwayrī, who had firsthand experience in managing the waqfs. In discussing the different administrative details of the complex, without any pressure to write a celebratory account ascribing a specific pietistic motivation to the complex and its founder, al-Nuwayrī may have expressed what was thought to be the real expressive intent of the complex. Al-Nuwayrī's view was evidenced when the next sultan, al-Ashraf Khalīl b. al-Manṣūr Qalāwūn, received oaths of allegiance from the Mamluk emirs at his father's mausoleum – as opposed to al-Ṣāliḥ Ayyūb's, as the previous Mamluk sultans had done.[63]

In the previous accounts, an unmistakable connection was created between the bīmāristān, on one hand, and the political career of the founding sultan, on the other.[64] In their accounts, Ibn ʿAbd al-Ẓāhir and Shāfiʿ b. ʿAlī' linked the benevolence of the sultan and his desire to build a large charitable institution with a huge endowment directly to his role as a sovereign and in a manner that was intended to solidify his legitimacy and legacy. Al-Nuwayrī's account, on the other hand, was aimed explicitly at solidifying the sultan's legacy by describing him as following the tradition of the last Ayyubid sovereign but in a more magnificent manner that transformed the memorial shrine into a rich charitable bīmāristān. The tomb occupied the discursive center of the complex as a testament to the magnificence of the sultan (now a source of legitimacy for his sons),

[62] Al-Nuwayrī, *Nihāyat al-'Arab*, 31: 106. The list of properties given by al-Nuwayrī here must only be taken as literary flourish, intending to show how rich and magnificent the complex's *waqf* was. The complex *waqf* document survived along with other annexes that added more properties, all of which fall within the larger categories explained by al-Nuwayrī. However, the document, which will be discussed later, should be considered the most reliable source for the *waqf* and the endowed properties due to its legally binding nature.

[63] Al-Maqrīzī, *al-Sulūk;* Al-Harithy, "Space in Mamluk Architecture," 83.

[64] On the rise of al-Manṣūr Qalāwūn and his connection to the Baḥarī mamluk corps, see Northrup, *From Slave to Sultan*.

his piety, and care for his people.[65] The bīmāristān, regardless of its metaphorical place in the complex, became proof of the sultan's power and dignity. Conversely, the dignity, the magnificence, and the piety of the ruler became the conditions upon which a bīmāristān of this size could be established. It appeared inconceivable that a lesser lord or a less magnificent sovereign would be able to undertake a similar project and have it be worthy of mention. In either case, the bīmāristān played a significant role through its being part of a larger architectural plan that also expressed specific political goals and views. Much like Nūr al-Dīn Zankī, al-Nāṣir Ṣalāḥ al-Dīn, and al-Ṣāliḥ Najm al-Dīn Ayyūb, al-Manṣūr Qalāwūn's constructions were part of a larger process of architectural or built patronage intended to channel the sultan's benevolence but also to commemorate his reign and immortalize his memory.

Location and Political Architecture

Regardless of the original motivation behind the building of the complex or its main expressive intent, the choice of its placement was a clear message that echoed the choice of the placement of Fāṭimah Khātūn's mausoleum built less than a year earlier. Just as his wife's mausoleum was built opposite that of his master's wife, Qalāwūn built his complex, including his mausoleum, opposite that of his master. The place chosen for his complex was previously occupied by one of two Fatimid caliphal palaces that faced each other, forming the "Bayn al-Qaṣrayn (between the two palaces)" square and giving the avenue its name. This palace was originally known as Dār Sitt al-Mulk in reference to Sitt al-Mulk, the daughter of the Fatimid Caliph al-ʿAzīz (r. 975–996) and sister to al-Ḥākim (r. 996–1021). After the fall of the Fatimids, the palace was given by Ṣalāḥ al-Dīn to his emir and lieutenant Fakhr al-Dīn Jihārkas (d. 1211). After Jihārkas's death, the palace went to al-Afḍal Quṭb al-Dīn, son of the Ayyubid Sultan al-ʿĀdil I (d. 1218), hence the name al-Dār al-Quṭbīyyah. Quṭb al-Dīn's offspring continued to live in this palace until Qalāwūn bought it in order to build the bīmāristān.[66] Although the purchase appeared to be legitimate and from the sultan's own purse, Sanjar al-Shujāʿī was accused of forcing the inhabitants out too hastily in a manner unworthy of nobility. This appears to have marred the entire project and to have tainted the place and the process of its selection, prompting Ibn ʿAbd al-Ẓāhir (Qalāwūn's

[65] See Sabra, *Poverty and Charity in Medieval Islam*, 99.

[66] Al-Maqrīzī, *al-Khiṭaṭ*, 4: 406. See also Ibn ʿAlī, Lewicka, *Biography of Qalāwūn*, 409–10.

biographer) to claim that there was no other place available at the center of the city and that the palace was too big for its inhabitants anyway.[67] Although the second point might be true, the first is blatantly false because the *waqfs* dedicated to the bīmāristān were almost all on Bayn al-Qaṣrayn avenue and contained shops and gardens, any of which the bīmāristān could have easily replaced.

In addition to the precedent of Fāṭimah Khātūn's mausoleum, the accounts describing the inauguration of the complex leave no doubt as to Qalāwūn's explicit intention to build his mausoleum opposite his master's. When Qalāwūn visited the complex after its completion, he was quick to show his dismay. He addressed al-Shujāʿī saying "O ʿAlam al-Dīn, haven't I instructed you that when you build this tomb (*al-qubba*; lit. the dome) that you build it facing (*qubalat*) the tomb of my master (*qubbat usthādhī*)?"[68] Although the entire complex was facing that of al-Ṣāliḥ Ayyūb, the two domes were not exactly facing one another; the madrasa, which was to the south of the complex, faced al-Ṣāliḥ Ayyūb's *qubba*, whereas Qalāwūn's *qubba* was now more aligned with Baybars's madrasa, which the latter had built beside al-Ṣāliḥ's mausoleum likely to show his loyalty as well. Qalāwūn wanted the two mausoleums to be directly facing one another in a clear simultaneous expression of his loyalty to his master and of his succeeding his master. As the madrasa came to occupy this position opposite al-Ṣāliḥ's mausoleum, Qalāwūn might have seen his objective unrealized and grew frustrated with his emir.

Qalāwūn's huge complex literally overshadowed those of his master and also of his esteemed predecessor (Baybars) and transformed the symbolic sites of power and legitimacy. In a way, building this new complex served to effectively symbolize the legitimacy of the new Mamluk state and the new Qalawunid dynasty.[69] According to Northrup,

> By erecting his monument on a site facing the tomb of his master, Qalāwūn without a doubt sought to emphasize his relationship with al-Ṣāliḥ Ayyūb. While he may have wished to symbolize his personal devotion to his master or perhaps to emphasize the achievements of the Ṣāliḥīyyah,[70] who had been the dominant political and military force in Egypt since the days of al-Ṣāliḥ, Qalāwūn's principal aim must have been to strengthen his claim, and

[67] Ibn ʿAbd al-Ẓāhir, *Tashrīf al-Ayyām*, 56.
[68] Tārikh Qirṭāy cited in Northrup, *From Slave to Sultan*, 119, note 409.
[69] Al-Harithy, "Space in Mamluk Architecture," 83.
[70] The Mamluk corps acquired by al-Ṣāliḥ Ayyūb.

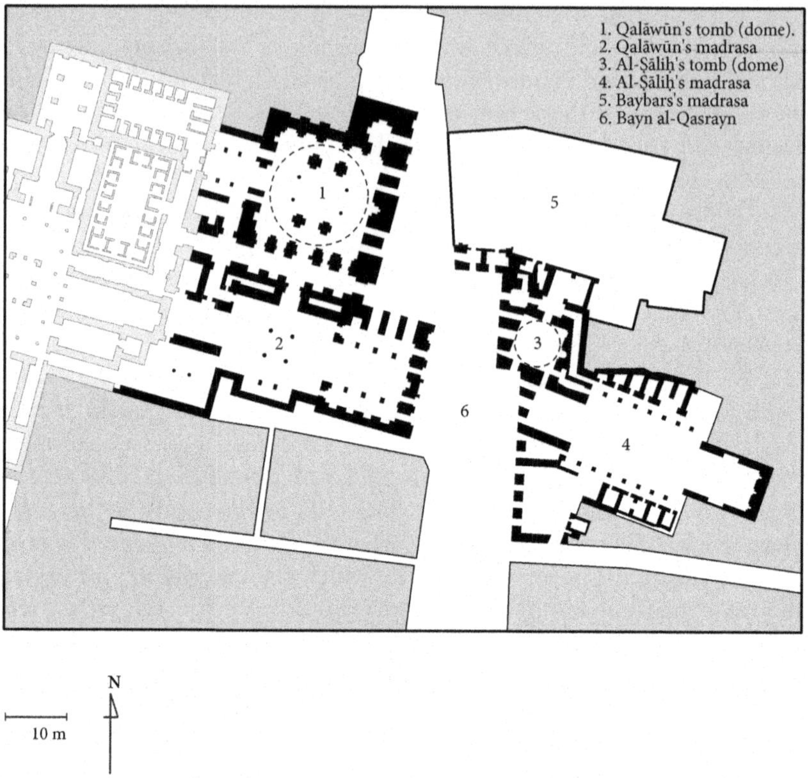

Figure 2.2: The relation between the two complexes (Al-Manusri and Al-Salihi)

perhaps that of his heir (his son, also named al-Ṣāliḥ) to being the legitimate successor(s) to the Ayyubid ruler.[71]

The architectural relationship between the complex and the mausoleum of al-Ṣāliḥ Ayyūb remodeled the space of the Bayn al-Qaṣrayn square, creating what Huwayda al-Harithy calls "an urban pocket":

> The siting of the complex of Qalawun [sic], the placement of significant architectural elements, and the treatment of the facade define both the form and character of this open space, or pocket, a space without boundaries of its own. The projection of the *madrasa* section of the complex of Qalawun [sic] into al-Mu'izz [sic] street complements the mausoleum of al-Salih [sic] and

[71] Northrup, *From Slave to Sultan*, 119.

> gives the space between the two complexes a sense of enclosure. Through contraction and expansion the building makes a clear distinction between the street and the urban pocket, but does not obstruct the flow along the path. The complementary relationship the complex establishes with the two institutions across this space is reinforced by the similar treatment of their facades, which lends the space further definition.[72]

As mentioned before, Al-Shujāʿī was accused of ordering the palace's inhabitants to vacate the palace immediately, before they were ready to move, in a manner that might have been unworthy of the Ayyubid nobility. He was also accused of using force and intimidation to acquire the palace at a fraction of the price. Furthermore, he forced every passerby in the neighboring streets to help with the physical construction by carrying some stones, assisting workers, or by donating money to the construction, which relied on forced and underpaid labor to boot:

> The majority of people ceased to pass close to the bīmāristān. After the construction [was concluded] and the *waqf* created, they asked the *faqīhs* for a *fatwa* [to the question]: "What do the *faqīhs* of the nation have to say about a place whose owners were forced to evacuate and which was built by supervisors (*nuẓẓār*) who did not pay the workers and [who used] materials brought from other buildings that they destroyed? Is it permissible to pray in such a place?" A number of *faqīhs* replied that it was not permissible to pray there.[73]

Al-Shūjāʿī was informed of this *fatwa*, which threatened the fate of the bīmāristān, and he tried to obtain a contrary *fatwa* by sending a request to the concerned *faqīhs* who had issued the earlier *fatwa*, but he was unable to convince them to change their minds. He then invited Shaykh Muḥammad al-Murjānī, who was the most vocal of the aforementioned *faqīhs*, to give a sermon in the complex. Al-Murjānī agreed but delivered a fiery sermon condemning both the forced evacuation of people from their houses and forced labor as impermissible under Islamic law, essentially repeating his *fatwa*, but this time inside the complex itself.[74] As a last resort, Al-Shujāʿī, now worried about his master's anger, discussed the issue with the famous Shāfiʿī Judge Ibn Daqīq al-ʿĪd. He explained that the sultan wanted to follow the example of Nūr al-Dīn but only received blame. The judge repeated the story about Nūr al-Dīn paying for his bīmāristān with ransom money from Crusader nobles captured in his

72 Al-Harithy, "Space in Mamluk Architecture," 84.
73 Al-Maqrīzī, *al-Khiṭaṭ*, 4: 407.
74 Ibid., 4: 407–08.

wars in 1154. He added, "'But the sultan [Qalāwūn] wanted to create good by [building the bīmāristān], and I wish him well. As for you, if you did this [supervising the construction, forced labor, and forced evacuation] to benefit people, you deserve God's reward. But if you did it to please your master, you will receive nothing.' Al-Shujāʿī said 'God knows the intentions' and appointed Ibn Daqīq al-ʿĪd a professor in the mausoleum,"[75] thereby ending the controversy. Here, the connection to Nūr al-Dīn's bīmāristān is significant in revealing the metaphorical genealogy that Qalāwūn and his men had in mind; they sought to portray Qalāwūn as a fighter of Crusaders, a uniter of the realm, and a builder of public relief institutions and madrasas, similar to Nūr al-Dīn, who also had a complex relationship with the Ayyubids.

About a century later, when al-Maqrīzī was writing his account, the controversy acquired different meanings and lost much of its political and legal relevance. Al-Maqrīzī questioned not only the proper acquisition of the palace by Qalāwūn and his emir, but also its acquisition by the Ayyubids who resided there. Directly addressing his reader as he rarely did when attempting to express his own opinion, he wrote: "If you look closely and know what indeed had taken place, you will find that these people were not but thieves who stole from other thieves, and aggressors who assailed other aggressors."[76] Although al-Maqrīzī was known for his pro-Fatimid sympathies, his view of the question showed that the elapsed century and the physical reality of the bīmāristān had added more shades to the issue and rendered the controversy largely insignificant. The physical "injury" inflicted by Qalāwūn against the Ayyubid city by his demolition of al-Dār al-Quṭbīyyah and by his confrontation with and literal overshadowing of the last Ayyubid monument – the mausoleum of al-Ṣāliḥ Ayyūb – was no longer relevant; the bīmāristān was now just another layer in a developing city. In relation to forced labor, al-Maqrīzī used the same logic adding, "I pray to you by God to inform me for I do not know: who, among them [men of power] did not use these methods for carrying out their affairs; only that some inflict more harm than others!"[77]

As opposed to the bīmāristān, which continued to be the central component of the complex, the madrasa appears to have not been part of Qalāwūn's plan. Shāfiʿ ibn ʿAlī, another author of Qalāwūn's regnal histories, wrote that when Qalāwūn inaugurated the bīmāristān, he was

[75] Ibid., 4: 408.
[76] Ibid.
[77] Ibid.

intent on not entering the madrasa, which he disliked. Ibn ʿAlī considered it to be an unwarranted addition by al-Shujāʿī that angered his master, and it was placed at a site where Qalāwūn had wanted his own tomb to be. Considering the style of construction of the Qalawunid complex might give us some ideas about al-Shujāʿī's original plans or desires that were in conflict with his master's. The complex was indeed built to be very similar to al-Ṣāliḥ Ayyūb's complex, with similar facade and even a similar L-shaped corridor connecting al-Ṣāliḥ's tomb with the two madrasas in his complex.[78] The only difference was that Qalāwūn's complex had only one madrasa and a bīmāristān. Al-Shujāʿī, who was Qalāwūn's chief building supervisor, and who might have had architectural experience of his own,[79] may have had a preference for madrasas similar to the one he built for Qalāwūn's wife. He probably desired to add such an important piece to his master's complex, or he may have been in favor of replicating al-Ṣāliḥ's complex with two madrasas, as opposed to a bīmāristān. Qalāwūn, as will be explained later, did not think much of madrasas and thought that his predecessors had built enough of them. Probably as a result, the madrasa did not have enough endowments supporting it and seems to have suffered from limited funds, as explained by al-Nuwayrī.

Conclusion

In 1285, Qalāwūn had already established himself as the unrivaled ruler of the empire, dismantled the power of his rivals and enemies, and consolidated a loyal corps of Mamluks that would eventually ensure his sons' succession and create the longest lasting dynasty in Mamluk history. At the height of his glory, he inaugurated his complex, which was composed of the bīmāristān, his shrine, and a madrasa. The complex was part of the sultan's earlier built patronage and also linked him to the traditions of other patrons. Choosing a location for the new bīmāristān was an act that carried many practical and symbolic ramifications. It modified the urban scene and the city's organization, removing existing structures and replacing them with others. It also modified the flow of movement of people and things both at the immediate local level and at the citywide or even regional level. The way the Qalawunid complex was built created a new

[78] Al-Harithy, "Space in Mamluk Architecture," 88.

[79] See Rabbat, "Architects and Artists in Mamluk Society." Rabbat argues that the emirs occupying the position of *shād al-ʿamāʾir* (construction supervisors) in the Bahari Mamluk period had significant architectural experience and played an important role in shaping their patron's architectural projects.

"square" that would interrupt the regular movement in Bayn al-Qaṣrayn avenue and create a moment to stop, observe, and recognize. At another level, the bīmāristān attracted people from the poorer suburbs and neighborhoods of the capital to the center of the city, thus creating new sites for interactions and completing the Ayyubid project of opening up the heart of the Fatimid city to the populace. At the symbolic level, building the bīmāristān as part of the Qalawunid complex reflected a specific social, political, and historical order and expressed particular narratives of power and authority. As a monument, the bīmāristān was a site for remembrance, for producing and codifying history, and for symbolizing the power and prestige of the sovereign.

As a new physical reality in the heart of Cairo, the complex stood literally to overshadow al-madrasah al-Ṣāliḥīyyah, built by the sultan's own master and the last Ayyubid sovereign. The new construction erased one of the last pieces of the city's Fatimid imprint, which had already been claimed by the Ayyubids, and destroyed in the process other Ayyubid monuments that contributed parts and materials to the now rising Mamluk edifice. The new complex came with a network of properties that both financed it and enforced its presence. The garden and the two existing roofed markets were located within a network of much older properties belonging to other *waqfs*. In essence, the complex, with all its properties, was carefully positioned in the fabric of the "endowed" city in order to testify to the piety, wealth, and magnanimity of its founders. The physical realization of a monument of that size not only derived its meaning from the history of the bīmāristān as an institution or from the influences of neighboring institutions in the Levant and Egypt, but also relied on a history of monuments in which the meaning of a monument, regardless of its form, was rooted in its ability to initiate and regulate memory and remembering. In establishing al-Bīmāristān al-Manṣūrī, Qalāwūn and his entourage were drawing on a history of building memories within towns and of memorializing victories in buildings. His complex and *waqfs* were, in a way, replicating other types of institutions built by other sovereigns like Nūr al-Dīn Zankī, Ṣalāḥ al-Dīn al-Ayyūbī, Najm al-Dīn Ayyūb, and al-Ẓāhir Baybars. At the same time, the new bīmāristān tapped into a host of meanings and concepts that were rooted in the *waqf* institution with its variable roles and evolving history.

Building the Bīmāristān changed the urban structure of part of the city not only by replacing an old palace with a bīmāristān for the poor but also by bringing new visitors to the city, as a new destination for the sick-poor. A site of service to visitors of the saints of Cairo and students of masters within the growing capital, the Bīmāristān was embedded in the map of visitation (*ziyārah*) as a new "stop" on a continuous trip. Here, the Sultan's shrine stood not only as a testimony to his patronage but also to his personage as an effective saint performing miracles through the acts of physicians and caretakers. It is no accident that people used oil from the shrine's lamps to cure their ailing eyes five centuries after the bīmāristān was built and a century after it was last renovated.[80] The complex, with its bīmāristān, shrine, and madrasa, was establishing new acts of remembrance, whether intentional, patronized, and designed or implicit in the making of such a monument. The *waqf* and the sultan's offspring would sponsor Qur'an reciters to read in the sultan's shrine during ceremonies attended by the madrasa's students and teachers; these ceremonies were heard, if not also attended, by those being cared for in the bīmāristān. The festivities marking religious holidays and political occasions began or ended in the sultan's shrine and bīmāristān, with the poor, now accustomed to this trip, becoming major audiences to these events. The ritualized *fātiḥah,* or prayer of intercession, that Nūr al-Dīn Zankī reportedly coveted from his patronized poor and mystics, were also expected from the sultan's patronized sick. In this view, the new bīmāristān was a new place for old practices of remembering that kept Qalāwūn's name and memory alive within the fabric of the city.

80 ʿĪsá, Tārīkh al-Bīmāristānāt fī al-Islām, 68.

CHAPTER 3

"The Best of Deeds": Medical Patronage in Mamluk Egypt

Qalāwūn as a Patron of Medicine

In his history of Qalāwūn's life and reign, Shāfiʿ ibn ʿAlī described the ceremony inaugurating the bīmāristān. The sultan rode to the bīmāristān, sat in its southern *iwān*, and announced his *waqf* in front of the four chief judges of the empire. The sultan then bestowed robes of honor on all the attendants and moved to the madrasa:

> This *madrasa* was added by emir ʿAlam al-Dīn al-Shujāʿī, and our lord the sultan did not order its [construction], nor did he want but a bīmāristān, and gaining the divine reward [due for its construction]. When he exited the bīmāristān, he almost did not enter [the *madrasa*]; turning away from it, and being done with it. Then, he entered it . . ., since not every secret should be announced, and sat in its prayer's niche.[1]

Qalāwūn, as shown in his regnal history written by Ibn ʿAlī, did not approve of the madrasa and did not want it built. He may have been particularly disappointed because he wanted his own mausoleum to face that of his master. Instead, al-Shujāʿī had placed the madrasa facing al-Ṣāliḥ's mausoleum. Yet his frustration with the building arrangement and its design, which Qirṭāy reported, was not the only reason for his near-decision to avoid entering the madrasa. After the large controversy that had surrounded the complex and the *fatwa* prohibiting prayers in the madrasa or mausoleum, his refusal to enter the madrasa would have had disastrous implications.

In the decrees written to appoint the chief physician of the bīmāristān, promulgated only few days after the event described by Ibn ʿAlī, the sultan's scribe Ibn al-Mukarram explained the sultan's agenda in relation to building the bīmāristān:

> We saw that every king who preceded us, even if he followed the best path in managing the flock, had been interested in the science of religion and

[1] Lewicka, *Safi Ibn Ali's Biography of the Mamluk Sultan Qalawun*, 408.

> neglected the science of bodies, and each of [our predecessors] built a *madrasa* and did not care for a bīmāristān, and neglected [the prophet's] saying science is [of] two [types], and did not admonish any of his flock to be occupied with the science of medicine that is necessary, nor endowed a *waqf* for the students of this science, mentioned [in traditions], nor prepared a place of attendance for those occupied with this art, nor appointed a *shaykh* for [those] occupied [with medicine]. We have known of this what they had been ignorant of, and remembered of this nearness [to God] what they neglected, and connected of these religious and earthly means what they separated, and built a bīmāristān that dazzled the eyes with joy.[2]

The predecessors to which he referred may well have been al-Ṣāliḥ Ayyūb and Baybars I. Both figures were well-respected by the sultan, and both had built a madrasa across the street from where Qalāwūn was building his bīmāristān and mausoleum.[3] Qalāwūn's previous acts of patronage clearly represented his interest in bīmāristāns and lack of interest in madrasas: he did not build any madrasas (except for one dedicated to his wife), but he built a bīmāristān in Hebron, as explained in the previous chapter. Qalāwūn also renovated al-Bīmāristān al-Nūrī in Damascus and added to its *waqfs*. But his preference for bīmāristāns cannot explain entirely his particular dislike of the madrasa built in his own complex. We could also attribute this dislike to his perception of the madrasa as redundant or perhaps to his fear that it suggested competition with his master, which he did not seem to desire. As Ibn al-Mukarram's decree explained, the sultan thought that medicine was not patronized sufficiently and that there were many madrasas but not enough bīmāristāns. This position toward madrasas and bīmāristāns, or rather toward law and medicine, can also be detected in the writings of Ibn al-Ukhuwwa (d. 1329), a market inspector in Cairo, who complained that most physicians were Christians and Jews and that few Muslims took on the profession.[4] Ibn al-Ukhuwwa explained this phenomenon by the

[2] Ibn al-Furāt, *Tārīkh Ibn al-Furāt*, 8: 25, "*Wa ra'aynā kullaman [sic] taqaddamanā min al-mulūk, wa in salaka fī siyāsat al-ra'iyyah aḥsan sulūk, qad ihtamma bi-'ilm al-adyān wa ahmal 'ilm al-abdān, wa ansha'a kullun minhum madrasatan wa lam yaḥfal bi-Bīmāristān, wa ghafala 'an qawlihi ṣallā Allāh 'alayhi wa sallam al-'ilm 'ilmān, wa lam ya'khudh aḥadan min ra'iyyatihi bi-l-ishtighāl bi-'ilm al-ṭibb al-muḍṭarri illayhi, wa lā waqafa waqfan 'alāṭalabat hādhā al-'ilm al-manṣūṣi 'alayh, wa lā a'addā lahu makānan yaḥḍuru man yashtaghil bihādhā al-fann fihi, wa lā naṣṣaba lahu shakhṣan yata-maththalu hādhā al-mushtaghil ladayhi, 'alimnā naḥnu bi-ḥamd Allāh ta'ālā min dhalik mā jahilūh, wa dhakharnā min hadhihi al-qurbah mā ahmalūh, wa-waṣalnā min hādhih al-asbāb al-dīniyyah wa al-dunyawiyyah mā faṣalūh, wa ansha'nā Bīmāristānan yubhiru al-'uyūn bahjah.*"

[3] Northrup, "Qalawun's Patronage of the Medical Sciences in Thirteenth-Century Egypt," 129–30.

[4] Ibn al-Ukhūwah, *Ma'ālim al-Qurbah fī Aḥkām al-Ḥisbah*, 166.

fact that law was a vehicle for gaining money and a higher position in the society, whereas medicine was not. With the spread of madrasas since the early Ayyubid period, places for teaching and also for employing these students increased this imbalance noted by Ibn al-Ukhuwwa and others. The decree appointing the chief physician of the bīmāristān reflected the priority of teaching more Muslims the medical art and warned the chief physician twice against denying education or certification to those who deserved it, a possible reference to Muslim students who did not come from medical families.

As the decrees of appointment indicate, Qalāwūn's patronage of medical sciences was premised on its status as a necessary science (*muḍṭarrun ilayhi*). As such, its patronage was a duty of the sovereign and its learning was a communal obligation for Muslims (*farḍ kifāyah*). The sovereign was therefore required to facilitate its learning and practice. Qalāwūn's medical patronage did not involve any specific relations with physicians but was focused mainly on bīmāristāns, including his two bīmāristāns in Hebron and Cairo and his renovations of al-Bīmāristān al-Nūrī in Damascus. While the Hebron bīmāristān was dedicated to visitors and pilgrims to the Abrahamic Sanctuary, the Cairo bīmāristān was meant to be the main bīmāristān of the capital and to serve the local population of and visitors to Cairo and al-Fusṭaṭ. In this way, Qalāwūn's medical patronage was not directed toward the profession-qua-profession or toward the practitioners of the science, but rather toward the poor, his flock, by fulfilling their need for medical care. In the same vein, the inclusion of regular lessons and the appointment of teachers in al-Bīmāristān al-Manṣūrī in Cairo were meant to provide Muslims a chance to learn medicine to further supply the needs of the flock and to facilitate the execution of God's demands. This educational policy would eventually collide with a perceived reluctance on the part of non-Muslim practitioners to teach Muslim students from nonmedical families. This perception, which was embedded in part in the rise of anti-Christian narratives in Mamluk Egypt, was also a reflection of sociointellectual and socioprofessional norms in which certain practices persisted in specific families, and students without the requisite family heritage found it difficult to find their way into a new profession.

In this chapter, we will analyze the three surviving documents of Qalāwūn's medical patronage; namely, the *waqf* document and the two decrees appointing the chief physician and the chief of the bīmāristān.

The *Waqf* Document: The Voice of Place

Establishing a Language of Charity

Al-Bīmāristān al-Manṣūrī's *waqf* document was a testimony to the perception of the bīmāristān and its role in society. The document is kept in the Cairo National Archives' (Document No. 15, *Maḥfazah 2*). Document 15 comprises two *waqf* documents promulgated by al-Manṣūr Qalāwūn for the bīmāristān, each created nine days apart. The first is the original *waqf* document, which includes the original endowment and the stipulations and details related to the administration and functioning of the bīmāristān.[5] The second added more revenues to the original endowment but did not include any details or stipulations about the institution's functioning; it refered instead to the first document for these details.[6] The archives of the Egyptian Ministry of Awqāf keeps a second copy of National Archives' Document 15 under the number 1010. The Ministry's archives also have another document (No. 1011), also promulgated by al-Manṣūr Qalāwūn, which added even more revenues to the bīmāristān's endowment. Similar to the second part of Document 15, Document 1011 did not include any details related to the management or administration of the bīmāristān.

The *waqf* document has been studied only twice. The first was by Aḥmad ʿIsā in his book, *Tārīkh al-Bīmāristānāt fī al-Islām,*[7] in which the author described the bīmāristān using details mentioned in the document along with accounts from other historians. The second study was done by M. M. Amīn and S. A. ʿAmmār of Cairo University in 1976, in their edition of al-Ḥasan b. ʿUmar b. Ḥabīb's *Tadhkirat al-Nabīh fī Ayyām al-Manṣūr wa Banīh.* In an appendix to the first volume of their edition, Amīn and ʿAmmār edited and published all the previously mentioned *waqf* documents of the bīmāristān. They also edited and published other important waqf documents of al-Nāṣir Muḥammad and al-Nāṣir Ḥasan in the appendixes of the second and third volumes, respectively.[8] In the coming pages, we will rely on their edition in our analysis of the document.

[5] The manuscript mentioned earlier is actually an autographed copy of the original document that was "compared to the original copy according to traditions *qubalāt bi-niskhat al-aṣl ḥasab al-uṣūl*"; Ibn Ḥabīb, *Tadhkirat al-Nabīh,* 1: 310.

[6] Ibid., 1: 391.

[7] ʿIsā, *Tārīkh al-Bīmāristānāt fī al-Islām.*

[8] Ibn Ḥabīb, *Tadhkirat al-Nabīh.*

The document opens with an introduction that spans roughly 67 lines out of the document's total of 329 lines, excluding autographs of the authors and legal witnesses; it is therefore about one-fifth of the document's active text.[9] This introduction to the bīmāristān's document, one of the earlier *waqfs* of this size, opens an interesting window onto early perceptions of the waqf system itself and the way religious and intellectual elites conceived of it. Moreover, the introduction of what was the biggest architectural achievement of Qalāwūn's reign included important titles for the sultan that expressed his status and showed the priorities of his reign.

After the formulaic *basmalah* (opening with the name of God) and *ḥamd* (thanking God), in the fifth and sixth lines, the author continued to praise God by enumerating the divine attributes related to the acceptance of offerings and the reward of good-doers. He wrote: "[God] opens the gates of mercy by facilitating nearness and easing good-doing (*taysīr al-qurubāt wa-tashīl al-mabarrāt*)."[10] Here, the term *qurubāt* is connected to the legal reasoning behind the *waqf*; it connotes a manner of gaining nearness to God by doing good that is not necessarily mandated. The author expanded on this theme of nonobligatory beneficence by explaining that the deeds described in this document were among "the best of deeds after duties (*wājibāt*)."[11] He then enumerated a number of examples perceived as among the best of nonobligatory deeds and also as the justification for the bīmāristān as an institution: "dispelling distress (*tafrīj al-kurubāt*), and succoring those with plight and needs (*ighāthat dhawī al-iḍṭirār wa-l-ḥājāt*), satisfying the deficiency of those with poverty and need (*sadd khillāt ahl al-faqr wa-al-fāqāt*), and giving refuge to strangers whose means were severed (*īwā᾽ al-ghurabā᾽ alladhīna taqaṭaʿat bihim al-asbāb*)."[12]

Perpetual charity, or *al-ṣadaqah al-jāriyah*, remained an important part of the religious and legal underwriting of the project. The document begins its discussion of *al-ṣadaqah al-jāriyah* at line twelve with Muḥammad's tradition: "Our prophet Muḥammad ... said that if the servant (*al-ʿabd*) dies, his [good] deeds are cut from this world except for three and counted among them perpetual charities (*wa ʿadda minhā al-ṣadaqāt al-jāriyāt*)."[13]

9 Ibn Ḥabīb, *Tadhkirat al-Nabīh fī Ayyām al-Manṣūr wa Banīh*, 329–37. On introductions and their role in texts, see P. Freimark, "Mukaddima."
10 Ibn Ḥabīb, *Tadhkirat Al-Nabīh*, 1: 329.
11 On this question, see Bonner, Ener, and Singer (eds.), *Poverty and Charity in Middle Eastern Contexts*, 31–48.
12 Ibn Ḥabīb, *Tadhkirat Al-Nabīh*, 1: 330.
13 Ibid.

Another *hadīth* follows that returns the narrative to the question of need and aid. In this tradition, Muḥammad said, "God is in the help of a servant so long as the servant is in the help of his brother (*Allāh fī ʿawn al-ʿabd mādām al-ʿabd fī ʿawn akhīh*)." The document explained the tradition: "Money is [all God's] money and He, in his magnanimity, borrows from his own money (*yastaqrid min mālihi*), and the creatures are his children (*wa al-khalq ʿiyāluhu*), and the most loved by God among his servants is the [greatest] benefactor to his children by finding comfort [for them] and providing means (*bi-ījād al-rāḥāt wa-tawfīr al-ṣadaqāt*)."[14]

As a *khuṭbah* or sermon, the introduction to the document was formulated around three fixed formulas that provided important transition points from one part of the introduction to the next. The first formula, "thanking and praising God (*ḥamd Allāh wa al-thanāʾ ʿalayhi*)," is found at line two. The second, the pronouncement of faith (*shahādatān*), proclaims that there is only one God and that Muḥammad is his prophet. The third prays for and praises Muḥammad, at which point the introduction ends with the formulaic *ammā baʿd* ("then"). Each of these three occasions or narrative moments allowed the writer to provide important glosses that would explain and elaborate on the other functions of the document and on its original subject. In these glosses, the author referenced prophetic traditions and verses from the Quran, but not through the use of quotations or fixed, borrowed blocks of texts. Rather, the author recalled textual elements of these prophetic traditions by borrowing their words, structures, and even meanings, thereby relying upon the audience's memory of these texts to recall the references immediately and without difficulty.

The first part of the introduction, the longest in the case of al-Manṣūrī's *waqf* document, follows the formulaic thanksgiving to God ("*al-ḥamd lil-lāh*") and alludes to prophetic and Quranic texts that recall the language of charity. Here, the author made two references to God's doubling of rewards for *sadaqāt* that relied on a number of verses from the Quran, among them 2: 276: "God blots out usury, but freewill offerings He augments with interest. God loves not any guilty ingrate." This verse was referenced twice in the introduction to indicate the divine promise of multiplying the reward for charity, and it functioned to highlight the impressive size of this institution. More importantly, the text also recalls 9: 103–104, verses that instructed Muḥammad to take the obligatory alms and linked his acquisition to purification, but with an emphasis on God's acceptance of charity: "Take of their wealth a freewill offering, to purify

[14] Ibid., 1: 330–31.

them and to cleanse them thereby, and pray for them; thy prayers are a comfort for them; God is All-Hearing, All-Knowing. (103) Do they not know that God is He who accepts repentance from His servants, and takes the freewill offerings, and that God – He turns, and is All-Compassionate? (104)." Finally, the document recalls a prophetic tradition in which Muḥammad said: "No one gives a charity (*taṣadaqa bi-ṣadaqah*) but God would take it in his right hand, grow it, as one of you would grow his foal or calf, so it [the charity] grows in God's hand until it is bigger than a mountain." In all these examples, the document constructed a network of references connected to charity, God's acceptance of charity, and his multiplication of the reward. All these verses located the *waqf* within this environment. When explaining the targets of charity and its main audience, the document did not reproduce the dominant verses on the subject but instead stressed the need of the sick as well as of strangers and wayfarers. It recalled the tradition about God's assistance to those who help others, one of only two traditions mentioned explicitly, along with the tradition on *al-ṣadaqah al-jāriyah.*

The Sultan

Following the traditional *ammā baʿd* (then), the author commenced with the description of the *waqf* by establishing the legal act of endowment (*ḥabs*) through reference to the name of the *wāqif*, al-Manṣūr Qalāwūn, and his legal representative (*wakīl*), Aybak al-Afram, who promulgated the act on the sultan's behalf. The mention of the sultan's titles along with his name allowed for an important opportunity to infuse the document with more meaning in relation to the sultan's reign and his legitimacy, as well as to provide the text with more details about the role played by the bīmāristān in the region's political cosmology. Danielle Jacquart and Françoise Micheau explain: "la création des *madrasas* servait la politique menée alors au sein du monde sunnite: renforcement de l'orthodoxie, lutte contre le Chiisme, réarmement moral. Les hôpitaux les plus importants ont été fondés dans ce contexte. . . . le Sultan Mamluk, al-Mansour Qalawun, fit construire au Caire un ensemble architectural prestigieux, comprenant une madrasa, un mausolée, un hôpital; il inscrivit explicitement cette fondation dans le cadre du *gihad*."[15] Similarly, Ulrich Haarmann, in his analysis of a document produced close to the end of the Mamluk empire, explains that the justification of the rule of the "Turks" in the Mamluk

[15] Jacquart and Micheau, *La Médecine Arabe et l'Occident Médiéval*, 245–46.

empire relied on their ability to provide protection to the nation and to wage the holy war against the enemies of Islam.[16] In spite of its stress on charity and assistance of those in need, this document was also rooted in a language of warfare and jihad that manifested itself especially in the honorary epithets given to the Sultan.

Epithets and honorary titles given to sovereigns, whether in documents or inscribed on the inaugural plaques of different buildings, usually carried important messages about the sovereign, the perception of his work, and the legitimacy of his reign. In al-Bīmāristān al-Manṣūrī's *waqf* document, the epithets and honorary titles occupy nine lines, from line 35 to line 43, at which point his name is mentioned and then followed by thirteen more lines of prayers and praise to the sultan, in which his reign and his domain are described in equally elaborate terms. In addition to his original title "*al-Manṣūr*" ("victorious"), the document includes more titles related to war, conquest, and *jihād* such as: warrior [of holy war] (*mujāhid*), garrisoned (*murābiṭ*), triumphant (*muẓaffar*), and gallant (*humām*). The document also elaborates in relation to specific events, enemies, or foes, a testimony to their centrality in the imaginary surrounding al-Manṣūr Qalāwūn's reign. For instance, he is described as *qāhir al-khawārij wa al-mutamaridīn* (vanquisher of kharijites and rebels) and *mubīd al-firinj wa al-arman wa al-tatār* (Annihilator of the Franks, Armenians, and Tatar), and he is also identified as *ṣāḥib al-Qiblatayn* (the sovereign of the two *qiblas*) in reference to Mecca and Jerusalem.[17] He is also described as the sovereign of lands, regions, and inlets (*thughūr*); the *Sultan* over the Arabs, Persians, and Turks; "Alexander of his time (*Iskandar al-zamān*)"; and "the partner of the Prince of the Believers (*qasīm amīr al-mu'minīn*)." By referencing his wars against the Crusaders (Franks), the Mongols, the Armenians, and the "rebels" – in a possible reference to his successive wars against Mamluk insurgents in the Levant – al-Manṣūr Qalāwūn was legitimized as a warrior and a patron of jihad.

Although the opening lines of the *waqf* document included few details about the institution itself, they provided an important narrative about the place of the institution in its social, political, and cultural context. The introduction, with its embellished mention of the sultan and his titles and its emphasis on questions of perpetual charity and divine reward, gave voice to the symbolic significance of the structure itself. In different acts of

[16] Haarmann, "Rather the Injustice of the Turks than the Righteousness of the Arabs: Changing the Attitudes of Ulama towards Mamluk Rule in the Late Fifteenth Century," 61–77.

[17] Ibn Ḥabīb, *Tadhkirat al-Nabīh*, 1: 334.

public reading, the document's introduction served to locate the bīmāristān historically and to establish al-Manṣūr's ownership of the institution and of the earthly and divine rewards it might procure. The *waqf* document, however, was also a detailed administrative manual intended to regulate and organize the workings of the institution, its finances, and its different affairs. In the remainder of this chapter, we will analyze the different components of the *waqf* document in relation to patients, physicians, administrators and will locate these discussions within their larger context.

Funding the Bīmāristān

After the introductions, the *waqf* document proceeded to enumerate the properties and the sources of revenue that funded the bīmāristān. Although all contemporary accounts, such as those of al-Nuwayrī, attested that the bīmāristān's *waqfs* were remarkably rich and more than sufficient to provide for its expenses, the actual properties endowed were limited in number. The *waqf* document enumerated only six sites: an orchard, three roofed markets (*qaysārīyah*), one bathhouse, and a number of dwellings for rent. One of the three roofed markets and the bathhouse were new and built especially for the bīmāristān: the roofed market was not yet completed when the document was promulgated, and the bathhouse was meant as part of the bīmāristān, for the use of the patients and others. The six properties, however, were all located in the center of Cairo either overlooking or very near Bayn al-Qaṣrayn Avenue, making them some of the most valuable pieces of real estate in the entire empire. This explains why so small a number of properties could provide the huge income needed by the bīmāristān. "These properties were without a doubt among the most valuable and lucrative sites available. That the sultan controlled these properties – including shops, baths, dwellings and orchards – is some indication for the degree of economic and political power he had acquired at this point in his reign. It should also be remembered that, although these properties had been set aside as *waqf*, the sultan retained the right to administer them during his lifetime and reserved that privilege for his sons after his death."[18]

The orchard (*bustān*) measured about 21.5 *feddans* (about 22.37 acres) and included a well and waterwheel. It was located not too far from the

[18] Northrup, *From Slave to Sultan: The Career of al-Mansour Qalawun and the Consolidation of the Mamluk Rule in Egypt and Syria (678–689 A.H/1267–1290 A.D)*, 121.

bīmāristān itself, immediately outside the major gates of Cairo and overlooking the extension of Bayn al-Qaṣrayn Avenue. The document explained that it was surrounded by the *waqfs* of the Ẓāhirī mosque on both its southern and eastern borders and was also bordered by other *waqfs* on the east and north, such as that of Ibn Sinmār and of al-Zaytūn mosque, along with the estate of emir Qushtumur al-ʿAjamī. The orchard was located among a number of other endowed properties that supplied funds for mosques and madrasas surrounding the bīmāristān itself.[19] The rest of the endowed properties were even closer to the bīmāristān, and some were even part of the bīmāristān's building. The larger roofed market (*qaysārīyah*) was located to the north of al-Ṣāliḥīyah madrasa at the beginning of Bayn al-Qaṣrayn Avenue and had sixty-three shops of different sizes that were available for rent to the benefit of the *waqf*.[20] The second *Qaysārīyah* had thirty-six shops and was also on Bayn al-Qaṣrayn Avenue, surrounded by properties endowed to al-Kāmilīyyah madrasa and al-Muẓaffariyyah madrasa. A third *Qaysārīyah* was being built just beside the bīmāristān and would contain fifty-two shops of different sizes, of which one could see "the signs (*maʿālim*) of shops and dwellings (*maqāʿid*) that are not completed, counting twenty-four."[21] Finally, the bathhouse, also yet to be completed, was actually part of the bīmāristān and would be available for the patients.

Although these properties were supposed to be endowed for perpetuity, it appears that at least one of the roofed markets fell into decay and another was significantly changed by the time al-Maqrīzī (d. 1442) was writing his famous *Khiṭaṭ* of Cairo. In his description of roofed markets, he explained that one of the three markets had been destroyed, namely *Qaysārīyat al-Ḍiyāfah*, likely the one north to al-Ṣāliḥīyyah madrasa on the other side of Bayn al-Qaṣrayn from the Bīmāristān.[22] Another market, *Qaysārīyat al-Afḍal*, is mentioned in al-Maqrīzī's *Khiṭaṭ* as part of the bīmāristān's *waqf* and may have been the new market under construction when the document was originally written. The third market, located close to the *waqf* of al-Kāmilīyyah madrasa, was originally a book market but later became a place for leather manufacturing and selling in 1398, at the orders of the emir supervising the bīmāristān's *waqf*.[23] The bathhouse, called "*ḥammām al-Sābāṭ*" or "*ḥammām al-māristān al-Manṣūrī*," seemed

[19] Ibn Ḥabīb, *Tadhkirat al-Nabīh*, 338–41.
[20] Ibid., 341–42.
[21] Ibid., 347.
[22] Al-Maqrīzī, *al-Khiṭāṭ*, 3: 86.
[23] Ibid., 2: 375.

to have survived. Al-Maqrīzī described it as close to the bīmāristān's back door (*bāb al-sirr*) on a street parallel to Bayn al-Qaṣrayn. Al-Maqrīzī also mentioned that there were benches located underneath the windows of the Qalawunid complex occupied by jewelers and ring-sellers. There was a water basin for animals in this area, right beneath the complex windows on Bayn al-Qaṣrayn avenue, which was removed and replaced with a *sabīl* from which people could drink by the emir Jamāl al-Dīn Āqūsh al-Ashrafī (d. 1335; known as *Nāʾib al-Karak*, the viceroy of al-Karak), who supervised the bīmāristān around 1330.[24] Because the emir's actions were part of his duties as the bīmāristān's supervisor, it is not unlikely that the benches or stalls in front of the bīmāristān were seen as part of its properties.

Qalāwūn's sons and grandsons added new *waqfs* to the complex. Al-Ashraf Khalīl, Qalāwūn's son and immediate successor (r. 1290–1293), added four large estates in Acre and Tyre, which he had conquered from the Crusaders, to the *waqf*. Al-Ashraf's additions were dedicated mainly to the madrasa and the mausoleum and paid less attention to the bīmāristān, which probably had all its large *waqfs* intact at the time.[25] Qalāwūn's grandson, al-Ṣāliḥ Ismāʿīl (r. 1342–1345), had another *waqf* added in his name to the mausoleum to support lessons in Islamic law. Al-Maqrīzī explained that al-Ṣāliḥ Ismāʿīl intended to build a madrasa of his own but died before doing so; his father-in-law the emir Arghūn established these lessons in his name in Qalāwūn's mausoleum.[26] There is evidence that other emirs contributed to the *waqf* and endowed their own properties to support the bīmāristān. At the end of the inauguration ceremony, Qalāwūn's chamberlain or major-domo (*amīr jandār*), the emir ʿIzz al-Dīn al-Afram, approached the sultan, greeted him, and presented documents testifying that he had endowed two properties for the bīmāristān. One of the two properties was close to the bīmāristān itself and was therefore a highly valuable property, whereas the other in Zuwayla Lane (*ḥarat zuwayla*) was close to the eastern gate of the city. The sultan accepted the gift. Ibn ʿAbd al-Ẓāhir explained that others followed the emir with similar gifts.[27] Similarly, when the emir Jamāl al-Dīn Āqūsh was appointed supervisor of the bīmāristān, he renovated the bīmāristān, repainting its walls and adding a new hall out of his own money.[28] When the Mamluk historian Ibn al-Furāt (d. 1405) described the bīmāristān, he mentioned that Qalāwūn had endowed villages and real estate in the Levant for

[24] Ibid., 4: 407.
[25] Ibid., 4: 381.
[26] Ibid., 4: 380.
[27] Ibn ʿAbd Al-Ẓāhir, Tashrīf al-Ayyām wa al-ʿUṣūr fī Sīrat al-Malik al-Manṣūr, 129.
[28] ʿĪsā, Tārīkh al-Bīmāristānāt fī al-Islām, 62 (citing al-Fayyūmī's Nathr al-Jammān).

the bīmāristān.[29] Because there is no contemporary or documentary evidence that any such properties were endowed by Qalāwūn, Ibn al-Furāt may have been referring to the *waqfs* endowed by Qalāwūn's son al-Ashraf Khalīl or to *waqfs* added by other emirs over the intervening century. Some of these may have been retrospectively identified with Qalāwūn himself. In all cases, the bīmāristān's *waqfs* were not stable but rather in a state of continuous dynamism: they were added to and modified over time.

The document stipulated two conditions that regulated the management of the *waqf* properties and were intended to protect the bīmāristān's finances and maintain its role. The first condition made the maintenance, renovation, and improvement of the *waqf* properties themselves the first expense priority. This included the restoration and renovation of buildings, the improvement of irrigation in the orchard, and other maintenance efforts. The second prohibited the *nāẓir* (supervisor) from renting the properties of the *waqf*, such as buildings and shops, to "a pauper, a poor, a man with immense power, or a dishonest man."[30] The two conditions were meant to protect the bīmāristān and to ensure permanence and prosperity of its *waqfs*. They also reflected the experience gained by al-Manṣūr Qalāwūn and his entourage from observing the conditions of the Ayyubid *waqfs*, including the ones used to support the decaying al-Bīmāristān al-Nāṣirī of Salāḥ al-Dīn. In fact, in prioritizing the maintenance of the *waqf*, Qalāwūn's *waqf* document charted a new tradition: Qalāwūn's sons and successors followed his example in establishing their own *waqfs*. This policy may have enabled many of these huge establishments to survive over time.[31] The permanence of the *waqf* became one of its central goals and a concept key to the perception that a *waqf* ensured the perpetual remembrance of its founder.

The prohibition against renting the *waqf* properties to men of power reflects Qalāwūn's awareness of the political environment in which he exercised power. To put this prohibition in context, it is instructive to remember that Qalāwūn was himself the supervisor of the *waqf* and had reserved this right to his sons, as the sultans of the realm. Should his progeny become extinct, the sultan of Egypt would assume the position of supervisor, followed by the Shāfiʿī judge of the realm. After the fall of the last Qalawunid sultan, al-Manṣūr Ḥājjī, and the assumption of al-Ẓāhir Barqūq (r. 1390–1399), Barqūq became the supervisor of the *waqf* and

29 Ibn al-Furāt, *Tārīkh Ibn al-Furāt*, 8: 22–24.
30 Ibn Ḥabīb, *Tadhkirat al-Nabīh*, 1: 361.
31 See al-Harithy, "The Concept of Space in Mamluk Architecture," 73–93; Sabra, *Poverty and Charity in Medieval Islam: Mamluk Egypt 1250–1517*, 95–100.

appointed his grand emirs as his deputies in the bīmāristān, although Qalāwūn's progeny survived.[32] In all these cases, the supervisor of the bīmāristān would have occupied the highest position in the state and would have had nothing to fear from men of power. Qalāwūn himself, however, was among the more powerful men in the realm before occupying the throne. In the first years of his reign, there were a number of other emirs whose might he had to counteract. In a way, the *waqf* document attempted to steer the bīmāristān as far away as possible from the power struggles with which Qalāwūn and his entourage were all too familiar.

The Bīmāristān's Spending Priorities

An analysis of the *waqf* document's spending priorities, along with its instructions on equipping the bīmāristān to undertake its duties, gives further insight into the authors' perceptions of the facility's charitable objectives. Anticipated expenses were chosen and formulated, first, in relation to the perceived role of the bīmāristān in the extended genealogy of similar institutions and, second, in relation to the needs and requirements of its intended patients. The document arranged the spending categories in two different lists. The first list comprised all legitimate expenses, which it placed in four categories:[33]

- *Maṣāliḥ al-Bīmāristān*, or the benefits of the bīmāristān, which included all issues related to maintenance, administration, expansion, and so forth
- Those who cared for the patients, such as physicians, oculists, surgeons, and cooks of syrups and medications ("*man yaqūm bi-maṣāliḥ al-marḍā bihi min al-aṭibbāʾ wa al-kaḥḥālīn wa al-jarāḥiyyīn wa-ṭabbākhīn al-sharāb wa al-rawand wa-ṣāniʿī al-maʿājīn wa-al-akḥāl wa al-adwiyah wa al-mushillāt al-mufradah wa al-murakkabah*")
- Caretakers (*qawamah*), janitors (*al-farrāshīn*), and employees responsible for storage and distribution of drugs, foods, and other necessities
- "What [is necessary] to support the treatment of patients (*mā yaqūm bi-madāwāt al-marḍā*)," such as medications, foods, and other materials needed for their preparations[34]

[32] Al-Maqrīzī, *al-Sulūk*, 1: 606.
[33] Ibn Ḥabīb, *Tadhkirat Al-Nabīh*, 1: 360–61.
[34] The four categories were not numbered in the document. However, each was distinguished by the author's repetition of the proposition *ḥarf al-jarr* "ʿalā" before each of the aforementioned categories while using a simple *ḥarf al-ʿaṭf* "wa" before every item within the category. This style would

Waqf revenues could be legitimately directed only toward these four categories. This list, however, was not sufficient to explain the intentions of the *wāqif* because it did not express any prioritization nor did it elaborate upon the four spending categories. The document's second list accomplished this by breaking the spending categories down into specific subcategories ordered by priority and relevance to the perceived purposes of the bīmāristān. The ordered list of priorities included the following:

1. The maintenance of the bīmāristān itself along with the *waqf* properties; this included renovations and the rebuilding of broken-down structures, which signified the intent to protect the bīmāristān's buildings and maintain or increase the productivity of the *waqf* properties[35]
2. The salaries of the bīmāristān's bureaucratic administration, which included the *nāẓir* himself, along with other administrators who were responsible for maintaining the properties, collecting rents, and supervising the different expenditures of the bīmāristān
3. The patients' needs in terms of furniture and other fixtures in the bīmāristān
4. Medications and the necessary tools and materials for their preparation and storage
5. Utensils for preparing and serving food and drinks to the patients
6. Salaries for two employees, one to supervise the distribution of medications and the other to supervise the kitchen and the distribution of food
7. Salaries for physicians, oculists, and surgeons
8. Additional salary for the chief physician in compensation for teaching a weekly lecture
9. Salaries for janitors and caretakers
10. Caring for the dead in the bīmāristān, including ritual washing, shrouding, and burial
11. Caring for the sick poor, including those in their homes (for whom medications were provided and, if they died from their maladies, burials arranged)
12. A garment given as a gift to those cured in the bīmāristān upon their exit

emphasize the similarities between the members of every category and the differences between them and members of the other categories.

[35] Ibid., 1: 362.

As mentioned before, by making the renovation and maintenance of the *waqf* the first spending priority, the authors of the *waqf* document intended to ensure the survival of the *waqf* for as long as possible. It is probable that this is why one of the markets was turned from a book to a leather market, thus allowing for more revenue. This category could also include renovations in the bīmāristān's buildings themselves.

The Nāẓir and the Bīmāristān's Administration

The second most important spending priority included the salaries of the top administrators, such as the *nāẓir*, the person responsible for renting the *waqf* properties; the supervisor of works and renovations (*mashadd*); a supervisor of workers; a notary; a scribe; and a treasurer. These positions were to be occupied by bureaucrats and administrators who belonged to "the people of the pen" (*ahl al-qalam*) and who represented the bureaucratic and legal management of the bīmāristān. The only exception would be the building supervisor (*mashadd*), although this position might have referred to a supervisor of construction workers in the bīmāristān. The document further emphasized the nature of education and training that these employees would need by adding that they should "be knowledgeable of the different [arts] of [administrative] writing (*anwā' al-kitābah*)" and that they must be known both for their piety and for their experience.[36] The only limitation placed on their salaries was that they be paid salaries commensurable to those in a similar position. This was a consistent formulation and was used in various *waqf* documents from the period to discuss many other salaries, yet it also allowed for a lot of discretion because the criterion of similarity could necessitate a similar *waqf* (and therefore similar responsibilities), which did not exist at the time or for decades to come. More importantly, since the *nāẓir* was the person responsible for appointing the rest of the bīmāristān staff (except for the teacher of medicine, as we will see below), he was the most influential figure in the administration and had a unique power to determine his and others' salaries.

The document was clear in determining the *nāẓir*: "[The sultan] decided that the *nāẓir* will be our lord, al-Sultān al-Manṣūr, who promulgated this *waqf*, during his life, and after [his death] the best of his sons, and his grandsons. If [his progeny] is extinct, then [the *nāẓir*] should be the best from the men emancipated by the Sultan."[37] In addition to maintaining his

[36] Ibid., line 251.
[37] Ibid., 1: 369.

control over the *waqf* and the complex, this stipulation would allow Qalāwūn, his progeny, and his *mamluks* to benefit financially from the *waqf* and to manage its different revenues.[38] Naturally, the sultan and his successors did not exercise their control over the bīmāristān personally but rather through a number of deputies, who managed their different *waqfs* and acted as the effective *nāẓirs* of the bīmāristān. Throughout the history of the bīmāristān during the Qalawunid dynasty (r. 1279–1382), the identity of the person occupying this position symbolized the power and dominance of the sultan, his ability to control his own finances and his family's *waqfs*, and his control of the emirs and high bureaucrats.

During the long, stable third reign of al-Nāṣir Muḥammad b. Qalāwūn (from 1309–1341), the sultan's personal treasurer (*nāẓir al-khāṣ*), a position introduced by al-Nāṣir Muḥammad himself in 1309, controlled the bīmāristān and became the most powerful bureaucrat in the entire empire.[39] During this period, the sultan, represented by his treasurer, exerted firm control over the bīmāristān and over the other rich *waqfs* of his predecessors. Al-Nāṣir also appointed an emir as a supervisor of the bīmāristān. This position, however, was reserved for respected emirs and was seen as a largely honorary post without any serious responsibilities. The first to be appointed to this position was Jamāl al-Dīn Āqūsh, known by the title "the Viceroy of Karak," in 1323. Al-Nāṣir had much respect for Āqūsh, so much that he used to stand up when Āqūsh entered the court.[40] The emir, however, had no real power and probably considered the position as an invitation to patronize the institution: he renovated the bīmāristān, removed the animal drinking basin in front of it, and put a sabil in its place. Even Āqūsh's appointment to a position in Tripoli did not necessitate the appointment of another emir as supervisor of the bīmāristān. A decade before his death, al-Nāṣir appointed a *nāẓir* for the

[38] On the financial implications of the *waqf*, see Amin, "Un Acte de Fondation de Waqf par une Chretienne (Xe Siècle H., XVIe S. Chr:)"; Al-Sayyid Marsot, "The Political and Economic Functions of the Ulama in the 18th Century"; Crecelius, "Incidences of Waqf Cases in Three Cairo Courts: 1640–1802"; Hathaway, "The Wealth and Influence of an Exiled Ottoman Eunuch in Egypt: The Waqf Inventory of Abbas Agha"; Hennequin, "Waqf et Monnaiedans l'Égypte Mamluke."

[39] Al-Qalaqashandī, *Ṣubḥ al-ʿAshā*, 4: 30–31. Al-Qalaqashandī (d. 1418) explained that after the creation of the position of Nāẓir al-Khāṣ (the sultan's treasurer), the position of the State Treasurer (*nāẓir bayt al-māl*), which used to be one of the highest ranking in the bureaucratic structure, lost its status. Bayt al-māl (the state treasury) itself continued to be called the Great Treasury (*al-khizānah al-kubrā*) but it only contained some vestments and honorary robes and little funds because the rest became part of the sultan's treasury.

[40] Al-Maqrīzī, *al-Sulūk*, 2: 193.

bīmāristān different from his own treasurer. Yet this *nāẓir* continued to report to the sultan directly, bypassing the emir appointed as supervisor.

Following al-Nāṣir's death and during the period of weak Qalawunid sultans, the position of the *nāẓir* continued to be occupied by an experienced bureaucrat, now supervised by the emir *nāẓir*. By 1354, with the rise of the emir Ṣarghatmish al-Nāṣirī, the position of the emir supervisor of the Bīmāristān became even more important at the political level. The majority of the emirs who occupied this position played significant roles in political conspiracies and factional wars, and the post became an effective prize for one of the highest ranking emirs in a victorious faction, along with other positions like the chief of the armies (*atābik*), and the deputy of the sultan (*nā'ib al-Salṭanah*). Ṣarghatmish and others following him supervised the bureaucratic *nāẓirs* and fired and punished them when necessary. The emir *nāẓir* soon became the guarantor of the proper functioning of the bīmāristān. Yet, the bureaucratic *nāẓir* continued to oversee the day-to-day operations.

Furniture, Food, and Medications

The following three spending priorities (the third, fourth, and fifth) focused on providing for the specific material needs of the patients, starting with furniture and other fixtures, followed by medications, foodstuffs, and the tools and utensils needed for food preparation. The presence of these items just after the salaries of the main administrators and before the physicians' salaries, as well as their specific order, are significant in understanding the sultan and his entourage's view of what actually constituted the bīmāristān and enabled it to perform its main roles and maintain its permanence. Following the actual structures and properties that established the material existence and financial viability of the bīmāristān, the document expressed the view that the *nāẓir* and the other top bureaucrats were the main figures necessary for running this institution or, for that matter, any institution. In a way, they were as important as the structures and properties themselves: their salaries had to be prioritized right after spending on renovation and maintenance of bīmāristān and its properties. Patients, with their needs, followed as the priority immediately after that. The most pressing patient need, however, was not for physicians who would serve them but rather for the material objects that would house, feed, and medicate them. Physicians and other medical practitioners, such as surgeons and oculists, remained significant to the bīmāristān's function, as we will see later. But the bīmāristān's central function remained first to house patients and provide for them and only second to provide top physicians to care of them.

There is no existing evidence that al-Bīmāristān al-Manṣūrī ever functioned without physicians, at least during the first five centuries of its life, and many guarantees were made in the document for hiring physicians and medical practitioners. These priorities do not suggest that the bīmāristān would function without physicians, but rather that the *nāẓir* was allowed and expected to reduce the salaries of physicians (and therefore to hire physicians of lower status) before attempting to reduce the bīmāristān's capacity to receive patients (by reducing the number of beds), to dispense medications, or to provide patients with food. Regardless of its pronounced medical nature, the *waqf* document showed clearly that the bīmāristān was not a public health project in the modern sense, but a monumental charity that intended to provide for as many people as possible. It was meant as a site of reference in the city even though it might not have provided the best medical care or have hired the best medical practitioners.

The order of the three patient-related priorities is equally significant. First came the furniture, which would be part of the bīmāristān's physical existence and would allow it to house patients, the disabled, and the sick poor, but also travelers, students, and others. Despite its avowed medical role, the bīmāristān was still a site for housing people. Its ability to house them remained central to its mission, as central as its own buildings and its top bureaucrats. Furniture and other fixtures in the bīmāristān included "iron or wooden beds . . ., quilts stuffed with cotton, throws stuffed with cotton as well, cotton covers, pillows and smooth covers."[41] The *nāẓir* could buy these items anew or commission their making, whichever was cheaper and more efficient. The document's authors linked these items to the patients' illnesses by instructing the *nāẓir* to distribute them so that "every patient [is] given, of beds and bedding, what is suitable for his condition and what is required for his illness (*'alā ḥasb ḥālihi wamā yaqtaḍīhi maraḍuhu*)."[42] It is not clear how specific types of beds and bedding would suit patients' conditions and diseases. The document's authors may have intended to rhetorically stress the centrality of medical care and medical practice to the bīmāristān by highlighting how all expenses were, in fact, linked to this care. In all cases, these items, and the care of providing individual beds, would have contrasted dramatically with the living conditions of the majority of the bīmāristān's audience.

[41] Ibn Ḥabīb, *Tadhkirat al-Nabīh*, 1: 363.
[42] Ibid.

Spending on medications, which occupied the fourth category, included spending on raw materials needed for making compound medications, tools needed for their making, and their storage.[43] The document grouped medications with foodstuffs as representing "what [is necessary] to support the treatment of patients" in the general list of eligible expenses mentioned earlier. In that list, the document's authors mentioned a number of examples for these medications, such as syrups, collyria, ophthalmics, and pastes. The grouping of medications together with foodstuff was consistent with the contemporary use of dieting (*ḥimyah*) as an important method of treatment; it was widely believed that recovery necessitated the providing of sufficient and well-arranged food to patients, as explained in Ibn Buṭlān's (d. 1075) famous tables "*Taqwīm al-ṣiḥah*" (Tacuinum Sanitatis).[44] Yet, the document appeared to have prioritized medications before foodstuff, contradictory to the known order of treatment as explained by physicians like Ibn al-Nafīs (d. 1290) and others.[45] As will be shown later, this shift in emphasis from using dieting as the primary method of treatment prior to medication to a more extensive use of medications and evacuations had been slowly taking hold since the beginning of the thirteenth century in the circles of physicians working in bīmāristāns.

The document instructed the *nāẓir*, in the fifth priority, to buy clay bowls for patients' food and glass or ceramic glasses for their drinks, as well as pots, jugs, jars, and so on. He was also instructed to buy lamps, oil for lighting, and water "from the blessed river Nile for their drink and food." Moreover, the *nāẓir* would buy straw covers for their food and straw hand-fans to use in the heat.[46] The document detailed how the clay bowls and the straw covers were to be used: every patient was to be given his or her food in a separate bowl, "without sharing [the bowl] with another patient," and it was to be covered with the straw cover.[47] The separate, clean, covered bowl, the straw fans, and even the clean water bought from water carriers from the Nile, not to mention the lamps and fuel oil, were

[43] Ibid., line 257.

[44] Although produced more than two centuries before this document was produced, it remained a popular text and a paragon of medical texts. For instance, the *Taqwīm* was mentioned in the decree of appointment of the chief physician of al-Bīmāristān al-Manṣūrī, composed only a few days after the inauguration of the Bīmāristān, as an example of a remarkable text that the chief physician should strive to emulate or exceed in value.

[45] Ibn al-Nafīs, *Al-Mūjaz fī al-Ṭibb*.

[46] Ibn Ḥabīb, *Tadhkirat al-Nabīh*, 1: 364.

[47] Ibid., 1: 365.

all novel to the daily lives of patients for whom such materials and luxuries were not easy to come by.

Access to freshly cooked food was a rarity in quotidian life, as Amalia Levanoni explains. Home-cooking was common only among the Mamluk and scholarly elites, in the institutions and establishments they sponsored, and in Mamluk army barracks in the citadel and elsewhere. For the majority of the populace, cooking at home was difficult because of the high prices of fuel and the inability to control fire or effectively extinguish it. Citing al-Maqrīzī, Levanoni explains that, after a huge fire in a crowded neighborhood in Cairo that burnt uncontrollably for five days, many abandoned cooking at home.[48] "Another difficulty in maintaining a kitchen was the high cost of cooking utensils. The ownership of pots and their quality were symbols of social status."[49] Although some people prepared food at home and had it cooked it in the market with the aid of professional cooks and bakers, this still posed significant financial difficulty and was not readily available to all or feasible on a daily basis.[50] But, as explained before, in having a kitchen the bīmāristān was not unique among other similar institutions or establishments, such as the Mamluk barracks, Sufi khānaqāhs, or even some madrasas, all of which included equipped kitchens that prepared food for the residents. It is not unlikely that the madrasa and the mausoleum shared the same kitchen with the bīmāristān, given the maintenance costs associated with keeping a functioning kitchen.

The types of food given to the patients are also significant in understanding how the document viewed the bīmāristān's intended clientele. The document mentioned "soup, rice, chicken, chicks, meat, etc. (*mara' waruz wa dajāj wa farārīkh wa laḥm wa ghayr dhālik*)"[51] as examples of food to offer patients. Although this list was not intended to be exhaustive, the food items mentioned and those omitted are significant when seen in relation to the common social meanings of specific foods at that time.[52] Meat and poultry were valuable and expensive food items quite difficult to

[48] Levanoni, "Food and Cooking during the Mamluk Era: Social and Political Implications," 204.

[49] Ibid., 205.

[50] Ibid., 206.

[51] Ibn Ḥabīb, *Tadhkirat al-Nabīh*, 1: 365.

[52] For more information on food and food consumption in the Mamluk period, see Isaac Israeli and Muḥammad Ṣabbāḥ, *Kitāb al-Aghdhiyah wa al-Adwiyah*; Van Der Veen, "When Is Food a Luxury?"; Lindsay, *Daily Life in the Medieval Islamic World*; Levanoni, "Food and Cooking during the Mamluk Era: Social and Political Implications." Also, Singer, "Serving up Charity: The Ottoman Public Kitchen"; Schofield, "The Social Economy of the Medieval Village in the Early Fourteenth Century"; Fleisher, "Rituals of Consumption and the Politics of Feasting on the Eastern African Coast, AD 700–1500"; Lewicka, *Food and Foodways of Medieval Cairenes: Aspects of Life in an Islamic Metropolis of the Eastern Mediterranean.*

obtain. Similarly, rice and white bread were expensive and more common in elite banquets than among the poor populace. Levanoni explains:

> The nutrition of the Egyptian rural masses in the Mamluk period was based mainly on locally-available crops. Upper Egypt was abundant in sugar cane and dates, so its inhabitants lived mainly on sweet foodstuffs (*ḥalāwah*). In Lower Egypt, taro (colocasia, *qulqās*) and peas *(jūlabān)* were staples of nutrition. The diet of the peasantry was based mainly on bread . . . Fish was also readily available, especially in the autumn, when the Nile tide brought this form of sustenance in large quantities. Fishing in this season was so easy that children could help provide food. Al-Maqrīzī testifies that milk and milk products were also important ingredients in the diet of the masses.[53]

Along with meat and poultry, the document also lists meat- or poultry-based soup (*mara*ʾ), which remained an important item in feeding the poor under the Mamluks and the Ottomans as well.[54] Bread, which unlike rice was a cheap and common food item, was not mentioned at all, and neither was fish or *ḥalāwah* (a crude sugar-based foodstuff prepared directly from cane sugar that was a common food item among poorer Egyptians). The document's list did not intend to provide elite foodstuff to the poor, nor was it attempting to erase the social and cultural differences that regulated food distribution. Instead, it intended to provide basic foodstuff that was available to the poor only upon special occasions, such as feasts and other elite-sponsored celebrations. Meat, poultry, soup, and rice were affordable to the lower strata of the scholarly elite, although probably not on a regular basis. Moreover, these foodstuffs were among those recommended by physicians, such as Ibn Buṭlān and Ibn al-Akfānī (d. 1348), as foods that can replenish a sick person's strength.[55] At the same time, the bīmāristān avoided common and cheap foods such as bread and fish as much as it avoided excessive luxuries and exuberant costs. The bīmāristān's kitchen was part of a more uniform charitable food landscape that included other kitchens in madrasas, khanāqāhs, or college mosques, where similar types of food items were offered, especially on Fridays, during the month of

[53] Levanoni, "Food and Cooking during the Mamluk Era: Social and Political Implications," 213.

[54] Singer, "Serving up Charity: The Ottoman Public Kitchen."

[55] Ibn al-Akfānī, *Ghunyat al-Labīb ʿinda Ghaybat al-Ṭabīb*, 78. Ibn al-Akfānī was a physician who served in al-Bīmāristān al-Manṣūrī. He was described by the Mamluk historian Khalīl b. Aybak al-Ṣafadī (d. 1363) as having "the best knowledge . . . of all that is needed for al-Bīmāristān al-Manṣūrī, so that nothing would be bought [by the Nāẓir] for the Bīmāristān except after his approval" (Al-Ṣafadī, *Kitāb al-Wāfī bi-l-Wafayāt*, 2: 26–27). Ibn al-Akfānī died in Cairo of plague during the Black Death. His nephew, al-Ḥāfiẓ al-ʿIrāqī, reported that Ibn al-Akfānī was so worried about the plague when it hit Cairo that "he withdrew to his home, took medicines that benefit from the epidemic, wore a red-yellowish garment, and stopped visiting with patients [in the Bīmāristān]. Yet, none of this helped him" (Ibn al-Akfānī, *Ghunyat al-Labīb ʿinda Ghaybat al-Ṭabīb*, 8).

Ramadan, and during different religious feasts. It is not possible for us to know how often the patients ate meats and poultry and whether or not some cheaper food items were presented. It is likely that meats, poultry, soup, and rice were presented only a few times or even once a week and that other items supplemented the menu. In all cases, the *waqf* document was clear in locating the bīmāristān on a specific charitable map tailoring these examples of food offerings to the bīmāristān's anticipated audience, who benefitted from similar food items in other similar institutions.

The delivery of food in clay bowls was not unique to the bīmāristān and was probably familiar to patients. Clay bowls were normally used to deliver food prepared in the market or bought from professional cooks and butchers, as well as food in feasts and charitable banquets: "This 'takeaway' food was sold in clay containers, while in the cooks' shops food was served in inexpensive clay utensils which often were not washed after use."[56] However, the document seemed intent on maintaining a certain level of cleanliness, which was a common trope in the *ḥisbah* manuals that discussed proper market practices. In these manuals, in addition to discussing different types of fraud in making food (such as using improper meats, like dog meat, rotten foodstuff, and masking these ingredients with spices and lemon), authors discussed cleanliness and instructed vendors to protect the food they sold against flies and other insects.[57] In the *waqf* document, these concerns, produced and propagated by the scholarly elites, found clear expression in the designation of a specific bowl for every patient and covers for the food to protect it from flies and insects. Both in the types of foods mentioned in the *waqf* document and the ways by which they were to be delivered, the *waqf* document represented the scholarly elite's views on proper living that should be followed by the masses and that should be supported by charitable institutions. These views were represented in this as in other charitable institutions designed and sponsored by these same elites.

Caretakers

The following four priorities (from six to nine) addressed the salaries of other employees in the bīmāristān, including medical practitioners. The first among these were two administrators who were given specific tasks in the day-to-day management of the bīmāristān. The first was a stockist (*khāzin*) responsible for storing all materials that would be distributed to

56 Levanoni, "Food and Cooking during the Mamluk Era: Social and Political Implications," 207.
57 See Ibn al-Ukhūwah, *Maʿālim al-Qurba*, 112–21.

patients daily, including foods and medications. He would be responsible for delivering and distributing these materials to the other caretakers, who were in turn to take them to the patients. The second was a secretary (*amīn*), who would supervise the kitchen and the distribution of cups and bowls, which may have been subject to theft or embezzlement.[58] The secretary's job description shows that the stocker would have concerned himself primarily with medications, their raw ingredients, and raw foodstuffs, whereas the secretary took care of cooked food and drinks and the utensils attached to their distribution. The document specified that these would be two Muslim men, but gave the *nāẓir* the right to hire more people if he thought it necessary.[59] Here again, the document betrayed the complex bureaucratic system from which it was born by emphasizing the importance of administrators, even at the second-tier level, over physicians, surgeons, and oculists. The document would deal with them only after all such administrators were accounted for.

The following spending priority considered salaries for physicians, surgeons, and oculists.[60] There is little information about the salaries that the bīmāristān gave to its medical practitioners or even how many practitioners there were. Some evidence suggests, however, that physicians generally received modest salaries in bīmāristāns. For instance, Raḍiyy al-Dīn al-Raḥbī (d. 1233), a well-known Damascene physician and one of the most senior physicians at al-Bīmāristān al-Nūrī, received only fifteen dinars in stipend for his service in the bīmāristān around 1218.[61] At the same time, his colleague al-Muhdhdhab al-Dakhwār received about a hundred dinars every month for serving in the court, in addition to many other rewards and payments for specific occasions.[62] When al-Maqrīzī (d. 1442) was writing his *Khiṭaṭ* and describing what he considered the most important bīmāristāns in history, he focused on how patrons established sufficient *waqfs* to pay for physicians.[63] Although al-Maqrīzī's accounts about ancient hospitals were largely mythical, they showed how he, a scholar, a *muḥtasib*, and a supervisor of bīmāristāns in Cairo and Damascus, understood the difficulties facing bīmāristāns in attracting the highest echelon of physicians in part due to the low salaries they offered.

58 Ibn Ḥabīb, *Tadhkirat al-Nabīh*, line 268.
59 Ibid., line 274.
60 Ibid., line 275.
61 Ibn Abī Usaybi'ah, *'Uyūn al-Anbā'*, 4: 189.
62 Ibid., 4: 320.
63 Al-Maqrīzī, *al-Khiṭaṭ*, 408.

Biographical dictionaries confirm al-Maqrīzī's fears and that the more famous and important physicians in Egypt did not serve in al-Bīmāristān al-Manṣūrī.[64] Members of the medical dynasty of Banū Ṣaghīr, which included some of the most distinguished physicians of fourteenth-century Egypt, hardly served in al-Bīmāristān al-Manṣūrī. Al-Sadīd ibn Kujak, who was Ibn al-Nafīs's assistant in the court, became the court physician after the latter's death and never served in the bīmāristān.[65] Faraj Allāh ibn Ṣaghīr, the true founder of the dynasty's glory, was also a student of Ibn al-Nafīs alongside his father and was appointed by the Mamluk Sultan al-Nāṣir Muḥammad to serve the sultan's harem but never served in al-Bīmāristān al-Manṣūrī.[66] In contrast, Muḥammad ibn Faraj Allāh ibn Ṣaghīr (fl. before 1341), who did not achieve a reputation close to his father's, served in al-Manṣūrī but never the sultan, although the latter knew him through his father.[67] Muḥammad's son, also named Muḥammad, studied Quran and Arabic with the famous Judge Burhān al-Dīn ibn Jamāʿah (d. 1388), who supervised the bīmāristān at the time and taught in the Qalāwūnid madrasa. Little is known about the son's medical practice.[68] Other physicians who served in al-Bīmāristān al-Manṣūrī include a physician from Safed by the name of Aḥmad ibn Yūsuf (d. 1337) who worked in the bīmāristān and served the court briefly. He was also a herbalist in Cairo.[69] Rukn al-Dīn al-Jaʿfarī al-Tunusī was another émigré who came to Cairo from Tunis in 1291. He worked as a deputy of the Mālikī judge and taught medicine in al-Bīmāristān al-Manṣūrī and the Ṭūlūnid mosque.[70] Muḥammad ibn Ibrāhīm al-Sanjārī (d. 1348) was a physician and a herbalist and worked in the bīmāristān assisting the *nāẓir* in acquiring drugs and herbs.[71] The most famous of this group is Ibn al-Akfānī (d. 1348). He was a scholar of *hadīth* and of law, and he also served in the bīmāristān.[72] The majority of these physicians did not achieve any significant prestige, and many of them had other professions in

[64] On biographical dictionaries, see al-Qadi, "Biographical Dictionaries as the Scholars' Alternative History of the Muslim Community"; Cooperson, *Classical Arabic Biography: The Heirs of the Prophets in the Age of Al-Ma'mun.* See also Brentjes, "The Study of Geometry According to Al-Sakhāwī (Cairo, 15th C) and Al-Muhibbī (Damascus, 17th C)."
[65] Al-ʿUmarī, *Masālik al-Abṣār fī Mamālik al-Amṣār*, 9: 508.
[66] Ibid., 9: 509–10.
[67] Ibid., 9: 512–13.
[68] ʿĪsā, *Tārīkh al-Bīmāristānāt fī Al-Islām*, 163.
[69] Ibid., 159.
[70] Ibid., 160.
[71] Ibid., 160–61.
[72] Ibn al-Akfānī, *Ghunyat Al-Labīb ʿinda Ghaybat al-Ṭabīb*.

addition to medicine. This indicates their limited reputation as physicians and also their limited income from medical practice.

The Lecturer of Medicine

At the end of its description of the medical practitioners and their different roles, the *waqf* document instructed the *nāẓir* to appoint a master of medicine (*shaykh*) who would be available to teach medicine to students: "[he should] sit on the large bench (*al-maṣṭabah al-kubrā*) . . . to work on the science of medicine in its different [branches] (*lil-ishtighāl bi-ʿilm al-ṭibb ʿalā ikhtilāf awḍāʿihi*) at the times designated by the *nāẓir*."[73] This *shaykh* was to be one of the practitioners in the bīmāristān "without increase in [the practitioners'] number" and would receive his salary from the *waqf* as usual. Although the document did not assign any administrative roles to this master physician nor is there any evidence that he performed any administrative roles, he was likely at the top of the bīmāristān's medical hierarchy: he was the highest paid practitioner because he was a *shaykh* (i.e., a senior respected practitioner) and because he received two salaries, one for teaching and one for practice. A similar arrangement was reported by Ibn Abī Uṣaybiʿah in al-Bīmāristān al-Nūrī where his masters taught and led the medical staff there whether officially or unofficially.

Qalāwūn chose to appoint the chief physician of the empire to the bīmāristān's teaching position. "On Wednesday the eleventh [of Rabīʿ al-Ākhir], al-Muwaffaq Aḥmad ibn al-Rashīd Abī Ḥulayqah came to the sultanic ceremonial hall (*dihlīz*), converted to Islam and called himself Aḥmad. The sultan [al-Manṣūr Qalāwūn] endowed him with honorific robes (*khalaʿa ʿalayhi*) and decreed (*rasama*) that he be equal to his brothers in the sciences (*bi-musawātihi bi-akhawayhi fī al-ʿulūm*)."[74] The Abī Ḥulayqah brothers, referenced here, were three of the most celebrated and talented physicians in the Mamluk capital of al-Manṣūr Qalāwūn, and they served the Sultan for a number of years as his personal physicians. Although they served in this capacity while Christian, the sultan asked them to convert in 1285 so that they could continue to hold their position at the top of the medical hierarchy. The two older brothers, Muhadhdhab al-Dīn Muḥammad and ʿAlam al-Dīn Ibrāhīm, converted and continued to occupy their positions, while Muwaffaq al-Dīn, the youngest and closest to the sultan, refused and lost his position as the chief physician, but he continued to serve as the sultan's

[73] Ibn Ḥabīb, *Tadhkirat al-Nabīh*, 1: 366.
[74] Al-Maqrīzī, *al-Sulūk*, 1: 722.

personal physician. When he converted, he was reappointed a chief physician equal to his brothers "in the sciences." The request for his conversion and the subsequent consequences of his refusal were largely new phenomena in the history of medical practitioners because non-Muslim physicians continued to constitute the majority of physicians during this period.[75] The development at hand was in part due to the bīmāristān's *waqf*, which prohibited hiring non-Muslims, and which in itself was part of a larger pattern of Mamluk anti-non-Muslim policies.[76] Since the chief physician became ex officio an employee at the bīmāristān, the condition of being a Muslim, which applied to the bīmāristān, extended to cover the position of the chief physician as well. It appears that the reappointment of the younger brother eventually happened in the same ceremony and with the same letter that appointed the two older brothers to the position of chief physician of the realm. The Mamluk historian Ibn al-Furāt (d. 1405) did not report the conversion story reported by al-Maqrīzī, but he copied both decrees of appointment, one to the position of chief physician (henceforth the chief physician decree) and the other to the teaching position in the bīmāristān (henceforth the bīmāristān decree). Both were promulgated on the eleventh of Ramaḍān 684/November 10, 1285, about nine to ten months after the sultan had inaugurated the bīmāristān in Dhū al-Qiʾdah 683/January-February 1285, according to Ibn al-Furāt's dating.

Both decrees used the previously mentioned *ḥadīth* "science is of two types; the science of religion and the science of bodies (*al-ʿilm ʿilmān ʿilm al-adyān wa ʿilm al-abdān*)" to locate the sultan's patronage of medicine within a pietistic, traditionalist landscape. The sultan saw it "incumbent upon [himself] to look carefully in these two sciences (*taʿayyan ʿalayna an nuḥsin fi hadhayn al-ʿilmayn al-nadhar)*"[77] as part of his duties and his following of Muḥammad's commandments. The bīmāristān figured in both decrees, and the position of the chief physician was intractably linked to the bīmāristān and included specific duties in the sultan's new establishment. The chief physician decree instructed Muhadhdhab al-Dīn, the eldest brother, to reside in Cairo and to be "relieved from travels and ceremonies (*li-yakun ... murfahan min al-asfār wa al-bayākīr*) and dedicated to what is peculiar to him of teaching in al-Bīmāristān al-Manṣūrī

[75] This actually would continue to be the case for the following two centuries at least. See Lewicka, *Medicine for Muslims? Islamic Theologians, Non-Muslim Physicians and the Medical Culture of the Mamluk Near East.*

[76] Ibn Ḥabīb, *Tadhkirat al-Nabīh.* See also, el-Leithy, "Sufis, Copts and the Politics of Piety: Moral Regulation in Fourteenth-Century Upper Egypt"; Little, "Coptic Conversion to Islam under the Baḥrī Mamlūks, 692–755/1293–1354"; Zaborowski, "Arab Christian Physicians as Interreligious Mediators: Abū Shākir as a Model Christian Expert."

[77] Ibn al-Furāt, *Tārīkh Ibn al-Furāt,* 8: 23.

and this distinguished position [of chief physician] (*mutawafirran ʿalā mā huwa makhṣūṣun bihi min tadrīs al-Bīmāristān al-Manṣūrī wa hādhā al-manṣib al-athīr*)."[78] Before that, the decree had already arranged the relationship among the three brothers: Muhadhdhab al-Dīn was clearly the superior among the three, and the document admonished the younger brothers to "recognize for al-Qāḍī[79] Muhadhdhab al-Dīn the privileges of precedence, age, and virtue . . . and respect the sanctity of brotherhood in [treating] him."[80] More concretely, they were required to abide by his decisions and to make no decisions of their own without his presence and approval. In case of disagreement, Muhadhdhab al-Dīn's decisions were to overrule his brothers. With this arrangement, Muhadhdhab al-Dīn was the effective chief physician, while his brothers, who served also as court physicians and traveled with the sultan, were given the title in recognition of their prestige, reputation, and service in the court. As such, the administrative requirements of the position and the newly added teaching duties were to be borne by the resident chief physician, Muhadhdhab al-Dīn.

The decree of appointment in the bīmāristān, issued at the same time as the chief physician decree, intended not only to appoint Muhadhdhab al-Dīn as the teacher of medicine in the bīmāristān, but also to emphasize the link between the bīmāristān's teaching position and that of the chief physician of the realm. The dignity and high status of this new position in the bīmāristān was construed to recognize none other than the chief physician as worthy of its honor:

> [We] created [in the bīmāristān] a place for the study of the science of medicine (*lil-ishtighāl bi-ʿilm al-ṭibb*) . . ., and [we] wanted [to appoint in it] one [who is] fit to give lessons, and from whom [both] a chief in this art and a follower [student] would benefit, who would be entrusted with the health of bodies and the preservation of selves. So we did not find but the chief of this faction (*ṭāʾifah*) worthy of this rank, and we would not be satisfied [to fill] this position with one who did not achieve this privilege.[81]

The link between the two positions, and the high regard in which the teaching position was portrayed, reveal that Qalāwūn thought very highly of his new bīmāristān, considered it the cornerstone of his medical patronage, and desired to ensure for it the service of the empire's best and most highly regarded physicians. The bīmāristān decree contained many details on the

78 Ibid., 8: 24.
79 The term "*qāḍī*" (Judge) was used as a sign of respect. The three physicians, who were not judges and did not have any education in the law, were called *qāḍīs* throughout the decrees.
80 Ibid.
81 Ibid., 8: 26. The word "faction" refers to physicians.

duties of the chief-physician-cum-medical-instructor. The decree instructed the chief physician to divide the students into groups of physicians, oculists, surgeons, bone-setters and iron workers, and herbalists or pharmacists.[82] He was to order each group to memorize what their profession required and to supervise them as they worked on their arts.[83] Qalāwūn's priorities and his intentions for the bīmāristān were clear: "so that people after people of these sciences are [qualified] in this blessed place, and [so that] tomorrow there [will be] from them many times who are there today."[84] As will be shown later, these new practitioners were to add more Muslims to a market dominated by non-Muslims. Qalāwūn, following on anti-Christian Mamluk policies, intended for the bīmāristān and its teaching program to create opportunities for Muslims to become physicians by bypassing the family-based training that dominated medicine and other professions as well.

The lectures and the way they were arranged betrayed a specific view of medical practice, the role of physicians, and their relations to other medical practitioners. While the chief physician gave lectures to physicians along with other practitioners, there is no evidence that he would be required or able (let alone desire) to grant *ijāzah*s (learning certificates) to the students of surgery or to future oculists or bone-setters. Instead, the decree suggested that these lectures would be a form of instruction (*tarbiyyah*; lit. upbringing) that could precede professional training and Ijaza. It explained: "[He should teach his students] so that it will be said about each of his students, when he is given *ijāzah* and is recommended [for practice or teaching], that his master (*shaykh*), with whom he was cultured, did well."[85] The verb *ta'addab* (cultured) was generally used to describe refinement of character and morals but not necessarily specific instructions or professional training (although the latter should not be excluded), and so its use here suggests that this type of bīmāristān instruction was only the beginning of more detailed training and education.[86] As such, the bīmāristān's lectures reflected the primacy of physicians and responded

[82] Ibid.
[83] Ibid., 8: 27.
[84] Ibid. (*"li-yatayassar fī hadhā al-makān al-mubārak min arbāb hādhihi al-'ulūm qawmun ba'd qawmin wa yaẓhar minhum fī al-ghad ... aḍ'āf man huwa ẓāhirun minhum al-yawm"*).
[85] Ibid. (*"li-yuqāl li-kullin min ṭalabatihi idhā shuri'a fī ijāzatihi wa tazkiyatihi, la-qad aḥsana shaykuhu alladhī 'alayhi ta'adab").*
[86] The decrees' author, Ibn al-Mukarram, also authored, almost at the same time, a decree appointing the instructor of Maliki jurisprudence, Ibn Shās, in the madrasa. There, he used a different formula to describe the potential praise that he would receive: "there is no reputation better than the saying ... about a judge or a mufti 'this is [one] of Ibn Shās' students'" (Ibid., 8: 28.). Here, the reference to Ibn Shās as the teacher and master of judges and muftis leaves no ambiguity about his role in the madrasa: he was to educate and "graduate" (or give *ijāzahs to*) these muftīs and judges.

to their consistent complaints about how other practitioners were ignorant of the basics of Galenic theory and of the proper manners necessary for medical practice. For physician-students, the bīmāristān may well have been the place where they received their *ijāzah*s; however, there is no evidence to support this claim or others.

Caretakers

Patients required others, besides medical practitioners, to care of them:

> The *nāẓir* spends from the revenues of this *waqf* on caretakers (*qawamah*) and janitors (*farrāshīn*) of men and women, what he sees [fit] to spend for each of them depending on his [or her] work, provided that each of them serves the ill and the disturbed [the mad] (*al-mukhtallīn*) of men and women in this bīmāristān; and washes their clothes, cleans their places, fixes their affairs (*iṣlāḥ shuʾūnihim*) and cares for [what brings] their benefits (*al-qiyām bi-maṣāliḥihim*).[87]

The *nāẓir* was again given permission to determine the appropriate number of caretakers and janitors but was warned, for the first time, against hiring too many: "so that the number [of caretakers and janitors] and [their] salaries would not exceed need depending on time." The caretakers and janitors were also the only category for which the *nāẓir* was required to hire both men and women in order to provide proper service to the patients and the disturbed. The document suggested that they would "serve" the patients in different ways, such as washing their clothes and cleaning their beds and wards. It also added two vague tasks: "fix their affairs" and "care for [what brings] their benefits." These two phrases were formulated in general terms to refer to any matter that the *nāẓir* judged necessary. The *nāẓir* was responsible for judging the need and, therefore, the number of people required to fill these positions. The number of caretakers may have increased during pilgrimage seasons as caravans passed through Cairo en route to Mecca or during other feasts when the city's shrines received their visitors.

Exiting the Bīmāristān

The tenth priority of spending dealt with those dying in the bīmāristān. For those "from among the sick [or] the disturbed; [of] men and women" who died in the bīmāristān, the *nāẓir* was required to pay for their ritual

[87] Ibn Ḥabīb, *Tadhkirat al-Nabīh*, 1: 366–67.

washing, preparation, and burial, including the fees for the washer and the grave digger, "according to prophetic *sunna* and [in] a satisfactory manner."[88] Funerary expenses were placed immediately after expenses related to caring for patients, a reflection of the common practice of providing charity for the burial of the poor.[89] It also indicates that the bīmāristān was probably a major site for the many destitute who could not afford their own burial and for many sick poor who did not have enough family support for the arrangement of their funerary rites. Those who were cured and were healthy enough to leave the bīmāristān would receive a garment as a means of congratulating them. Gifting vestments to show appreciation was a common practice among the Mamluk and scholarly elites; it signaled approval and support, or it marked new appointments, new positions, and important events. On any occasion, any person could be gifted specific types of vestments that matched his or her social and political position. The *waqf* document authors showed awareness of this custom, instructing the *nāẓir* to give vestments suitable to the person's status: "[For those] who become cured and healthy (*man ḥaṣal lahu al-shifāʾ wa al-ʿāfiyah*) from among those residing in this blessed bīmāristān, the *nāẓir* [buys] from this *waqf* revenues a vestment similar to that of his ilk (*kiswat mithlihi*)."[90] By ensuring that these vestments and garments were comparable to what was worn by those belonging to the patients' social, cultural, and economic ilk, the bīmāristān intended not to honor its patients but rather to provide further assistance as they exited the facility cured and healthy. At the same time, the giving of garments recalled and symbolized the honor and distinction of the sultan, his favor, and his generosity to his flock.

The details of living conditions, types of furniture, and foods available to the patients in the bīmāristān, as well as the different types of services made available to them, were oriented in many ways to the needs of the bīmāristān's perceived patients. The document's audience, whether the imagined one or the real one present at public readings of the document (mainly scholars and members of the Mamluk elites), would have had a clear idea of who the bīmāristān's patients were. The document would have reminded them several times of the pietistic narratives that explained the sultan's intentions and desires. The relatively luxurious set-up, with proper

88 Ibid., 367.

89 Bonner, Ener, and Singer (eds.), *Poverty and Charity in Middle Eastern Contexts*; Sabra, *Poverty and Charity in Medieval Islam: Mamluk Egypt 1250–1517*.

90 Ibn Ḥabīb, *Tadhkirat al-Nabīh*, 1: 367.

beds, stuffed soft beddings, expensive foods, water, and even fans and individual bowls stood in contrast to the lives of the expected patients and was possibly fashioned from the lifestyles of the document's authors and some of its audience. As members of the scholarly elite, the authors carried, protected, and propagated particular views and regulations concerning food preparation and specific expectations about food items. They consequently tailored the bīmāristān to resemble their own views and to provide to those poor patients an opportunity for propriety and good-living. The bīmāristān was not there simply to provide people access to physicians and free medications, although it did do this. Rather, it also made available a different quality of life that was not possible in the homes of the sick. The sick poor were either students, travelers, and visitors who had arrived in the capital with little ability to provide for themselves and subsequently had fallen ill with no one to care for them, or they belonged to the scores of riffraff who lacked the income or stable environment necessary to support themselves. The bīmāristān attempted to provide family-like care by hiring different employees to assist the patients and maintain their cleanliness. This form of care was normally carried out by family members, slaves, or servants, who may not have been available to many of those confined in the bīmāristān.

The bīmāristān's central role, however, remained the provision of medical care to patients, whether through consulting physicians or through free medications. All other provisions, from nourishment to bedding to services, were, at least discursively, formulated within a medical framework. As discussed earlier, the bīmāristān was not intended to turn away the needy or to carve out an exclusionary space that privileged one particular group of poor while refusing others. Instead, it functioned within a landscape of charity that allowed each institution to build its own audience in a manner that complemented the others and that helped form a larger social network of charity. The bīmāristān's facilities and the services that it offered were tailored to meet the perceived needs of specific groups of people who were seen as its primary audience. Along with physicians and free medications and treatments, the bīmāristān admitted patients in need of food and clean beddings, and it hired staff who offered the basic services that they lacked outside the bīmāristān. Those who could afford their own food and had family care available could still seek medical care while at home and without having to leave their families because the bīmāristān was able to send them medications, or their family members sought medical advice and medications (as well as funerary expenses) on their behalf.

Conclusion

At the end of the long discussion of spending priorities, the *waqf* document concluded by instructing the *nāẓir* to prioritize what he sees as more important: to privilege the poor and to put first what would bring divine reward to the sultan.[91] The patron's priority was clear, and the charitable nature of the bīmāristān could not have received greater emphasis. Throughout the entire document, the rules laid out were meant to preserve the bīmāristān as a charitable monument that would both immortalize the sultan's name and provide him with divine reward. The document would accomplish these two goals, first, by providing funds for the maintenance and renovation of the bīmāristān and its *waqfs* and also by providing sufficient funds for its main administrative staff and, second, by providing for patients' needs ranging from sleeping materials, to foods and medications, to money for medical care. Medical care, at least with respect to the therapeutic arts performed by specific practitioners, continued to be the pronounced function of the bīmāristān, although not its main spending priority. Its medical function was an integral part of a comprehensive care that provided help to the poor, the hungry, and the fatigued.

Al-Bīmāristān al-Manṣūrī symbolized Qalāwūn's wealth, power, and his magnanimity. It put him in a position close to other sovereigns and patrons whose power, wealth, and piety enabled them to accomplish such difficult feats, like building huge charitable institutions. The *waqf* document showed clear awareness of this dimension as it narrated the unrivaled and unique status of the bīmāristān. In fact, it was precisely because it had all these relevant precedents (each built with much effort and difficulty and only by great sovereigns) that it came to acquire its unparalleled position. Each of these institutions, standing to symbolize its patron, was likewise without a rival, and it was, in part, this similarity in dissimilarity that made such a project attractive to these patrons. Qalāwūn was clearly interested in patronizing bīmāristāns as opposed to madrasas. Although he built a madrasa for his wife, he did not intend to build a madrasa in his own complex. He had demonstrated his interest in bīmāristāns by building another in Hebron and by renovating al-Bīmāristān al-Nūrī in Damascus. Yet, Qalāwūn's interest in medicine was limited to these two bīmāristāns. He showed no interest in any other aspect of the medical sciences: he was not known to have had a specially close relationship with his physicians nor was he known to have bestowed significant gifts on them. He also did not

[91] Ibid., 1: 368.

attempt an overhaul of medical care in general, which would have involved renovating some of Cairo's or Fusṭaṭ's other bīmāristāns, many of which were falling into decay at the time. Even his interest in medical teaching was limited to its place within the bīmāristān as evident in the fact that he did not establish any additional medical lessons or lectures, whether in his madrasa or in any other place. Neither did he encourage the creation of medical madrasas, institutions that had begun a few decades earlier in the Levant.[92]

Peter Pormann's analysis of the bīmāristāns in Baghdad during al-Muqtadir's reign (908–932) finds an important example of medical patronage in the works of the *vizir* Ibn al-Jarrāḥ, one that contrasts with Qalāwūn's model.[93] Although Ibn al-Jarrāḥ did not build as huge an institution as al-Bīmāristān al-Manṣūrī, his interest in medicine was far more pervasive than Qalāwūn's. He had a close relation with the chief physician Sinān b. Thābit, helped protect the *waqf* of at least one old bīmāristān, and renovated others. He also instructed Sinān to create medical missions to prisons and to poor areas in Iraq in response to either famines or epidemics associated with political uprisings. Ibn al-Jarrāḥ's interests, which were likely as pietistic in motivation as were Qalāwūn's, extended to medicine and medical practice well beyond the walls of a specific bīmāristān or two. His efforts, which may well have been influenced by the charismatic and talented physician and courtier Sinān b. Thābit, improved several different bīmāristāns and aimed at providing more medical care to people who did not have access to it. Qalāwūn's interest was rooted in the charitable role played by the bīmāristān as an institution that offered much more than care delivered by medical practitioners (physicians, surgeons, and oculists). The priorities of spending as outlined in the *waqf* document show the expansive charitable role that the bīmāristān attempted to perform as it carved into the charitable landscape a niche dedicated to those with diseases, much as sabils delivered water but not food and kitchens delivered food but did not serve as places of abode.

[92] Ibn Muḥammad Nuʿaymī, *Al-Dāris fī Tārīkh al-Madāris*, 100–08.
[93] Pormann, "Islamic Hospitals in the Time of al-Muqtadir."

PART II

Physicians and Patients

CHAPTER 4

Theory and Practice: The Reign of the Bīmāristān Physicians

Introduction

After inaugurating al-Bīmāristān al-Manṣūrī in 1285, al-Manṣūr Qalāwūn issued a decree appointing Muhadhdhab al-Dīn ibn Abī Ḥulayqah, who was Qalāwūn's physician, to the teaching position of the new bīmāristān.[1] As explained earlier, Muhadhdhab al-Dīn ibn Abī Ḥulayqah was also appointed the chief physician, along with his two brothers, but he was expected to reside in Cairo and perform his duties in the bīmāristān while his brothers accompanied the sultan on his various trips.[2] Muhadhdhab al-Dīn came from a well-known medical family, one whose members served the Ayyubid and Mamluk Sultans of Egypt for more than a century. His father, Rashīd al-Dīn (b. 1195–d. before 1277), who was also his master in medicine, served the Ayyubid courts of al-Kāmil (r. 1218–1238) and of al-Ṣāliḥ Ayyūb (1240–1249), as well as the Mamluk court of al-Ẓāhir Baybars (r. 1260–1277).[3] Alongside Muhadhdhab al-Dīn and his brothers, two other physicians, also in the service of the Mamluk court, were equally if not more well-known and respected: Shahāb al-Dīn b. Abī al-Ḥawāfir and Alā' al-Dīn ibn al-Nafīs (d. 1288). The latter was, in fact, one of Muhadhdhab al-Dīn's teachers.[4] These five physicians (the three Ḥulayqah brothers, Ibn Abī al-Ḥawāfir, and Ibn al-Nafīs) belonged to a single medical genealogy directly linked to a circle formed around al-Bīmāristān al-Nūrī in Damascus about a century earlier.

Around al-Bīmāristān al-Nūrī, a growing circle of physicians read new texts, rediscovered others, and wrote summaries and commentaries

[1] For an analysis of this decree, see Northrup, "Qalawun's Patronage."
[2] Ibn al-Furāt, *Tārīkh Ibn al-Furāt*, 8: 27–28.
[3] Ibn Abī Usaybi'ah, *'Uyūn al-Anbā'*, 3: 479–80. Ibn Abī Uṣaybi'ah wrote a long biography of Rashīd al-Dīn b. Abī Ḥulayqah, which was mostly congratulatory. Muhadhdhab al-Dīn was, in fact, able to acquire Ibn Abī Uṣaybi'ah's book and sent a letter to the latter congratulating him on the book. This probably indicates that the biography of Rashīd al-Dīn was to the liking of his son.
[4] Al-'Umarī, *Masālik al-Abṣār fī Mamālik al-Amṣār*, 9: 151.

in new and largely unique ways. Their intellectual genealogy extended to the famous al-Bīmāristān al-ʿAḍudī in Baghdad linking them to a longer bīmāristān tradition that colored their work and the works of their students. The rise of this circle coincided with the rise of the new, bigger bīmāristāns in the Levant and Egypt, such as al-Nūrī, al-Ṣalāḥī, al-Nāṣirī, and al-Manṣūrī. Many members of this circle served in these bīmāristāns, whereas others who did not remained committed to the viability of the project and donated their money to different bīmāristāns. At the same time, the more distinguished members of this circle served in the courts of the Zangids and Ayyubids, who replaced the Seljuks, Fatimids, Crusaders, and other polities in Egypt and the Levant, replacing in turn previous medical elites and influencing medical thought and practice in the region. The study and analysis of the formation of this medical circle around al-Bīmāristān al-Nūrī at the end of the twelfth century, along with their writings and the books and texts they used in their teachings, provide important insights into medical practice in Levantine and Egyptian bīmāristāns in the eleventh and twelfth centuries and into medical thought and education during that period. This chapter will follow the formation of this Nūrī circle, analyze the medical texts and traditions that emerged there, and examine their influence on the medical thinking and practice in the thirteenth century. This will pave the way for a discussion of the sources of medical practice in al-Bīmāristān al-Manṣūrī in the following chapter.

Al-Dakhwār and His Circle: Medical Luminaries of Twelfth- and Thirteenth-Century Levant

To my knowledge, none of the writings of Muhadhdhab al-Dīn al-Dakhwār (d. 1231) is extant, which explains the dearth of works on the famous Damascene physician.[5] Al-Dakhwār's name and his lost works, however, figure prominently in the vitae of all major medical figures in the Levant and Egypt in the thirteenth century: he was either their teacher, the teacher of their teacher, or the author of the writings on which they worked.[6] Al-Dakhwār was a student of the famous Ibn al-Muṭrān

[5] The only exception is a commentary on Hippocrates' *The Foreknowledge,* composed by one of al-Dakhwār's favorite students, Ibn Qāḍī Baʿlabak, from his master's lectures. Al-Dakhwār and Ibn Qāḍī Baʿlabak, *Kitāb Sharḥ Tuqaddimuhu Al-Maʿrifah lil-Dakhwār.*

[6] To my knowledge, there is no scholarly study of Muhadhdhab al-Dīn al-Dakhwār and his works. For a brief mention of al-Dakhwār's intellectual circle in Damascus, see Gannagé, "Médecine et

(d. 1191),[7] who served in al-Bīmāristān al-Nūrī and in the court of Ṣalāḥ al-Dīn.[8] Before accompanying Ibn al-Muṭrān, al-Dakhwār started his medical education with another famous and influential Damascene physician and medical teacher, Raḍiyy al-Dīn al-Raḥbī (1140–1234), who also worked in al-Bīmāristān al-Nūrī.[9] With al-Raḥbī, Al-Dakhwār read only al-Majūsī's *al-Kitāb al-Malakī* (Latin: *Liber Regalis*).[10] Later in his career, al-Dakhwār served alongside al-Raḥbī in al-Bīmāristān al-Nūrī and seemed to have liked al-Raḥbī's son whom he appointed as chair of his medical madrasa. We do not have much information about the relation between Ibn al-Muṭrān and al-Raḥbī, except that they probably were both students of Muhdhdhab al-Dīn al-Naqqāsh (d. 1178), who came to the service of Nūr al-Dīn Zankī in Damascus and worked in al-Bīmāristān al-Nūrī when it was first inaugurated, and both probably served in al-Bīmāristān al-Nūrī.[11] Al-Naqqāsh was at the origin of this new medical genealogy, which came to be centered in Damascus around al-Bīmāristān al-Nūrī and served the Zangid court of Nūr al-Dīn (r. 1146–1174) and then the Ayyubid courts of Damascus starting with Ṣalāḥ al-Dīn (r. 1174–1193).

Philosophie à Damas à l'Aube du XIIIème Siècle: Un Tournant Post-Avicennien?" 250, and Lewicka, *Medicine for Muslims?*, 8.

7 Ibn Abī Usaybi'ah, *'Uyūn al-Anbā'*, 4: 318.

8 Ibid., 4: 131.

9 Ibid., 4: 188. Also, Lewicka, *Medicine for Muslims?*, 9.

10 Ibn Abī Usaybi'ah, *'Uyūn al-Anbā'*, 4: 318.

11 Ibn Abī Uṣaybi'ah was conspicuously silent on the relation or connection between the two physicians, although they coincided in al-Nūrī and had the same teacher in Muhadhdhab al-Dīn al-Naqqāsh (d. 1178). Moreover, Ibn Abī Uṣaybi'ah reported that al-Naqqāsh introduced al-Raḥbī to Ṣalāh al-Dīn in Damascus and that the latter invited him to serve in his court when Ibn al-Muṭrān had been serving there. The silence is probably due to the professional competition between the two and al-Raḥbī's self-professed hatred of *dhimmis* (non-Muslims). Al-Raḥbī told Ibn Abī Uṣaybi'ah that he always refused to teach medicine to non-Muslims, with only two exceptions: 'Imrān al-Isrā'īlī and Ibrāhīm al-Sāmirī (on this, see Lewicka, *Medicine for Muslims?*, 9, and Ibn Abī Uṣaybi'ah, *'Uyūn al-Anbā'*, 4: 190). Ibn Abī Uṣaybi'ah was very loyal to al-Raḥbī and his family and considered his piety and his austere living to be an ideal. He wrote: "If one considers the majority of the physicians of the Levant, one finds that they either read with [al-Raḥbī] or with someone who read with him. Among those who read with him in the beginning [of their education] is al-Shaykh Muhadhdhab al-Dīn 'Abd al-Raḥīm ibn 'Alī [al-Dakhwār] before he accompanied Ibn al-Muṭrān." (4: 190). In my reading, Ibn Abī Uṣaybi'ah greatly exaggerated al-Raḥbī's importance and impact and tried to link him to the majority of Levantine physicians in his dictionary. However, most of these connections were very limited in time and scope, similar to his connection to al-Dakhwār. Ibn Abī Uṣaybi'ah failed to back his claim with any examples (except for al-Dakhwār), and his dictionary contained only two physicians who read with al-Raḥbī: Kamāl al-Dīn al-Ḥimṣī (d. 1215), who was also a merchant and who also read with al-Makhzūmī (4: 209), and Fakhr al-Dīn al-Sā'ātī (d. 1218), who earned his living as a clock-maker and read medicine with Fakhr al-Dīn al-Mardīnī. Al-Raḥbī did not make a huge fortune, as did al-Dakhwār, nor was he able to maintain a court position. He also worked as a merchant, a dimension of his character downplayed by Ibn Abī Uṣaybi'ah. Al-Dakhwār's connection to al-Raḥbī's son, a more prolific and capable physician, is related to the son being one of al-Dakhwār's students and protégés.

Al-Naqqāsh, a recent émigré from Baghdad, descended from a long tradition of bīmāristān practice in the Abbasid capital and introduced this tradition to the Levant's new and biggest bīmāristān. He was a student of Amīn al-Dawlah ibn al-Tilmīdh (1074–1165), who was the head of a number of bīmāristāns in Baghdad, such as al-Bīmāristān al-ʿAḍudī,[12] where al-Naqqāsh was probably trained. Al-Naqqāsh probably brought to Damascus's new hospital the then-new dispensatory of his teacher "Aqrabādhīn Ibn al-Tilmīdh," which would become the one most frequently used in al-Bīmāristān al-Nūrī. He might have also brought Ibn al-Tilmīdh's shorter *Aqrabādhīn*, which was designed for the use of al-Bīmāristān al-ʿAḍudī. The Baghdadi tradition, from which al-Naqqāsh descended, showed specific interest in particular texts that were discussed and commented on by the famous Ibn al-Tilmīdh. These texts, and the practices they conditioned, became the backbone of the bīmāristān practice in the Levant and Egypt for the coming centuries. For instance, Ibn al-Tilmīdh wrote a commentary on Avicenna's *al-Qānūn* (Canon) and on Ḥunayn ibn Isḥāq's (Latin: *Johannitius*) *masāʾil* (Questions on Medicine). He also wrote a summary of Galen's commentary on the Aphorisms and another summary of al-Rāzī's *al-Ḥāwī*, although none of these writings has survived.[13] As will be shown later, these texts became influential in the circle of al-Dakhwār and his students, although not in other circles in the region. Eventually, al-Naqqāsh's tradition, his students and followers, among whom al-Dakhwār stood as the most important, dominated the medical scene in the Levant and Egypt.

As mentioned earlier, al-Dakhwār started working on medicine by reading *al-Kitāb al-Malakī* with al-Raḥbī. He also read parts of Ibn Sīnā's *al-Qānūn* with Fakhr al-Dīn al-Mardīnī. His main teacher remained Ibn al-Muṭrān, whom he accompanied and deeply respected, as evident from the accounts that al-Dakhwār reported about his teacher.[14] He also studied philosophy (*al-ʿulūm al-Hikmīyah*) with al-Āmidī; this provided another connection to Ibn Sīnā because al-Dakhwār memorized al-Āmidī's book *Kashf al-Tamwīhāt fī al-Ishārāt wa al-Tanbīhāt* (the revelation of

[12] For a biography of Ibn al-Tilmīdh, see Meyerhof, "Ibn al-Tilmīḏh"; Ibn al-Tilmīdh and Kahl, *The Dispensatory of Ibn at-Tilmīḏh: Arabic Text, English Translation, Study and Glossaries*, 7–19.

[13] Ibid., 14. Kahl distinguishes these writings as "Nonindependent writings." Emilie Savage-Smith mentioned that BL MS Or. 9202 contains four summaries of parts of the Canon and that "MS Or. 9202 also has an important collation note stating that the volume was read before and corrected by Ibn al-Tilmidh (d. 1165)" (Savage-Smith, "Galen's Lost Ophthalmology and the Summaria Alexandrinorum," 131, n. 26).

[14] Most of Ibn Abī Uṣaybiʿah's biography of Ibn al-Muṭrān was based on accounts reported by al-Dakhwār.

allusions in "Remarks and Admonitions"), a commentary on Ibn Sīnā's "Remarks and Admonitions."[15] Al-Dakhwār amassed enormous wealth and became one of the more important physicians in Ayyubid circles. His service to Al-ʿĀdil I (r. 1200–1218) earned him the trust of the sovereign, and he became the sovereign's boon companion and trusted adviser.[16] Even as a young physician, al-Dakhwār's remarkable intellectual genealogy and his reputed talent singled him out as one of the more sought-after physicians of his time. So confident was al-Dakhwār in his own abilities and worth that he initially refused to serve the court with a salary less than that of the famous senior court physician, Muwaffaq al-Dīn al-Salamī (d. 1204), all while living off only a small salary from al-Bīmāristān al-Nūrī. He may have regretted this decision especially when his friends and colleagues criticized him for missing such an important opportunity for financial gain and professional development. He was lucky enough, however, that al-Salamī died a few months later, and he was invited again to serve in the court with a salary similar to that of the late court physician.[17] However, one must recognize that the accounts of al-Dakhwār's brilliance are likely biased because they come from his student Ibn Abī Uṣaybiʿah and were read by al-Dakhwār himself.

True to his intellectual genealogy, al-Dakhwār's writings followed a pattern similar to the writings of Ibn al-Tilmīdh. He, too, composed a summary of *al-Ḥāwī* (*Liber Continens*) and engaged with Ḥunayn's *Questions*, composing a responsa to Ibn Abī Ṣādiq's commentary on it. He also wrote a treatise on evacuation (*al-istifrāgh*), along with a collection of commentaries and questions on medicine likely based on his experience.[18] Al-Dakhwār's students followed in his footsteps. In the following pages, we will look at the major works that animated this medical circle and see how such texts influenced the practice in the different bīmāristāns of the Levant and Egypt.

"Rediscovering" al-Rāzī

Both al-Rāzī's *al-Ḥāwī* and Ḥunayn's *Questions* continued to figure prominently in the writings of al-Dakhwār's students in a manner not seen in earlier generations or different contemporary circles. Whereas *The Question*'s popularity may have been due to its brevity and therefore its

15 Ibid., 4: 330.
16 Ibid., 4: 320.
17 Ibid. Part of al-Dakhwār's rejection of the appointment with a lower salary might have been due to the fact that al-Salamī was also a student of Ibn al-Muṭrān, albeit from an earlier generation than al-Dakhwār.
18 Ibid., 4: 337.

usefulness for students and practicing physicians alike, the growing popularity of *al-Ḥāwī*, a long complex text, in this environment is more difficult to understand. To Ibn Abī Uṣaybiʿah, a member of this circle and its effective historian, *al-Ḥāwī* was not seen as a complex, difficult text but rather as a useful collection of all the opinions of important medical authors on all diseases: "*Kitāb al-Ḥāwī*: It is [al-Rāzī's] greatest book in medicine. This is because he collected in it all that he found disparate in the mention of diseases and their treatments in all the medical books of the ancients, and who came after them until his time, and attributed every thing that he copied to its sayer, notwithstanding that al-Rāzī died and did not edit the book."[19] We can find nothing similar to this praise of *al-Ḥāwī* in al-Qifṭī's (d. 1248) biography of al-Rāzī,[20] or in Ibn al-Nadīm's (d. 990) listing of his books.[21] More significantly, Ibn Abī Uṣaybiʿah chose to list *al-Ḥāwī* as the first of al-Rāzī's books. This was unusual: not only was *al-Ḥāwī* an unfinished book, but this also represented a departure from the listings in al-Qifṭī and Ibn al-Nadīm, both of whom listed al-Rāzī's *al-Manṣurī* first, as the author's most famous completed medical text. Ibn Abī Uṣaybiʿah had a lot of praise for *al-Manṣurī* as well, and he included the titles and described the contents of its various treatises. Yet he still chose to place it well after al-Ḥāwī.[22] For Ibn Abī Uṣaybiʿah and his circle, *al-Ḥāwī* was a book of practice; it was valuable because it was devoted to diseases and their treatments, with little to no discussion of the theoretical aspects of medicine. Moreover, the fact that *al-Ḥāwī* was made of a collection of quotes from different medical authorities about these diseases made it all the more essential. Instead of viewing it as a huge, voluminous book, Ibn Abī Uṣaybiʿah saw it as the ultimate summary of practical medicine.

A closer look at al-Rāzī's vita in Ibn Abī Uṣaybiʿah and in comparison to al-Qifṭī and Ibn al-Nadīm reveals that Ibn Abī Uṣaybiʿah's *al-Ḥāwī* was probably different from what the other two authors were referring to under the same title. Both Ibn al-Nadīm and al-Qifṭī explained that *al-Ḥāwī* was also called *al-Jāmiʿ* ("The Collector") and *al-Ḥāṣir* ("Encompasser") and that it was composed of twelve sections, which Ibn al-Nadīm enumerated.[23] Ibn Abī Uṣaybiʿah did not mention that *al-Ḥāwī* was called *al-Jāmiʿ* or *al-Ḥāṣir*. Instead, he had a separate book named *al-Jāmiʿ*,

[19] Ibid., 3: 29.

[20] Al-Qifṭī, *Tārīkh Al-Ḥukamā'*, 274.

[21] Ibn Al-Nadīm, *Fihrist*, 417. Ibn al-Nadīm explained the parts of the book in great detail and enumerated its different chapters, as was his habit with long books, but he did not mention any of Ibn Abī Uṣaybiʿah's remarks about its value or about the fact that al-Rāzī mentioned those whom he cited.

[22] Ibn Abī Uṣaybiʿah, *ʿUyūn al-Anbā'*, 3: 36.

[23] Ibn al-Nadīm, *Fihrist*, 417.

"which is also called *Ḥāṣir al-Ṣināʿah al-Ṭibbiyyah* (the "Encompasser of Medical Art")," and enumerated the twelve sections that composed that book.[24] Table 4.1 compares the sections of the two books, which appear largely similar yet with meaningful differences.

Table 4.1: *Comparing the contents of* "al-Ḥāṣir *(The Encompasser)" in Ibn al-Nadīm's* Fihrist *and Ibn Abī Uṣaybiʿah's* Uyūn

Ibn al-Nadīm's Fihrist	Ibn Abī Uṣaybiʿah
On the treatment of the sick and [on] diseases	On the preservation of health, the treatment of diseases, bone-setting and procedures
On the preservation of health	
On bone-setting and surgeries	
On the powers of medications, foods, and all the substances needed in medicine	On the powers of foods and medications and what is needed for treatment in the craft of medicine
On compound medications	On compound medications including a mention of what needs [to be known] about them in the manner of an *aqrabādhīn*
On the craft of medicine	On what is needed in medicine including grinding drugs, burning, distilling, washing, extracting their powers, preserving them, . . . and the like
On pharmacopia; [including] medications, their colors, tastes, and smells	On pharmacopia; [including] the composition of drugs, their colors, tastes, and smells . . .
On substitutions (*al-ibdāl*)	On substitutions; mentioning what can substitute for each drug or food
On weights and measures	On explaining terms, weights, and measures of drugs, and the names of organs and diseases in Greek. Syriac, Persian, Indian, and Arabic; similar to the books known as *Shaqshamāʾī*
On anatomy and the benefits of organs	On anatomy and the benefits of organs
On the natural causes in the craft of medicine	On natural causes explaining the natural causes of illnesses
On the introduction to the craft of medicine; [composed of] two treatises: the first on medical terms and the second on the firsts in medicine	On the introduction to the craft of medicine; [composed of] two treatises; the first on natural things and the second on the firsts of medicine
	On a collection of treatments and recipes
	On what he knew of the writings of Galen and was not mentioned by Ḥunayn or was in Galen's *fihrist*

[24] Ibn Abī Uṣaybiʿah, *ʿUyūn al-Anbāʾ*, 3: 37–38.

The last section (on the writings of Galen) in Ibn Abī Uṣaybiʿah's enumeration was, in fact, listed as a separate book by both al-Qifṭī and Ibn al-Nadīm. It was mentioned incidentally right after the enumeration of sections in Ibn al-Nadīm, which could suggest that Ibn Abī Uṣaybiʿah might have confused it with part of *al-Jāmiʿ*. Although al-Qifṭī did not enumerate any sections, he followed Ibn al-Nadīm in mentioning the book on the writings of Galen as a separate text.[25] Ibn Abī Uṣaybiʿah took issue with Ibn al-Nadīm's and al-Qifṭī's assertion that this book was indeed *al-Ḥāwī*:

> I say: this division mentioned here is not for his book known as *al-Ḥāwī*, nor is it a satisfactory division. It is told that these are drafts of books that were found after al-Rāzī's death collected in this order, so they were thought to be one book. To this day, I have never seen a copy of this book nor have I seen someone who said that he saw it.[26]

Although it is possible that the book described by Ibn al-Nadīm did not survive in its entirety and that another book dedicated to diseases (or perhaps the first section mentioned in Ibn al-Nadīm's description) survived to be read and studied by Ibn Abī Uṣaybiʿah and his circle, it is hard to imagine that al-Qifṭī had access to texts that were not available to Ibn Abī Uṣaybiʿah or vice versa. Al-Qifṭī was born in Qifṭ in Upper Egypt in 1172 and was educated in Cairo until 1187, after which he went to Jerusalem accompanying his father. He was put in charge of finance in Aleppo by al-Ẓāhir Ghāzī (r. 1186–1216) and died in Aleppo in 1248.[27] Ibn Abī Uṣaybiʿah was familiar with al-Qifṭī's dictionary of physicians and cited him several times. It is inconceivable that al-Qifṭī (in Aleppo) had access to this book and that Ibn Abī Uṣaybiʿah (in nearby Damascus) had access neither to the book nor to anyone familiar with it. More significantly, had al-Qifṭī seen the *al-Ḥāwī* to which Ibn Abī Uṣaybiʿah referred, he would have realized that it was different from the supposed *al-Jāmiʿ*. The more plausible explanation of this discrepancy is that al-Qifṭī copied al-Rāzī's writings from Ibn al-Nadīm, a proposition supported by the fact that the two vitae are in the same order, with al-Qifṭī's essentially summarizing Ibn al-Nadīm's. More importantly, the circles of physicians surrounding al-Qifṭī must have had little interest in the writings of al-Rāzī, especially his voluminous *al-Ḥāwī*, unlike the

25 Al-Qifṭī, *Tārīkh al-Ḥukamāʾ*, 274.
26 Ibn Abī Uṣaybiʿah, *ʿUyūn al-Anbāʾ*, 3: 38.
27 Dietrich, "Ibn al-Ḳifṭī."

circles to which Ibn Abī Uṣaybiʿah belonged in Damascus and in Cairo, as will be shown later.

Al-Dakhwār's circle in Damascus, to which Ibn Abī Uṣaybiʿah belonged, was indeed interested in al-Rāzī, and especially *al-Ḥāwī*. Ibn Abī Uṣaybiʿah himself read al-Rāzī's writing "in relation to practice,"[28] as well as his writings on nourishment.[29] One of Ibn Abī Uṣaybiʿah's students, Abū al-Faraj al-Quff (d. 1286), read Galen and al-Rāzī with Ibn Abī Uṣaybiʿah himself.[30] In addition to al-Dakhwār's summary of *al-Ḥāwī*, Kamāl al-Dīn al-Ḥimṣī (d. 1215), a student of al-Raḥbī and a colleague of al-Dakhwār in al-Bīmāristān al-Nūrī, also wrote a summary of *al-Ḥāwī* but did not complete it.[31] Finally, another student of al-Dakhwār's, Rashīd al-Dīn Abū Saʿīd (d. 1249), who was "a Christian from Jerusalem"[32] and served the Ayyubid court in Cairo until his death, wrote a commentary on *al-Ḥāwī* as well.[33] Earlier in Ibn Abī Uṣaybiʿah's bio-bibliography of al-Rāzī, he mentioned twelve books, which were not mentioned in either al-Qifṭī or Ibn al-Nadīm and which he called "the twelve books of the art (*al-ithnā ʿashr kitāban fī al-ṣanʿah*)."[34] The designation of the books as "the books of the art" pointed to the use of the books for instruction in a manner similar to the designation and use of the sixteen books of Galen. This helps illuminate the meaning of Ibn Abī Uṣaybiʿah's references to "al-Rāzī's books, especially the practical part," which he read with al-Raḥbī and which he did not explain in detail and shows how this circle relied on al-Rāzī for medical instructions.

This interest in al-Rāzī and in *al-Ḥāwī* was hard to detect in the Levant or Egypt outside of or prior to this group. For instance, ʿAlī ibn Sulayman (d. after 1021), the chief physician of Cairo under the Fatimids, wrote a summary of *al-Ḥāwī*,[35] but none of his students seemed to have continued with similar writings. The famous Fatimid physician ʿAlī ibn Riḍwān (d. 1061), also the chief physician in Cairo, mentioned in his own vita

[28] Ibn Abī Uṣaybiʿah, *ʿUyūn al-Anbāʾ*, 4: 191.
[29] Ibid., 4: 192.
[30] Ibid., 4: 409.
[31] Ibid., 4: 210.
[32] Ibid., 4: 496.
[33] Ibid., 4: 498.
[34] Ibid., 3: 31. The books are (1) On the instructional introduction; (2) On the logical introduction; (3) Book of proof; (4) Book of management; (5) Book of quarantine; (6) Book of the elixir, in ten treatises; (7) Book on the honor of the art and its privilege; (8) Book on arrangements; (9) Book on treatments; (10) Book on symptoms and signs; (11) Book on passion; and (12) Book on tricks. None of these books survived.
[35] Ibid., 3: 370.

that he read *al-Ḥāwī* along with Galen and Hippocrates, but he generally disliked al-Rāzī and his approach. In his writings, he wrote a response to al-Rāzī on the question of prophecy and a treatise on solving some of al-Rāzī's doubts on Galen.[36] Muwaffaq al-Dīn al-Baghdādī (d. 1231), a contemporary of al-Dakhwār's but not part of the latter's circle of colleagues and students, was interested in al-Rāzī's *Doubts on Galen* (al-Shukūk ʿalā Jālinūs), as was Ibn Riḍwān, and he wrote a treatise solving some of these doubts. Both Ibn Riḍwān and al-Baghdādī considered the *Doubts* to be presumptuous and devoted time and effort to refuting al-Rāzī's supposed attacks on Galen. In a way, their interest was not primarily in al-Rāzī but rather part of their dedication to Greek learning and rejection of al-Rāzī's sacrilegious writings, which included his book on "the faults of saints." The *Doubts,* however, did not seem to interest al-Dakhwār and his circle as much.

With this in mind, we can view Ibn Abī Uṣaybiʿah's congratulatory biography of al-Rāzī in a different light. He defended al-Rāzī against the attacks of Ibn Riḍwān and others when he mentioned al-Rāzī's book on "the faults of the saints (*ʿuyūb al-awliyāʾ*)":

> I say: this book, if it was indeed composed, and God knows better, then it may be that some vicious [people] who are enemies of al-Rāzī composed it and attributed it to him, so that those who see the book would insult al-Rāzī or think ill of him. Al-Rāzī is indeed more sublime (*ajall*) than to try such a thing, or to compose on this issue. Some of those who rebuke (*yadhimmu*) al-Rāzī, or even charge him of unbelief, such as ʿAlī ibn Riḍwān al-Miṣrī and others, name this book [as justification for their position] and call it al-Rāzī's book on the craziness of prophets (*makhārīq al-anbiyāʾ*).[37]

Al-Rāzī's book on "faults of the saints" was mentioned by al-Qifṭī[38] and Ibn al-Nadīm,[39] but neither of them expressed doubts about its existence or authorship.

[36] Ibid., 3: 417.

[37] Ibid., 3: 45. Al-Rāzī's book on prophethood did not survive except in long excerpts in a refutation composed by his compatriot, Abū Ḥātim Aḥmad b. Ḥamdān al-Rāzī (d. c. 933): "The Signs of Prophecy in refuting [the opinions] of the heretic Abū Bakr al-Rāzī" (Abū Ḥātim al-Rāzī, *Aʿlām Al-Nubuwwa*). It appears that the book did not survive to Ibn Abī Uṣaybiʿah's time either as evident from his doubts about whether it was ever composed (his doubts about its authorship may be part of his defense of Abū Bakr al-Rāzī). This doubt is reasonable because Abū Ḥātim's refutation recreated not only said excerpts of Abū Bakr al-Rāzī's book, but also what the former claimed to be conversations and communications. Abū Ḥātim was a well-known Ismaili theologian and missionary (*dāʿī*), and his books were well-known in Fatimid Cairo. It appears that Ibn Riḍwān and other Fatimid authors attacked Abū Bakr al-Rāzī based on Abū Ḥātim's book and recreation. For more information on Abū Ḥātim al-Rāzī, see Stern, "Abū Ḥātim al-Rāzī." See also Kraus, "Raziana II: Extrait du Kitāb Aʿlām al-Nubuwwa d'Abū Ḥātim al-Rāzī."

[38] Al-Qifṭī, *Tārīkh al-Ḥukamāʾ*, 276.

[39] Ibn al-Nadīm, *Fihrist,* 419. Ibn al-Nadīm called the book "on the faults of prophets."

In the Fatimid context in Egypt and parts of the Levant, al-Rāzī was well-known and his writings were known and read. His work, however, must have been perceived through the lens of the work of Abū Ḥātim al-Rāzī (d. ca. 933), an important and respected Ismaili theologian and missionary (*dāʿī*). Abū Ḥātim even became the chief missionary in the Rey region, one of the more important regions in the Persianate East and the birthplace of both Rāzīs.[40] To Abū Ḥātim, Abū Bakr al-Rāzī (the physician; Rhazes) was a heretic who criticized, if not rejected outright, the notion of prophecy. Philosophically, Rhazes was seen as an iconoclast who failed to understand Aristotelian philosophy properly. This prompted Ibn Sīnā and Maimonides, for instance, to reject his philosophical writings as unworthy of attention while simultaneously recognizing his importance as a physician.[41] Yet a closer look at al-Rāzī's (Rhazes) bio-bibliography in Ibn al-Nadīm's *Fihrist*, al-Qifṭī, and Ibn Abī Uṣaybiʿah reveals more information about how and why the great physician was perceived this way in Fatimid Ismaili circles. In addition to the book on prophethood, al-Rāzī (Rhazes) authored two other curious treatises. The first was "A book on the works of the Infallible Honorable Imām (*al-Imām al-Fāḍil al-maʿṣūm)*"[42] and is mostly about the writing of Jaʿfar al-Ṣādiq (d. 765), the sixth Imām for both Ismailis and Imami Shiites and known as *al-Imām al-Fāḍil*; al-Rāzī's (Rhazes) interests in alchemy must have brought him close to the writings of Jābir b. Ḥayyān (d. ca. 815), himself a student of Jaʿfar al-Ṣādiq. Calling Jaʿfar infallible, however, is a significant indication that al-Rāzī had Shiite tendencies. His other book entitled "The true Imām and [the truly] guided [nation](*maʾmūmīn*)" affirms this but also suggests that al-Rāzī (Rhazes) had Twelver Imami tendencies. His book might have implied doubts concerning the rising Fatimid Caliphate and the claims of the Fatimid Caliph to the title of the Shiite Imamate. Al-Rāzī's (Rhazes) presumed Twelver tendencies help us interpret Abū Ḥātim's severe attacks despite al-Rāzī's (Rhazes) laudatory book about the Sixth Imām and may also explain the interest that the Buyids, a Twelver dynasty that ruled over Iraq and Iran between 934 and 1055, had in his writings. It was the famous Buyid vizir Ibn al-ʿAmīd (d. 970), a literatus

40 On Abū Ḥātim al-Rāzī, see Daiber, "Abū Ḥātim Ar-Rāzī (10th Century AD) on the Unity and Diversity of Religions"; Daneshgar, "Abū Ḥātim Al-Rāzī: The Proofs of Prophecy: A Parallel English-Arabic Text (Review)"; Vajda, "Les Lettres Et Les Sons De La Langue Arabe D'après Abū Ḥātim Al-Rāzī."

41 Harvey, "Did Maimonides' Letter to Samuel Ibn Tibbon Determine Which Philosophers Would Be Studied by Later Jewish Thinkers?"

42 Ibn Abī Usaybiʿah, *ʿUyūn al-Anbāʾ*, 3: 45.

and *vizir* of Rukn al-Dawlah (d. 976), who commissioned the organization and publication of *al-Ḥāwī*.[43] In the Fatimid context, al-Rāzī (Rhazes) appeared as a heretic, and his writings in philosophy seemed confused and iconoclastic within the Aristotelian context.[44] The reception his writings received was worthy of an iconoclast, both in relation to philosophy and medicine. His *Doubts on Galen* offers perhaps the best example: Ibn Riḍwān wrote a responsa against it, along with another directed at al-Rāzī's book on prophethood.[45]

The new circle formed around al-Bīmāristān al-Nūrī had different views about al-Rāzī and engaged in a rediscovery of his writings. The group, built around the bīmāristān and the teachings of Muhadhdhab al-Dīn al-Naqqāsh (d. 1178), adopted a view of al-Rāzī that was more common in Baghdad in the circles around Amīn al-Dawlah ibn al-Tilmīdh (d. 1165) and possibly around al-Bīmāristān al-ʿAḍudī – the huge bīmāristān built in Baghdad by the Buyid ruler ʿAḍud al-Dawlah. It is likely that the revival and rediscovery of al-Rāzī and his writings, especially *al-Ḥāwī*, did not exceed the circle of al-Raḥbī and al-Dakhwār in Damascus and, later, in Cairo, as suggested by the absences in al-Qifṭī's dictionary composed in nearby Aleppo. Yet this rediscovery of al-Rāzī was not a recovery of his philosophical or even theoretical writings, such as the *Doubts* – no author in this circle engaged with these works. Instead, the circle rediscovered a practitioner and a practical corpus. Ibn Abī Uṣaybiʿah's understanding of *al-Ḥāwī* as a collection of different opinions arranged in a manner more suitable for practitioners (i.e., by diseases) reflects this point.

Al-Qānūn

Al-Rāzī was not the only significant author who figured prominently in the writings of this group. Ibn Sīnā was another important figure, and his *al-Qānūn* generated a significant amount of writing. Kamāl al-Dīn al-Ḥimṣī (d. 1215), student then colleague of al-Raḥbī and al-Dakhwār at al-Bīmāristān al-Nūrī, read and wrote a commentary on its *Kulliyyāt* (the Generalities).[46] Fakhr al-Dīn al-Sāʿātī (d. 1218), also a student of al-Raḥbī,

[43] On Ibn al-ʿAmīd and the literary context of the Buyid court, see Durand-Guédy, "Private Letters, Official Correspondence: Buyid Inshā' as a Historical Source," 125–54 and Naaman, "Sariqa in Practice: The Case of al-Ṣāḥib Ibn ʿAbbād."

[44] See, for instance, Ibn Ṣāʿid al-Andalusī's (d. 1070) on al-Rāzī's philosophical writings as deviations and misunderstandings of Aristotle. Ibn Ṣāʿid al-Andalusī, *Ṭabaqāt al-Umam*.

[45] Ibn Abī Usaybiʿah, *ʿUyūn Al-Anbā'*, 3: 417.

[46] Ibid., 4: 210.

wrote a commentary on *al-Qānūn* and "completed the Book of Colics for Ibn Sīnā," the Book of Colics being one of Ibn Sīnā's unfinished books.[47] Al-Dakhwār's students were also prolific in relation to *al-Qānūn*. One of his more prominent students, Najm al-Dīn al-Labūdī (1210–1268), who worked in the court of Homs and in Alexandria, wrote a summary of the *Kulliyyāt* of *al-Qānūn*. He also wrote a summary of Ibn Sīnā's *al-Ishārāt wa al-Tanbīhāt* (Remarks and Admonitions),[48] a book that figured in al-Dakhwār's philosophical education. Similarly, Sharaf al-Dīn al-Raḥbī (d. 1269), Raḍīy al-Dīn al-Raḥbī's son and one of al-Dakhwār's favorite students, also wrote marginalia on *al-Qānūn*.[49] Najm al-Dīn ibn al-Munfākh (1197–1254), another student of al-Dakhwār, likewise wrote a book on "the neglected [parts] of *al-Kulliyyāt*."[50] *Al-Kulliyyāt* of *al-Qānūn* was so popular in this circle that one of al-Dakhwār's students was nicknamed *al-Kullī* (of the *Kulliyyāt*) because he memorized it so proficiently and remarkably.[51]

The most important commentator on Ibn Sīnā was undoubtedly Ibn al-Nafīs (d. 1288), a member of this group in Damascus and one of al-Dakhwār's more talented and recognized students. Ibn al-Nafīs wrote a commentary on *al-Qānūn*'s anatomy,[52] as well as a commentary on the entire book, and his famous *al-Mūjaz* was a summary of *al-Qānūn*.[53] Although the other commentaries authored by his colleagues in the circle did not survive, Ibn al-Nafīs' works on *al-Qānūn* became one of the most important commentaries on the book.[54] Most of Ibn al-Nafīs' colleagues in al-Dakhwār's circle focused on the first book (*al-Kulliyyāt*) of *al-Qānūn*, but he decided to write both a commentary and a summary of the whole book, as well as a commentary on *al-Qānūn*'s anatomy. In his commentary on the anatomy of *al-Qānūn*, Ibn al-Nafīs gathered one part from *al-Qānūn*'s first book with another part from the third book, effectively creating "the anatomy of *al-Qānūn*" before commenting on it.[55] The group's interest in Ibn Sīnā continued the legacy of Ibn al-Tilmīdh, who also wrote commentaries on *al-Qānūn*. Yet the group seemed all the more

47 Ibid., 4: 160.
48 Ibid., 4: 165.
49 Ibid., 4: 207.
50 Ibid., 4: 390.
51 Ibid., 4: 385.
52 Ibn al-Nafīs, *Sharḥ Tashrīḥ al-Qānūn*.
53 Ibn al-Nafīs, *Mūjaz al-Qānūn*.
54 See Fancy, *Science and Religion in Mamluk Egypt: Ibn Al-Nafis, Pulmonary Transit and Bodily Resurrection*.
55 Ibn al-Nafīs, *Sharḥ Tashrīḥ al-Qānūn*, 1–2.

interested in Ibn Sīnā's theoretical medical writings. It appears that they used his writings as a source for theoretical training, in contradistinction to al-Rāzī's practice-oriented writings.

Questions *and* Aphorisms

Two other works loom large in the bio-bibliographies of the authors in al-Dakhwār's circle, and these are not as commonly cited or studied in the Levant and Egypt outside this circle: *al-Masāʾil* (*The Questions*) by Ḥunayn ibn Isḥāq (Latin: Johannitius) and Hippocrates' *Aphorisms*. The former represented an important summary of the important theoretical and practical aspects of medical practice, and a number of authors in the circle commented on and summarized it. They include Kamāl al-Dīn al-Ḥimṣī (d. 1215),[56] Shams al-Dīn al-Labūdī (d. 1224),[57] his son Najm al-Dīn (1210–d. after 1268), and Ibn al-Nafīs (d. 1288).[58] Ibn Abī Uṣaybiʿah described *al-Masāʾil* as "the introduction (*al-madkhal*) to the art of medicine, because he [Ḥunayn] collected in it general [rules], which function as the principles of this science."[59] As was his custom with books in which he had a special interest, Ibn Abī Uṣaybiʿah continued to describe the book in detail, mentioning how it did not all belong to Ḥunayn but that parts of it were composed by Ḥubaysh, Ḥunayn's student and nephew. Ibn Abī Uṣaybiʿah's extensive discussion of the book was copied from a well-known commentary on *al-Masāʾil* composed by Ibn Abī Ṣādiq al-Nisābūrī (active eleventh century). The circle used Ibn Abī Ṣādiq's commentaries extensively. For instance, Al-Dakhwār himself wrote a responsa to Ibn Abī Ṣādiq's commentary on *al-Masāʾil*,[60] and Sharaf al-Dīn al-Raḥbī wrote a commentary on Ibn Abī Ṣādiq's same commentary.[61]

Despite the interest in Ibn Abī Ṣādiq's works, the details of his life and career were not known to Ibn Abī Uṣaybiʿah: he wrote a short, laudatory biography of the physician in which he suggested that Ibn Abī Ṣādiq may have been a student of Ibn Sīnā, a historical inaccuracy.[62] Not only was this

[56] Ibid., 4: 209.

[57] Ibid., 4: 163. Shams al-Dīn al-Labūdī was not a student of al-Dakhwār or al-Raḥbī but rather their colleague at al-Bīmāristān al-Nūrī, and his son Najm al-Dīn (1210–d. after 1268) was al-Dakhwār's student.

[58] Ibn Al-Nafīs, *Sharḥ Fuṣul Abuqrāṭ*, 43.

[59] Ibn Abī Usaybiʿah, *ʿUyūn al-Anbāʾ*, 2: 150–51.

[60] Ibn Abī Usaybiʿah, *ʿUyūn al-Anbāʾ*, 4: 337.

[61] Ibid., 4: 207. To my knowledge, Ibn Abī Ṣādiq's commentaries were not published.

[62] Ibid., 3: 126. On Ibn Sīnā's immediate students, see Al-Rahim, "Avicenna's Immediate Disciples: Their Lives and Works."

connection between Ibn Abī Ṣādiq and Ibn Sīnā untrue, but Ibn Abī Uṣaybiʿah also did not suggest any evidence for it. In his view, the fact that Ibn Abī Ṣādiq was Persian and was highly valued and appreciated for his erudition suggested the possibility that he was indeed a student of the Chief Master (*al-shaykh al-raʾīs*) Ibn Sīnā. More than anything, this assumption of Ibn Abī Ṣādiq's relation with Ibn Sīnā and the reasoning that likely underlay it are only indicative of how the circle valued Ibn Abī Ṣādiq's work along with Ibn Sīnā's but at a different – lower – level.

In brief, and as mentioned before, the circle's interest in *al-Ḥāwī* was unique in the Levantine environment, as suggested by al-Qifṭī's lack of familiarity with the text (or at least the text this circle was using). This unusual interest in *al-Ḥāwī* had its origins in the works of Ibn al-Tilmīdh, who presided over al-Bīmāristān al-ʿAḍudī and wrote a summary of *al-Ḥāwī*. The fact that the Buyid *vizir* Ibn al-ʿAmīd commissioned the collection of *al-Ḥāwī* might have brought *al-Ḥāwī* to the attention of the physicians in al-Bīmāristān al-ʿAḍudī, from which the book made its way, in its new garb, to the Levant. The circle's interest in the *Aphorisms* and Ḥunayn's *Questions* appeared equally novel in the Levantine environment and could have had its roots with Ibn al-Tilmīdh as well. The most celebrated commentary on these two books at the time was almost a century old and composed by the otherwise unknown physician or author Ibn Abī Ṣādiq, about whom Ibn Abī Uṣaybiʿah failed to acquire sufficient information. The circle engaged repetitively with Ibn Abī Ṣādiq's commentaries. For instance, al-Dakhwār wrote "Response to Ibn Abī Ṣādiq on Ḥunayn's *Questions*,"[63] and Sharaf al-Dīn al-Raḥbī wrote marginalia on Ibn Abī Ṣādiq's commentary on the *Questions*, as well.[64] Ibn al-Nafīs' commentary on the *Aphorisms* also engaged with Ibn Abī Ṣādiq's commentary, although he did not mention his name directly.[65]

In addition to Ibn Sīnā's *al-Qānūn* (particularly its first book on *al-Kulliyyāt*); al-Rāzī's *al-Ḥāwī*, along with other practical texts of al-Rāzī; Ḥunayn's *Questions* (influenced to some extent by Ibn Abī Ṣādiq's commentary) and Hippocrates' *Aphorisms* (also influenced by Ibn Abī Ṣādiq's commentary), al-Dakhwār's circle at al-Bīmāristān al-Nūrī also focused on Galen's book on *al-ʿilal wa al-amrāḍ* (causes and diseases), on which Najm al-Dīn ibn al-Munfākh (d. 1254)[66] and al-Sadīd ibn Abī al-Bayān both commented. The latter was not directly part of this group

[63] Ibid., 4: 337.
[64] Ibid., 4: 207.
[65] Ibn al-Nafīs, *Sharḥ Fuṣul Abuqrāṭ*.
[66] Ibn Abī Usaybiʿah, *ʿUyūn al-Anbāʾ*, 4: 390.

but worked with Ibn Abī Uṣaybiʿah and others in al-Bīmāristān al-Nāṣirī.[67] Both al-Dakhwār and Ibn al-Nafīs commented on Hippocrates' *Prognostikon* (*Taqdīmat al-Maʿrifah*).[68] Ibn al-Nafīs, who might have been the more theoretically talented and oriented member of the circle, composed a commentary on "The Nature of Man" as well.[69] These texts, all of which were already known but most of which were not valued as much as they were inside this circle, formed the foundation for this group's works and writings and their view of medical practice. As will be shown, the way these texts were arranged, discussed, and studied show a new emerging practice-oriented tradition that started at al-Bīmāristān al-Nūrī to dominate the medical scene in the Levant and Egypt.

Theory, Practice, and a (New) Disease-Oriented Approach

Every member of this circle, except for Sharaf al-Dīn al-Raḥbī, composed treatises on their own practice and experience, including what seemed to be selections from different medical texts related to their practice. The connection to *al-Ḥāwī* and its arrangement is clear: these writings followed al-Rāzī's example of selecting quotes from medical texts and linking them to practice. Although writing on practice was not unprecedented, most of such writings were in the form of a *kunnāsh*, a large endeavor that included summaries of theoretical and practical matters.[70] These writings, however, were rather small treatises that did not even hold a distinctive name apart from "commentaries in medicine (*taʿālīq fī al-ṭibb*)"[71] or "commentaries on what occurred with him through experience."[72] Although these

[67] Ibid., 3: 463.

[68] Franz Rosenthal analyzed a list of Hippocratic writings composed by Alī ibn Riḍwān, in which he identified "*Taqdīmat al-Maʿrifah*" as *Progonstikon*. The English translation of the Arabic title is Rosenthal's: see Rosenthal, "An Eleventh-Century List of the Works of Hippocrates," 157. Al-Dakhwār's commentary on *Progonstikon* was composed by his student Ibn Qāḍī Baʿlabak, who explained in his introduction that al-Dakhwār was hesitant about writing the commentary and that he had entrusted Ibn Qāḍī Baʿlabak to write it from his notes and make it available to those who deserved it. See Al-Dakhwār and Ibn Qāḍī Baʿlabak, *Kitāb Sharḥ Tuqaddimuhu Al-Maʿrifah Lil-Dakhwār 565–628 AH-1160–1230 AD*, 143.

[69] Amr, "Ibn Al-Nafis: Discoverer of the Pulmonary Circulation," 385. Ibn al-Nafīs' theoretical interests were evident in his commentary on *al-Qānūn* and his engagement with Ibn Sīnā's and Ibn Ṭufayl's works. See Fancy, *Science and Religion in Mamluk Egypt.*

[70] See, for instance, Peter Promann's analysis of al-Kaskarī's *Kunnāsh*. Pormann, "Medical Methodology and Hospital Practice."

[71] This title occurs in the writings of al-Dakhwār (4: 337) and al-Ḥimṣī (4: 209).

[72] This title occurs in the writings of Najm al-Dīn ibn al-Munfākh (4: 390). Rashīd al-Dīn ibn Abī Ḥulayqah wrote "Diseases, their causes, signs and treatments with what was confirmed by experience" (3: 492).

practice-oriented notes and writings seemed to have little influence beyond this particular circle of physicians, they demonstrate a strong investment in practice and practical writings that was not seen with such consistency previously.

Apart from Ibn Sīnā's theoretical writings, al-Dakhwār's circle seemed genuinely interested in practical questions and in approaching texts like *al-Ḥāwī*, the *Aphorisms*, and *Questions* with a more practical and disease-oriented bent. For example, *al-Ḥāwī*, in Ibn Abī Uṣaybiʿah's description, acquired greater importance because of its anatomical division and its focus on diseases occurring in different parts of the body. This interest in anatomy was clearest in Ibn al-Nafīs novel commentary on the anatomy of *al-Qānūn*, in which he essentially rearranged *al-Qānūn* and brought together the anatomical parts from the first and third books to write a new, unprecedented anatomical commentary.[73] In this same vein, books on the preservation of health were glaringly absent from their writings, although they remained a staple in the writings of many physicians, such as Ibn al-Muṭrān. But none of the physicians in this circle wrote a single treatise on preservation of health. This is all the more remarkable in view of their successes in the courts, where most physicians composed treatises of this type.[74] The circle was also apparently uninterested in writing on philosophical debates despite their engagement with Ibn Sīnā.[75] Instead, their writings focused on strictly practical issues, such as evacuation, or on specific diseases, such as dropsy (*al-istisqāʾ*) and joint pain.

The fact that a number of the members of the circle were oculists before learning theoretical medicine may have contributed to anchoring the

[73] Sharaf al-Dīn al-Raḥbī (d. 1269) wrote a treatise entitled "The Creation of man (*Khalq al-Insān*)," which may have been a treatise on anatomy as well (Ibn Abī Usaybiʿah, *ʿUyūn al-Anbāʾ*, 4: 207). Also, the commentaries on the *Kulliyyāt* (first book) of *al-Qānūn* written by Kamāl al-Dīn al-Ḥimṣī (d. 1215) or Najm al-Dīn al-Labbūdī (d. after 1268) must have included sections on anatomy. However, Ibn al-Nafīs' work was unprecedented in its adding the anatomical parts in the third book to the first book in a single commentary.

[74] Treatises on dieting for the healthy and on the preservation of health were frequently dedicated to royal or courtly patrons by their physicians. For instance, Maimonides (d. 1204) dedicated his "On the regimen of health" to the Ayyūbid king al-Malik al-Afḍal b. Ṣalāḥ al-Dīn (Maimonides, *Moses Maimonides' Two Treatises on the Regimen of Health: Fī Tadbīr Al-Ṣiḥḥah, and Maqālah Fī Bayān Baʿḍ Al-Aʿrāḍ Wa-Al-Jawāb ʿanhā*). Also, Ibn al-Muṭrān (d. 1191) wrote a similar treatise dedicated to Ṣalāḥ al-Dīn entitled "*al-Maqālah al-Nāṣiriyyah fī Ḥifẓ al-Umūr al-Ṣiḥḥiyyah* (The Treatise [dedicated to] al-Nāṣir [Ṣalāḥ al-Dīn] on the preservation of health.)" (Ibn Abī Usaybiʿah, *ʿUyūn al-Anbāʾ*, 4: 131.) This conclusion about their writings is based on the bio-bibliographies composed by Ibn Abī Uṣaybiʿah, who was in close relation with this circle.

[75] An exception to that might be Ibn al-Nafīs, although his engagement with Ibn Sīnā's philosophical system was largely through his physiology. Fancy, *Science and Religion in Mamluk Egypt*.

circle's interest in practice. Al-Raḥbī and al-Dakhwār, along with Ibn Abī Uṣaybiʿah himself, were all oculists. Ibn al-Nafīs wrote a significant treatise on ocular medicine, which indicated a preference for practice and experimentation even in its title: "*al-muhadhdhab fī al-kuḥl al-mujarrab* (the well-arranged [book] on experimented ocular [medicine]."[76] This interest and experience in a more practical branch of medicine may have influenced their outlook on practice as a whole. The group's interest in theory, however, appeared to be informed by and limited to *al-Qānūn* and the easily readable *Questions* of Ḥunayn. Probably one of the more illustrative examples of this circle's practice- and disease-oriented approach can be seen in Ibn al-Nafīs's commentary on the *Aphorisms* – a book of practice in itself – in which he engaged with Ibn Abī Ṣādiq's commentary and showed his specific priorities and interests.

Ibn al-Nafīs' Commentary on the Aphorisms

Ibn Riḍwān's eleventh-century list of Hippocrates' works recognized the *Aphorisms* and the *Foreknowledge* as two texts that introduce the dogmatist physician to practice. According to Ibn Riḍwān, the dogmatist physician should memorize the "plain text" of the *Aphorisms*, then the *Foreknowledge*, after studying the *Nature of Man*.[77] The *Aphorisms* was most likely considered a practical text because of the little attention it gave to theoretical consideration or to physiological and anatomical consideration. Yet the text's focus on practice also meant that it considered questions of preservation of health, food and nourishment for the healthy, and differences in nourishment based on location and weather. Ibn Abī Ṣādiq explained in his commentary:

> This [first] treatise includes twenty-three aphorisms; one is the opening of the book (*muftataḥ al-kitāb*), one on a general rule (*qānūn kullī*), eleven aphorisms on arranging the nourishment of the sick, four aphorisms on the nourishment of the healthy, and six aphorisms on the rules of evacuation.[78]

Ibn al-Nafīs' commentary on the *Aphorisms* followed the Hippocratic text in its focus on practice. Ibn al-Nafīs had different views, however, on the arrangement of the text into treatises and on the ordering of the aphorisms themselves. He did not think the book was originally divisible into treatises: "The division of this book into seven treatises was not done

[76] Ibn Al-Nafīs, *Al-Muhadhdhab fī al-Kuḥl al-Mujarrab*.
[77] Rosenthal, "An Eleventh-Century List of the Works of Hippocrates," 159.
[78] Ibn Abī Ṣādiq al-Nīsābūri, "Sharḥ Fuṣūl Buqrāṭ," 3v.

by Hippocrates, in my view, as the beginnings of [each] treatise is connected to the end of the one before it. Rather, this [division] was done by the commentators and we will not follow it."[79] The common division of the text to which Ibn al-Nafīs objected divided the text into seven treatises: the first addressed nourishment and evacuation;[80] the second addressed crises (*al-buḥrān*), referring to crises at the end of diseases and disease symptoms;[81] the third addressed "airs and ages";[82] the fourth "evacuation and the mention of sweat and fevers";[83] the fifth "the signs of diseases, [as well as] the diseases of women";[84] the sixth "the symptoms occurring in [specific] diseases"; and the seventh "the signs forbearing good or bad [prognosis]."[85]

Ibn al-Nafīs' argument against the division had significant implications on the reading of the text and its overall value. For instance, let us consider that in Ibn Abī Ṣādiq's commentary, the third treatise was viewed as a discussion of general rules about the effect of different weathers and airs on health and disease, as well as the rules describing the healthy and diseased states of different ages.[86] By linking this third treatise with the previous one on the development of diseases and their symptoms and with the following one on evacuation and fevers, however, Ibn al-Nafīs saw the third treatise as focusing on diseases and treatments, modifying how aphorisms were understood to essentially remove issues related to healthy conditions. Consequently, in his commentary, the third treatise became the locus for a description of the effects of weather and its changes on diseases and on the different complexions of different ages. The focus was now specifically on the means of knowing what diseases affected people and at what times, rather than on the means of understanding how to preserve their health.

This different understanding of the third treatise can be further illustrated by comparing Ibn al-Nafīs's and Ibn Abī Ṣādiq's commentaries on the treatise's particular aphorisms. For instance, one aphorism reads: "Considering the conditions of weather in general throughout the year,

[79] Ibn al-Nafīs, *Sharḥ Fuṣul Abuqrāṭ*, 117. Although Ibn al-Nafīs was opposed to the division, at least two of the manuscripts used by Yusuf Zidan in the edition of the commentary on the aphorisms reverted to the original division into seven treatises.

[80] Ibn Abī Ṣādiq al-Nīsābūri, "Sharḥ Fuṣūl Buqrāṭ," 3v.

[81] Ibn al-Nafīs, *Sharḥ Fuṣul Abuqrāṭ*, 117. The subjects of the treatises were those used in a number of manuscripts of Ibn al-Nafīs' commentary that reverted to the original division, albeit while mentioning the author's dismissal of such division.

[82] Ibid., 153.

[83] Ibid., 191.

[84] Ibid., 241.

[85] Ibid., 321.

[86] Ibn Abī Ṣādiq al-Nīsābūri, "Sharḥ Fuṣūl Buqrāṭ," 32r.

less rain is healthier (*aṣaḥ*), and less mortal (*aqall mawtan*)." Ibn Abī Ṣādiq considered this aphorism a general rule about health and healthy behaviors and explained the aphorism in relation to how healthy organs thrive better in drier conditions.[87] For Ibn al-Nafīs, the aphorism was about diseases and how they become more frequent and more deadly during rainy weather. He centered his commentary on rottenness as the reason for the greater number of diseases and for the more mortal ones occurring during rainy seasons.[88]

Moreover, Ibn al-Nafīs' commentary was infused with his own experience and practice. For instance, in reference to an aphorism that states "If at one time during the year, in one day, [one finds] a time of heat and a time of cold, expect the occurrence of autumn diseases," Ibn Abī Ṣādiq's commentary was a single sentence that explained: "This is because it would be similar to the weather of the autumn, so generating the diseases generated by autumn [weather]."[89] Ibn al-Nafīs, conversely, had a much longer explanation that focused on how this aphorism indicated an expectation but should not be considered a rule. Motivated by his practice and his own observations, he continued to explain how these changes in weather must be severe and must last for an extended period, not just a day, for them to create the effects described by Hippocrates.[90] Ibn al-Nafīs's commentary was concerned with diseases and not with questions of health preservation, unlike Ibn Abī Ṣādiq's writing, which paid more attention to the discussion of health and its preservation. Although members of al-Dakhwār's circle read Ibn Abī Ṣādiq's work diligently and respected the author, they did not necessarily accept all his arguments, as evident by al-Dakhwār's response to the author and Ibn al-Nafīs's approach to the *Aphorisms*.

Other treatises in the *Aphorisms* seemed to have focused on different subjects for each author. Ibn Abī Ṣādiq explained that the first treatise concerned nourishment and evacuation and that it contained aphorisms on nourishment for the healthy and for the sick.[91] This identification and arrangement is similar to the contents of the well-known translation attributed to Ḥunayn ibn Isḥāq, on which both Ibn al-Nafīs and Ibn Abī Ṣādiq most probably depended in their commentaries. Ibn al-Nafīs, however, described the treatise as one addressing "the arrangements (*al-tadbīr*)

87 Ibn Abī Ṣādiq Al-Nīsābūri, "Sharḥ Fuṣūl Buqrāṭ," 36v.
88 Ibn al-Nafīs, *Sharḥ Fuṣul Abuqrāṭ*, 169.
89 Ibid., 33r–v.
90 Ibn al-Nafīs, *Sharḥ Fuṣul Abuqrāṭ*, 156.
91 Ibn Abī Ṣādiq Al-Nīsābūri, "Sharḥ Fuṣūl Buqrāṭ," 3v.

[in relation to] patients and diseases."[92] Consistent with this view, Ibn al-Nafīs considered all the nourishment-related aphorisms in the treatise to be related to diseases, to the nourishment of the sick, and to evacuations. Therefore, Ibn al-Nafīs chose to order the aphorisms differently from Ḥunayn and Ibn Abī Ṣādiq and in a manner that better served the treatise's purpose as Ibn al-Nafīs saw it.

Consider the fourteenth aphorism in Ibn Abī Ṣādiq, which he considered to be the first of four aphorisms discussing the nourishment of the healthy. The aphorism reads "The elderly (*al-mashāyikh*) are the most tolerant of people for fasting, followed by the seniors (*al-kuhūl*), and the young (*al-fityān*). The least tolerant of fasting are the children (*al-ṣibyān*), and whoever of them has more desire [for food], he will be less tolerant of [fasting]." Ibn Abī Ṣādiq explained, "He [Hippocrates] moves in this aphorism to the discussion of the nourishment of the healthy" and then proceeded to understand fasting as a decrease of food for the healthy.[93] Ibn al-Nafīs located the same aphorism in the middle of a discussion about nourishment for the sick. Although he admitted that it indicated a rule that is applicable to both healthy and diseased individuals, he moved quickly to explaining it in terms of feeding the ill, which fits with his general arrangement of the treatise.[94]

A more significant difference occurs in a discussion of the second aphorism, which Ibn Abī Ṣādiq read as the articulation of a general rule. The long aphorism starts by explaining that "the severe increase in body mass (*khuṣb al-badan*) for those [used to] sport [and exertion] is dangerous," and it continues to explain how such increase, which these people are not used to, can cause diseases and that their weight needs to be reduced rapidly to avoid such problems. The aphorism concludes that evacuation should be careful and gradual since "any evacuation that reaches the maximum is dangerous, and any nourishment that reaches the maximum is dangerous as well." Ibn Abī Ṣādiq explained that this is a general rule of medicine and indicated that extreme measures are dangerous and should be avoided.[95] In Ibn al-Nafīs' commentary, this aphorism is actually the third (not the second). Instead, the second aphorism is one that describes the general rules of evacuation: "If what is evacuated from the body through voluntary diarrhea or vomiting is of the kind from which the body should be cleansed, this [evacuation] will be useful and easy to

[92] Ibn al-Nafīs, *Sharḥ Fuṣūl Ibiqrāṭ*, 73.
[93] Ibn Abī Ṣādiq al-Nīsābūri, "Sharḥ Fuṣūl Buqrāṭ," 12r.
[94] Ibn al-Nafīs, *Sharḥ Fuṣul Abuqrāṭ*, 94.
[95] Ibn Abī Ṣādiq al-Nīsābūri, "Sharḥ Fuṣūl Buqrāṭ," 5v.

bear."[96] However, this aphorism on evacuation is the eighteenth aphorism in Ibn Abī Ṣādiq.[97]

Both Ibn al-Nafīs and Ibn Abī Ṣādiq shared the opinion that this aphorism laid out the general rule for evacuation. It is for this reason that the difference in arrangement is especially significant: in Ibn al-Nafīs' version, this aphorism, being the second in the first treatise and in the entire book, sets up the entire treatise to focus on the management of diseases and highlights the evacuation aphorisms as the central ones throughout the treatise. In Ibn Abī Ṣādiq, this aphorism, as Number Eighteen, opens a subsection on evacuation, thus allowing the beginning of the treatise to function as a discussion of nourishment for the healthy. In this way, Ibn al-Nafīs rearranged the entire treatise to tuck the aphorisms on healthy nourishment between those discussing evacuation and nourishment for the sick, thereby changing the outlook and the value of the entire treatise.

Ibn al-Nafīs was aware of the unique ordering of the aphorisms in his commentary and that this ordering was significant to the utility of the book. In the beginning of the commentary, he explained that "[As] we have mentioned in explaining this book, this book's copies are different based on the different aims of those seeking it. In this copy, we follow what we find most worthy of commentaries and best in composition."[98] In his explanation of his third aphorism, which is Ibn Abī Ṣādiq's second, Ibn al-Nafīs explained why the other commentators placed that aphorism earlier: "This aphorism was [mentioned] first [in other copies and commentaries] because it contained a general rule that should be brought forward, which is that excess is dangerous."[99] Although he understood why this aphorism was mentioned earlier in other commentaries, he chose to push it to the back to better serve the way he thought the entire book of *Aphorisms* should be read. As a result of this rearrangement, Ibn al-Nafīs'

[96] Ibn al-Nafīs, *Sharḥ Fuṣul Abuqrāṭ*, 76–7.

[97] Ibid., 14v.

[98] Ibid., 73. Yusuf Zidan, the commentary's editor, chose a version of the text that would read "[As for] our previous commentaries on this book, their copies [the commentaries] are different based on the different aims of those seeking it." He argues that this stands as evidence that Ibn al-Nafīs composed several commentaries on the *Aphorisms*. There is no other evidence that Ibn al-Nafīs composed more than one commentary on the *Aphorisms*, nor was it customary to do so, let alone to write commentaries that are admittedly different from one another. The more accurate reading, in my view, is the one just presented, wherein Ibn al-Nafīs commented on the different arrangement of his commentary compared to other known commentaries, such as Ibn Abī Ṣādiq's, or other copies, such as Ḥunayn's. This is consistent with similar notes in the beginning of the treatises and in the third aphorism, as will be seen later.

[99] Ibid., 80.

commentary, especially on the first chapter of the *Aphorisms*, was entirely dominated by evacuation and its rules and mentioned only infrequently nourishment for the healthy.

Ibn al-Nafīs constructed his work on the *Aphorisms* in a way similar to his commentary on the anatomy of *al-Qānūn*: he decided to rearrange the *Aphorisms* to deliver what he understood as the central point of the text more effectively, much like he rearranged *al-Qānūn* to deliver a coherent and clearer explanation of anatomy. In both cases, Ibn al-Nafīs' commentary revealed a significant practice-oriented bias, valuing the knowledge acquired through experience. Even more significantly, this practice-oriented approach was arranged around diseases; it valued anatomical knowledge that viewed diseases through their connection to the body's anatomy. We can see this tendency not only in Ibn al-Nafīs' writings but also in the writings of all the members of al-Dakhwār's circle, who came to dominate both bīmāristān and court practice in the Levant and Egypt from the second half of the thirteenth century. There is little doubt that Ibn al-Nafīs was more philosophically educated and more theoretically inclined than his colleagues – the other students of al-Dakhwār – as evident by his more philosophical writings such as "*al-Risālah al-Kāmiliyyah.*"[100] Yet different members of the circle appreciated al-Rāzī's works despite the latter's medical-theoretical differences with Ibn Sīnā, let alone his widely unpopular philosophical writings. A possible explanation of this admiration for al-Rāzī by a circle dominated by Ibn Sīnā's physiology and philosophy is al-Rāzī's emphasis on practice and his discussion of his cases and experimentations, which had no parallel in Ibn Sīnā. Together, the two writers formed a coherent body of medical knowledge, with al-Rāzī's inclination toward practice complementing the theoretical and philosophical Avicennian corpus.

Did al-Dakhwār's Circle Force the Islamization of Medical Practice?

In her paper "Medicine for Muslims?" Paulina Lewicka discusses the conditions of non-Muslim physicians from the eleventh to the fourteenth centuries, concluding:

> Doubtlessly, the theologians set the medical culture on a new course. Doubtlessly, they contributed to re-evaluating the notion of "*ṭibb*" which,

[100] On this question, see Fancy, "The Virtuous Son of the Rational: A Traditionalist's Response to Falāsifa" and *Science and Religion in Mamluk Egypt.*

> once free of theology and religion, now gained a religious attribute and lost its universal character. Moreover, their increased command of theoretical medical knowledge, combined with taking over a part of theoretical medical education and with the (presumed) promotion of the revised *al-ṭibb al-nabawī*, made it possible to introduce a religious segregation to medical culture.[101]

These changes, she argues, resulted in the fact that "medical practice was left to professionals who did not or could not, for various reasons, study medical theory." Yet these changes, she explains, did not result in any significant shift in the number of medical practitioners of different religious affiliations, and these same theologians continued to consult non-Muslim physicians up to the sixteenth century.[102] Lewicka's thesis that the Islamization of medical practice coupled with the decline of theoretical medical learning was due to the dominance of religious scholars rests on two main issues, both connected to the circle of physicians around al-Bīmāristān al-Nūrī and the socioprofessional context in which they practiced. The first of these issues is the influence of figures like Raḍiyy al-Dīn al-Raḥbī, who was said to have refused to teach medicine to non-Muslims. Second, she argues that the incorporation of medical education in the madrasa curricula and the creation of new medical madrasas such as that of al-Dakhwār limited access to medical education to Muslims only (since non-Muslims could not attend madrasas). These two processes, led by al-Raḥbī, al-Dakhwār, and their students, were in part responding to religious scholars' complaints against non-Muslims' dominating medical practice, such as those registered in Ibn al-Ukhuwwa's (d. 1329) *ḥisbah* manual, which explained that learning medicine was a communal religious obligations on Muslims (*farḍ kifāyah*).[103]

Indeed, al-Raḥbī did not teach medicine to non-Muslims except for only two: ʿImrān al-Isrāʾīlī (d. 1275), a Jewish physician who spent most of his career in al-Bīmāristān al-Nūrī, frequenting some of the Levantine Ayyubid courts but without any consistent service, and Ibrāhīm b. Khalaf al-Sāmirī, who did not receive much accolade either. Al-Raḥbī explained to his protégé and biographer Ibn Abī Uṣaybiʿah that these two non-Muslim physicians pressured him in many ways and used important figures as intermediaries until he acquiesced. Their persistence coupled with pressure from worthy friends apparently convinced al-Raḥbī of their talent and

[101] Lewicka, *Medicine for Muslims?*, 16.
[102] Ibid., 17; Ibn al-Ukhūwah, *Maʿālim al-Qurba*, 166.
[103] Lewicka, *Medicine for Muslims?*, 5.

dedication.[104] Al-Raḥbī's refusal to teach non-Muslims is remarkable seeing that one of his masters was, in fact, Ibn Jamīʿ al-Miṣrī, a Jewish physician. Yet, Ibn Jamīʿ did not seem to have helped al-Raḥbī advance his career, and al-Raḥbī did not establish any prominence until he became associated with Muhadhdhab al-Dīn al-Naqqāsh in Damascus, who introduced him to Ṣalāḥ al-Dīn's court. Before that, Raḍiyy al-Dīn al-Raḥbī practiced in a modest shop in Damascus and languished in obscurity. Why or how his relationship with Ibn Jamīʿ ended is not clear, although it is not unlikely that this unsuccessful association impacted al-Raḥbī's attitudes toward non-Muslims. While al-Raḥbī was studying with al-Naqqāsh, Ibn al-Muṭrān (a Christian) was also studying with the same master. Ibn al-Muṭrān, however, was likely closer to the master, as the former's father was a colleague of al-Naqqāsh himself in Baghdad under Ibn al-Tilmīdh.[105] Ibn al-Muṭrān's career advanced much more quickly than that of al-Raḥbī.

Ibn Abī Uṣaybiʿah explained that al-Raḥbī had taught a great many important physicians: "if [one] considered the majority of the physicians in the Levant, [he] would find that [they] either read with al-Raḥbī or read with someone who read with him." Moreover, "al-Shaykh Raḍiyy al-Dīn said to me one day, 'all those who read with me and accompanied me became prominent and people benefitted from them.' He mentioned to me the names of many of them who became prominent and famous in the art of medicine, some of whom died, and some were distant in life [from us]."[106] Based on these two statements, Lewicka concludes that al-Raḥbī's hatred of and reluctance to teach non-Muslims had probably spread throughout the Levant and Egypt with his numerous students. Yet Ibn Abī Uṣaybiʿah failed to report any of the names of Raḍiyy al-Dīn al-Raḥbī's students.[107] We have more evidence as to al-Raḥbī's stature in the Damascene medical scene in comparison with al-Dakhwār, who was presumably one of those who read with him. Ibn Abī Uṣaybiʿah reported that after al-Raḥbī was introduced to Ṣalāḥ al-Dīn in Damascus (around

[104] Ibn Abī Usaybiʿah, *ʿUyūn al-Anbāʾ*, 4: 190.

[105] Ibid., 4: 131.

[106] Ibid., 4: 190.

[107] Throughout Ibn Abī Uṣaybiʿah's dictionary, only three of al-Raḥbī's students are biographied: ʿImrān al-Isrāʾīlī (4: 256), who was mentioned earlier and worked at al-Bīmāristān al-Nūrī; Kamāl al-Dīn al-Ḥimṣī (4: 209); and Fakhr al-Dīn ibn al-Sāʿātī (4: 160). Al-Ḥimṣī was a merchant and practiced in the bīmāristān first with no salary but then was appointed with a salary. Ibn Abī Uṣaybiʿah mentioned that he read *al-Qānūn* with al-Makhzūmī, casting some doubt on the role al-Raḥbī played in his education. Like his father, Ibn al-Sāʿātī was, in fact, a clock-maker. He was also a student of Fakhr al-Dīn al-Mārdīnī, a far more prominent scholar than al-Raḥbī, and he worked in al-ʿĀdil's court.

1174), the latter liked him and ordered him a salary of thirty dinars to frequent the court and bīmāristān. This arrangement was renewed under al-ʿĀdil I, when he succeeded Ṣalāh al-Dīn in Damascus in 1193. When al-Malik al-Muʿaẓẓam b. al-ʿĀdil took over after his father's death in 1218, however, al-Raḥbī was asked to frequent the bīmāristān only, and his salary was reduced to fifteen dinars. This remained his salary until he died in 1234.[108] Conversely, in 1208, when al-Dakhwār was still at the beginning of his career, he was offered thirty dinars to frequent the castle alongside the famous physician Muwaffaq al-Dīn ibn ʿAbd al-ʿAzīz al-Salamī (d. 1208). Al-Dakhwār rejected the offer because al-Salamī's salary was a hundred dinars, in addition to other salaries, rewards, and gifts amounting to several hundred dinars. Al-Dakhwār added: "I know my stature in the science and I will not serve with [less than] his salary."[109] One month later, al-Salamī died and al-Dakhwār was appointed with al-Salamī's salaries, as he desired.

Al-Dakhwār's anecdote is significant in showing that payments and salaries were considered important in determining a physician's worth and a patron's appreciation of his knowledge and work. Even in Ibn Abī Uṣaybiʿah's world of biographies, where the ideal medical practitioner was always portrayed as pious, charitable, and with little care for material rewards, payments from the court or from rich patrons acquired different meaning than those from the bīmāristān or from poor patients, with whom the ideals of charity would most appropriately apply.[110] In this regard, al-Raḥbī's acceptance of a salary of fifteen dinars to attend the castle is remarkable and reflective of his stature in the medical environment of Ayyubid Damascus. In this context, where apprenticeship and connections to masters had important professional implications, it is hard to understand why so many Levantine physicians would take al-Raḥbī as their master and mentor, unless this mentorship was for a brief period and in connection to specific readings, much like al-Dakhwār's was early in his career.

Al-Dakhwār, who came from a family of oculists and was an oculist himself, started his medical education by reading al-Majūsī's *al-Malakī* with al-Raḥbī before attaching himself to Ibn al-Muṭrān, whom he followed and accompanied. Here, reading with al-Raḥbī, a modest yet known physician, introduced al-Dakhwār to medicine. However, al-Raḥbī's

[108] Ibid., 4: 189.
[109] Ibid., 4: 320.
[110] Here, it is important to note that Ibn Abī Uṣaybiʿah's biography of al-Dakhwār, his students, and other members of his circle was very flattering and intended to cast them in a very positive light because Ibn Abī Uṣaybiʿah belonged to this circle and because they had direct access to his writings, as he himself mentioned several times.

mentorship could not serve more than an introduction. Al-Dakhwār had to move to a more remarkable, better connected master, such as Ibn al-Muṭrān, to lead him through the field. It is likely that other physicians and students would have followed the same route. It appears that Ibn Abī Uṣaybiʿah, himself a physician who failed to attach himself to lucrative court positions and who showed in his writings great piety and knowledge of religious sciences, identified more with al-Raḥbī and exaggerated his influence and his importance. It is significant that the biographer failed to mention any of al-Raḥbī's students and tried to dismiss possible questions about them by claiming that they died a long time ago (and therefore were forgotten) or traveled far away. Although al-Raḥbī's attitude toward non-Muslims could indicate a more profound process of Islamization of medical practice, as will be discussed later, he might not have held as much influence in setting or spreading this attitude as Ibn Abī Uṣaybiʿah would have his readers believe. Contrary to al-Raḥbī, al-Dakhwār, whose influence was unquestionable, did not seem to hold such strong views about teaching non-Muslims, as he himself was a student of Ibn al-Muṭrān and had a number of non-Muslim students, such as Rashīd al-Dīn b. Abī Ḥulayqah (b. 1194), who eventually became the chief physician in Egypt.[111] Close to the end of his career, al-Dakhwār used considerable sums of the fortunes he accumulated in his court service to build a madrasa for teaching medicine in Damascus. Medical madrasas were not common, and, as such, the project showed al-Dakhwār's commitment to medicine and medical education. Al-Dakhwar appointed his favorite students to lead the madrasa and created a rich *waqf* to support its functioning. Although it is not clear whether non-Muslims were allowed to study in al-Dakhwār's madrasa, it is likely that they were not and that, similar to other law madrasas, which al-Dakhwār may have attempted to emulate, it allowed only Muslims to study there.

In 1223, shortly before al-Dakhwār opened his madrasa, al-Malik al-Ashraf (d. 1237) of Damascus decreed to restrict the scholars appointed in the madrasas to their own fields, effectively demanding they abandon the study of "ancient sciences." Lewicka argues that this decree had detrimental effects on the study of medical theory because it prevented medical students from learning philosophy and that it contributed to a shift to practice that led to the deterioration of medical knowledge in general. However, there is no evidence that this decree had any serious effects on

111 Ibid., 3: 489.

the ground, whether in general or in relation to medicine.[112] In fact, and as mentioned before, al-Dakhwār (d. 1231), who was close to the court and whose madrasa was supported by al-Malik al-Ashraf, studied philosophy close to the end of his life, most likely after 1223 and al-Ashraf's decision. His students continued to teach and learn these sciences throughout the second half of the thirteenth century under the auspices of al-Malik al-Ashraf himself. Recent studies had questioned the assumption that religious scholars were successful in launching a whole-sale attack on philosophy and "rational sciences" during the thirteenth century.[113] The shift toward practice could be hardly linked to any influence from Muslim conservative scholars and should not be seen apart from the enduring influence of Ibn Sīnā, who was, as seen earlier, the main source of theoretical medicine at the time. Ibn Sīnā became all the more popular in the fourteenth and fifteenth centuries, and his writings were even more influential. As discussed earlier, the shift toward practical medicine was not related to a rejection of philosophy or theoretical sciences but was rooted in the influence of certain circles of physicians, all of whom were theoretically trained and comfortable with theory and had little to do with any anti-philosophy tendencies. Instead, their connection to the bīmāristān marked their priorities and accentuated their interests in practice. The study of the fate of non-Muslim physicians needs to be located within the larger changes and measures affecting non-Muslims under the Mamluks, as well as the attempts at forced conversions and persecution that gradually resulted in major demographic shifts in the region over the thirteenth and fourteenth centuries, thus sealing its fate as a Muslim-majority region once and for all.

The complaint against Christians and Jews dominating medical practice in Islamdom was not new, by any means, and must have influenced al-Raḥbī, al-Dakhwār, and their students and patrons. We find such complaints in al-Jāḥiz's (d. 868) writings in the ninth century, just as Arabophone Galenism was starting to take off, ushered forward by the

[112] Lewicka, *Medicine for Muslims?*, 8. Lewicka cites Ibn Kathīr (d. 1373), who was a conservative scholar, a member of Ibn al-Qayyim's circle, and hardly an unbiased source in this regard, and who consistently highlighted similar decisions or measures and exaggerated their importance. Yet even Ibn Kathīr's reporting of this decision and its renewal in the annals of the Hijri years 626 (1223), 631 (1233), 635 (1237) is a telltale sign of the ineffectiveness of such a decision on the ground, prompting its supporters to demand its reissuance.

[113] Dimitri Gutas called this period "the Golden Age of Arabic philosophy": Gutas, "The Heritage of Avicenna: The Golden Age of Arabic Philosophy, 1000–ca. 1350." Also, Fancy, *Science and Religion in Mamluk Egypt*, 37–40.

translations carried out largely by non-Muslims.[114] Similarly, the communal religious obligation to learn medicine (*farḍ kifāyah*) was not new but can be traced back to the writings of Ibn Ḥanbal and al-Shāfiʿī in the ninth century.[115] These consistent complaints were perhaps behind Qalāwūn's interest in teaching medicine to Muslim students. As seen before, Qalāwūn's decrees to appoint the chief physician and the bīmāristān instructor recalled the obligation to teach medicine, lamented its neglect, and took on the responsibility for spreading medical learning. As such, the decrees compared the bīmāristān to a madrasa as a site of spreading useful knowledge and teaching. These public lectures were not new, as a lesson was given at Ibn Ṭūlūn's mosque, which was obviously restricted to Muslims, and which may have originated in al-Bīmāristān al-Ṭūlūnī and moved to the mosque after the bīmāristān fell into ruins.

As teaching in the bīmāristān became part of the duties of the chief physician, the chief physician had to be Muslim. The effect of the stipulation in al-Manṣūr Qalāwūn's *waqf* and bīmāristān was palpable immediately because the sultan's three physicians, preparing to assume the position of chief physician and to teach in the bīmāristān, were made to convert to Islam prior to assuming the office. In the centuries to come in the history of al-Bīmāristān al-Manṣūrī, there would be no non-Muslim chief physician: the position continued to be connected to the bīmāristān, and non-Muslims would have to convert to occupy it. However, this absence of non-Muslims from the top of the medical hierarchy contrasts with their consistent domination of medical practice in the streets and markets, as evident by Ibn al-Ukhuwwa's statement some decades after the inauguration of the bīmāristān. The restriction on employing non-Muslims in the bīmāristān should be read within the context of professional competition over positions, which gradually became the hallmark of the thirteenth- and fourteenth-century politics in the Levant and Egypt. In this context, bureaucrats and scholars occupying state positions were keen on removing non-Muslims as possible competitors for such positions. The same period, in which al-Bīmāristān al-Manṣūrī's *waqf* was promulgated, witnessed severe attacks on non-Muslim bureaucrats, who were forced to convert or be removed from office. We should read the stipulation in al-Bīmāristān al-Manṣūrī's *waqf* document in this same context: it was primarily a (largely successful) attack on non-Muslim bureaucrats and an

[114] On translations, see Gutas, *Greek Thought, Arabic Culture*. Also Sabra, "The Appropriation and Subsequent Naturalization of Greek Science in Medieval Islam: A Preliminary Statement."

[115] Lewicka, *Medicine for Muslims?*, 12.

attempt to institutionalize their expulsion from state and religious positions. These decisions influenced physicians, as the chief physician became necessarily a Muslim. There is little evidence, however, that this measure was directed toward physicians in particular or that it was followed up with any other similar decisions aimed at the elimination of non-Muslim physicians.

Perhaps we need to revisit Ibn al-Ukhuwwa's statement. Ibn al-Ukhuwwa explained that non-Muslims dominated the medical field not due to any active action on their part against Muslims; rather, it was due to the unwillingness of Muslims to pursue a field that was far less profitable than the religious sciences and law, which could lead to a position in a madrasa or a role in the expanding Mamluk bureaucracy. For Ibn al-Ukhuwwa, there was a religious need for Muslims to take up medicine. This communal obligation was not satisfied because medicine was largely a difficult and nonprofitable career. Apart from the very few physicians who acquired rich and influential clientele, the vast majority of practitioners languished in obscurity and poverty after prolonged years of study and apprenticeship. They had little access to permanent positions or stable lives, as did students of religious sciences who could, in the worst-case scenario, end up as preachers in small mosques or as teachers in small madrasas and *kuttābs*. The fact that non-Muslims continued to dominate medical practice was a sign of their continued marginalization and alienation from state positions, which left them with the less profitable medical practice, hardly the envy of anyone. That being said, another difficulty facing those who wished to pursue a medical career and who did not descend from medical families was securing a teacher. It is not unlikely that some non-Muslim physicians and teachers harbored sentiments similar to al-Rahbī's about teaching non-Muslims, although they would not have been able to express them so publicly. Qalāwūn's patronizing of public lectures given by no less than the chief physician and his admonition to the chief physician not to reject worthy students were ways to mitigate this difficulty and increase the ranks of Muslim physicians. Yet, the main difficulty that Ibn al-Ukhuwwa complained about was one related to medicine itself, not to its teachers.

The Other Baghdadi Émigré

A little more than ten years after Muhadhdhab al-Dīn al-Naqqāsh's death in 1178, the physician Muwaffaq al-Dīn ʿAbd al-Laṭīf al-Baghdādī (d. 1231) arrived in Damascus as another émigré from Baghdad. He represented a set of trends in the Baghdad medical communities that differed from those of al-Naqqāsh's and his students, such as Ibn al-Muṭrān (d. 1191). Muwaffaq al-Dīn ʿAbd al-Laṭīf al-Baghdādī left Baghdad for Mosul, Damascus, and Egypt in 1189,[116] and he spent the rest of his career in the same milieu as Ibn al-Muṭrān (d. 1191), al-Dakhwār (d. 1231), al-Raḥbī (d. 1234), and their students. Al-Baghdādī did not figure much in our story about the circles surrounding al-Bīmāristān al-Nūrī, al-Nāṣirī, and al-Manṣūrī because he did not serve in any of these bīmāristāns and was not associated with the physicians working there.[117] Al-Baghdādī's writings and activities are important, however, for they show the distinctive nature of al-Dakhwār's circle, and they enable us to better understand this circle's contributions within its context.

Al-Baghdādī's medical pedigree in Baghdad was not clear. He associated himself with Amīn al-Dawlah ibn al-Tilmīdh's estranged son and claimed to have studied with him. Ibn Abī Uṣaybiʿah found this claim unsustainable because this son was not known as a good physician or to have achieved any repute.[118] In fact, reports suggest that this son was deeply alienated from his famous father and had failed to rise up to his father's position. Some reports even suggested that he was mentally ill.[119] Because all these reports can be traced back to Ibn Abī Uṣaybiʿah, we must doubt their authenticity based on Ibn Abī Uṣaybiʿah's bias in favor of Ibn al-Tilmīdh and his line in the Levant, including al-Dakhwār. It seems very unlikely that al-Baghdādī, an otherwise famous physician and a prolific and proud author, would claim association with a person known to have been mentally ill or lacking any repute. What is more likely is that the son's estrangement from his father, which prompted the father to effectively disown his son and openly wish for his death, motivated the father's direct and indirect students such as al-Naqqāsh, Ibn al-Muṭrān, and eventually al-Dakhwār and al-Raḥbī, to claim that the son was unstable and unworthy of his father's favor. These figures were most definitely Ibn Abī Uṣaybiʿah's main sources. Al-Baghdādī's association with the son could indicate that his methods differed from those of Ibn al-Tilmīdh and his followers, as will be affirmed by other evidence.

[116] Ibn Abī Usaybiʿah, *ʿUyūn al-Anbāʾ*, 4: 220.

[117] Al-Baghdādī was a close friend to Ibn Abī Uṣaybiʿah's grandfather and knew his father. He told ibn Abī Uṣaybiʿah's father that he would want to teach the young Ibn Abī Uṣaybiʿah, but the latter, who was closely associated with al-Dakhwār and al-Raḥbī, never studied with al-Baghdādī (4: 213). In fact, Ibn Abī Uṣaybiʿah had some harsh criticism for al-Baghdādī.

[118] Ibid., 4: 218.

[119] Ibn al-Tilmīdh and Kahl, *The Dispensatory of Ibn al-Tilmīḏ*.

Al-Baghdādī was well known for his deep dislike of Ibn Sīnā, a fact that Ibn Abī Uṣaybiʿah attributed to al-Baghdādī's dislike of Persians and his bias to his Baghdadi and Iraqi compatriots.[120] But al-Baghdādī's dislike of Ibn Sīnā could have had deeper roots than his regional biases. For one, he was taught in philosophy, theology (*kalām*), and religious sciences by Baghdadi scholars associated with the al-Niẓāmiyyah madrasa and was impressed with al-Ghazālī and his writings.[121] Also, al-Baghdādī's father, himself a scholar of *ḥadīth*, made sure that his son began his education with *ḥadīth* scholars, many of whom did not appreciate Ibn Sīnā's philosophical writings. Then, in Egypt, al-Baghdādī was introduced to al-Fārābī's writings, as well as to the writings of the ancients, such as Aristotle, and he claimed to have finally found an appreciation for philosophy after reading Ibn Sīnā had made him doubt the usefulness of the entire endeavor.[122] This education left its markings on al-Baghdādī's prolific writings. He wrote profusely on *ḥadīth, tafsir*, and other religious sciences, including a book on "forty medical [prophetic] traditions."[123] He also wrote a number of commentaries and marginalia on al-Fārābī's works, such as *al-Burhān*, and two treatises on al-Fārābī's *al-Madīnah al-Faḍilah*.[124] In medicine, his writings engaged Galen and Hippocrates directly as he commented on a number of their treatises including the *Aphorisms* and the *Foreknowledge*.[125] He also wrote a number of commentaries on Aristotle's works.[126] His engagement with other Islamicate scholars was colored by his deep admiration of the ancients, which led him to write a response to al-Rāzī's doubts on Galen as well as a response to Ibn Riḍwān's treatise on contradictions between Galen and Aristotle.[127] Evidently, he engaged critically with some of Ibn Sīnā's writings and their commentaries, and his clear statements about Ibn Sīnā left no doubt about his feelings toward *al-shaykh al-raʾīs*.

Al-Baghdādī's works and intellectual trajectory stood in opposition to those of al-Dakhwār's circle. Whereas they considered Ibn Sīnā's writings as the main source for philosophical training and for theoretical medicine, al-Baghdādī claimed that they had no value, focusing on al-Fārābī, with whom the circle never engaged. Al-Baghdādī's position toward al-Rāzī seemed similar to that of other figures in the Fatimid Egyptian milieu, as explained

[120] Ibn Abī Usaybiʿah, *ʿUyūn al-Anbāʾ*, 4: 213.
[121] Ibid., 4: 214.
[122] Ibid., 4: 228.
[123] Ibid., 4: 243.
[124] Ibid., 4: 250.
[125] Ibid., 4: 246.
[126] Ibid., 4: 252.
[127] Ibid., 4: 249.

earlier, whereas al-Dakhwār's circle revived al-Rāzī's *al-Ḥāwī* and used it as a main source for their education. Even though al-Baghdādī and al-Dakhwār's circle shared an interest in such books as the *Aphorisms* and the *Foreknowledge*, the authors of al-Dakhwār's circle neglected al-Baghdādī's commentaries and engaged with the older commentaries written by (the Persian) Ibn Abī Ṣādiq, whom they understood to be a student of Ibn Sīnā's. Along with Ibn Abī Uṣaybiʿah's rebuke of al-Baghdādī, Najm al-Dīn al-Labbūdī (d. after 1268), one of al-Dakhwār's students and a member of a long-standing family of Levantine physicians, wrote a treatise entitled "Showing the absurd opinions in the writings of al-Muwaffaq ʿAbd al-Laṭīf [al-Baghdādī]."[128]

Conclusion

In the previous pages, we traced the intellectual interests and trajectories of a circle of physicians that was formed around al-Bīmāristān al-Nūrī under the guidance of Muhadhdhab al-Dīn al-Naqqāsh (d. 1178). The group witnessed its true success and prominence under the guidance of al-Dakhwār (d. 1231), whose distinguished court positions, bīmāristān service, and medical madrasa shaped the medical elite in the Levant and Egypt for more than a century. The connection of al-Dakhwār's circle to bīmāristāns and to bīmāristān practice is evident and played a significant role in their interest in practice. The character of the circle was based on al-Dakhwār and al-Raḥbī, and it had its roots in Muhadhdhab al-Dīn al-Naqqāsh (d. 1178), al-Raḥbī's teacher and connected to al-Dakhwār through Ibn al-Muṭrān. Al-Naqqāsh was the perfect product of Baghdad's most celebrated bīmāristān physician, Amīn al-Dawlah ibn al-Tilmīdh, and he received his training in al-Bīmāristān al-ʿAḍudī, over which Ibn al-Tilmīdh presided. Ibn al-Muṭrān's father was also a student of Ibn al-Tilmīdh, thus further connecting the famous Levantine physician and his student al-Dakhwār to Baghdad's famous bīmāristāns. This deep connection to bimāristāns was manifest not only in the practice of the circle's members but also in the commitment to the bīmāristān "project," evident even in the attitudes of those who did not practice regularly in the bīmāristān and spent most of their careers in courts. For example, Ibn Qāḍī Baʿlabak (d. 1272), one of al-Dakhwār's favorite students, spent most of

[128] Ibid., 4: 165. On Muwaffaq al-Dīn al-Baghdādī, see Pormann and Joosse, "Decline and Decadence in Iraq and Syria after the Age of Avicenna?: ʿAbd al-Latif al-Baghdadi (1162–1231) between Myth and History."

his career in court service until he came back to Damascus to preside over al-Dakhwār's school of medicine. Although he did not practice in al-Bīmāristān al-Nūrī for any extended period of time, he bought a number of houses surrounding al-Nūrī and donated them to the bīmāristān after his death.[129] The history of Ibn al-Nafīs' engagement with the bimāristāns in Cairo and Damascus is not clear. He died less than three years after the inauguration of al-Bīmāristān al-Manṣūrī and may not have been able to practice there at all on account of his old age. Yet he donated his library and his house to al-Bīmāristān al-Manṣūrī after his death, thus showing his commitment to this new bīmāristān.[130]

The interests of this group and their writings were different from other circles surrounding them. Most remarkably, their commitment to Ibn Sīnā's philosophical and theoretical writings never wavered and could have contributed to the rise of the philosopher's importance during the thirteenth and fourteenth centuries, culminating in Ibn al-Nafīs' important contributions to Ibn Sīnā's legacy. Similarly, this circle appeared to have "rediscovered" *al-Ḥāwī* in the Levantine and Egyptian contexts. As mentioned before, *al-Ḥāwī* was collected under the patronage of the Buyid *vizir* Abū al-Fatḥ ibn al-ʿAmīd (d. 976), *vizir* to the Buyid ruler Rukn al-Dawlah, perhaps a decade before Rukn al-Dawlah's son ʿAḍud al-Dawlah built the famous al-Bīmāristān al-ʿAḍudī in Baghdad around 981. It is unlikely that Ibn al-Nadīm (d. 998) was unaware of *al-Ḥāwī* or that he did not see the newly collected book, although he never mentioned the patronage by Ibn al-ʿAmīd. Regardless, we are faced with a particular version of *al-Ḥāwī* that was circulated in Damascus and used primarily by al-Dakhwār's circle in the beginning of the thirteenth century and that was not even known to al-Qifṭī (d. 1248) in Aleppo. It is possible that Ibn al-ʿAmīd's book was different from an earlier "*Ḥāwī*," one which was less organized and much larger in size. Likewise, the collection of the book patronized by Ibn al-ʿAmīd may have lasted for some years and never attracted the attention of Ibn al-Nadīm, all while surviving in al-Bīmāristān al-ʿAḍudī and traveling to the Levant and al-Bīmāristān al-Nūrī with al-Naqqāsh. It is also possible that the book described by Ibn al-Nadīm was later reorganized and summarized in al-Bīmāristān al-ʿAḍudī by Ibn al-Tilmīdh or others and that this new version circulated in Damascus among al-Naqqāsh's students. In addition to *al-Ḥāwī*, we also have twelve other treatises by al-Rāzī, which were used for teaching

[129] Ibn Abī Usaybiʿah, *ʿUyūn al-Anbāʾ*, 4: 375.
[130] Ibn Faḍl Allāh al-ʿUmarī, *Masālik al-Abṣār fī Mamālik al-Amṣār*, 9: 502.

medicine and which could not be found in al-Qifṭī or in Ibn al-Nadīm, thus indicating that they were a product of al-Dakhwār's circle and their associates.

In all cases, al-Dakhwār's circle rehabilitated or forced the dominance of the two authors, Ibn Sīnā and al-Rāzī, and placed more emphasis on practical writings derived from their own experience. They also renewed interest in books such as the *Aphorisms* and the *Foreknowledge*, which they used to stress practical, disease-oriented approaches. Although their interests were not always shared by their contemporaries, their successes and remarkable careers allowed their program of study and practice to dominate the medical scene in the Levant and Egypt throughout the thirteenth and fourteenth centuries. It came to replace the views of the Fatimid elites. In the following chapter, this program will help us better understand the medical practice in the bīmāristāns of the thirteenth and fourteenth centuries in institutions like al-Bīmāristān al-Manṣūrī.

CHAPTER 5

"A House for King and Slave": Patients and Medical Practice in the Bīmāristān

Introduction

Descriptions of the functioning of al-Bīmāristān al-Manṣūrī, available in the *waqf* document or in eyewitness accounts, indicate that the bīmāristān must have consistently produced a trail of paperwork. The *waqf* document required administrators to write down many of the details of their daily work, such as purchase orders for food; herbs and materials used for medications; budgets and money orders issuing funds; purchases of materials needed for patients, from clothes to beddings to food; and the like.[1] Physicians were expected to write down descriptions of patients' conditions and to keep these records close to patients' beds. They likewise had to write down the recipes or medications that they prescribed to patients confined in the bīmāristān.[2] Nonadmitted patients who only sought prescriptions probably received recipes in writing that they took either to local herbalists or to the bīmāristān's druggists.[3] Evidence from practice and eyewitness accounts suggests that this writing routine was not simply a regulation imposed by the *waqf* document and never implemented. Instead, Shihāb al-Dīn al-Nuwayrī (d. 1333), who presided over the bīmāristān for a number of years, described these writing practices as an integral part of the bīmāristān, the Qalawunid complex, and the *waqf* bureaucracy.[4] Ibn Abī Uṣaybiʿah's description of his own work with al-Dakhwār in al-Bīmāristān al-Nūrī indicated that al-Dakhwār wrote down his prescriptions especially if they contained dangerous drugs or unusual recipes.

[1] Ibn Ḥabīb, *Tadhkirat al-Nabīh*, 1: 363.

[2] Ibid., 1: 366.

[3] Evidence of this practice (writing recipes or prescriptions by physicians for patients to take to their herbalists) can be found in the Genizah collection where many such documents exist. See, for instance, Chipman and Lev, "Arabic Prescriptions from the Cairo Genizah" and "Syrups from the Apothecary's Shop: A Genizah Fragment Containing One of the Earliest Manuscripts of Minhaj Al-Dukkan."

[4] Al-Nuwayrī, *Nihāyat al-ʾArab*, 31: 108–09.

These supposedly numerous writings, however, did not survive, thus depriving us of sources to describe medical practice and day-to-day functioning in the bīmāristān. Al-Bīmāristān al-Manṣūrī endured a number of fires, at least one severe earthquake, and a number of renovation projects that may have inadvertently destroyed such records, had they really existed. In the middle of the eighteenth century, the Ottoman emir ʿAbd al-Raḥmān Katkhudā (d. 1778 at about seventy years of age) decided to renovate al-Bīmāristān al-Manṣūrī.[5] Katkhudā could not locate the bīmāristān's *waqf* document and was told that it was lost in a fire.[6] Although this particular document had in fact survived, the failure to find such an important document signified the total organizational disarray of the bīmāristān's "documents." Moreover, even assuming that those in the bīmāristān consistently produced this paperwork, there is no reason to believe it was kept or preserved, especially since most of these documents concerned daily activities that might not have been deemed worth keeping. It is likely that the paper was recycled, washed, or resold.[7] There is, therefore, little available in the way of bīmāristān documents. In this chapter, we will attempt to reconstruct the experience inside al-Bīmāristān al-Manṣūrī using these different sources and references.

Walking the Bīmāristān's Halls

The overall architectural structure of al-Bīmāristān al-Manṣūrī was similar to that of al-Bīmāristān al-Nūrī: a cruciform structure with four *īwāns* surrounding a courtyard. In al-Nūrī, one of the four *īwāns* served as the entryway into the courtyard; the other three were built as true cul-de-sac-like structures. The patients' halls and other rooms opened onto the courtyard beside the *īwāns*. In al-Bīmāristān al-Manṣūrī, a much larger structure, three of the four *īwāns* were true cul-de-sac structures, whereas the fourth opened through an arch into a larger hall. To enter the bīmāristān, patients and visitors had to go through the complex's huge

5 On ʿAbd al-Raḥmān Kathkhudā and his patronage, see Raymond, "Les Constructions de l'Emir ʿAbd al-Raḥmān Katkhudā au Caire"; Behrens-Abouseif, "The Abd al-Rahman Katkhuda Style in 18th Century Cairo"; and Crecelius, "Problems of ʿAbd al-Raḥmān Katkhudā's Leadership of the Qazdughli Faction."

6 ʿIsā, *Tārīkh al-Bīmāristānāt fī al-Islām*, 64–65.

7 On medieval Arabic archives, see El-Leithy, "Living Documents, Dying Archives: Towards a Historical Anthropology of Medieval Arabic Archives." For an earlier context, see Sijpesteijn, *Shaping a Muslim State: The World of a Mid-Eighth Century Egyptian Official.*

portal. The portal was set in three recessed layers, fostering the same inviting appearance we saw in al-Bīmāristān al-Nūrī and setting the entrance off from the outside.

Whereas those entering al-Bīmāristān al-Nūrī through its portal would have passed through a domed vestibule, the entrance to the Qalawunid complex was more complex and intricate. The portal led to a main corridor, which functioned as an extension to the street. The mausoleum (on the right, northeast) and the madrasa (on the left, southeast) overlooked the corridor through windows similar to those that opened onto the street. The entrances to the mausoleum and to the madrasa were located at the far end of the corridor facing one another, marking the end of the corridor/street and ushering the entrance to the bīmāristān. A series of domes led those approaching the bīmāristān to their left then to their right through an L-shaped corridor, which in turn opened onto the main courtyard of the bīmāristān just beside the east *īwān* (and not through the *īwān* as in al-Bīmāristān al-Nūrī). The relatively long L-shaped corridor isolated the environment inside the bīmāristān from the outside, effectively dampening street noise and creating the feeling of a limited, well-organized environment within. The long corridor between the mausoleum and the madrasa, as well as the L-shaped corridor leading to the bīmāristān's courtyard, would have taken the patient or the visitor through a relatively dark or shaded pathway from the sunny street to yet another sunny courtyard inside the hospital. This courtyard had a basin at its center and possibly arranged plants on its sides (as was the case in al-Bīmāristān al-Nūrī). The contrast between the busy dusty street and the calm, well-manicured courtyard separated by the dark corridor must have served to emphasize the healing and transformative function of the bīmāristān.

To the right side of those entering the bīmāristān, at the beginning of the L-shaped domed corridor, there would have stood a large wooden gate, effectively forcing them to take a left-turn along the L-shaped corridor. The gate separated the main entrance to the bīmāristān from another section that lay right behind the mausoleum, separated from it by the continuation of the L-shaped corridor. The section was made of two halls: one opened onto the main corridor with a door facing the back of mausoleum, whereas the other, completely separate from the first, opened at the end of the corridor with a smaller gate and was located perpendicular to the corridor in a manner that protected its inhabitants from view. The *waqf* document informs us that these two halls were dedicated to the melancholics (or the mad), with one serving males and the other serving females.[8] The arrangement of the two halls suggests that the farther one was probably dedicated to females. Removed from the regular movement of patients and visitors, the halls of the melancholic were tucked away in the far end of the complex behind the mausoleum. The halls had only this single entrance, which lay effectively outside the bīmāristān itself. As al-Nuwayrī explained, the two halls for the melancholics had running water, in the form of a basin, itself probably surrounded by greenery.[9] These halls appeared to have been divided into small stalls or cells where the melancholics would have been kept. The separation of these halls from the rest of the bīmāristān prompted the Mamluk historian Aḥmad b. Muḥammad al-Fayyūmī (d. ca. 1368) to designate this section as "the bīmāristān of the mad" (*bīmāristān al-majānīn*).[10]

The four *īwāns*, similar to the *īwāns* in al-Bīmāristān al-Nūrī, surrounded a basin. Both the Eastern and Western *īwāns* were elongated in shape and narrower at the end. The Northern one opened into a larger hall with columns, which might have been a place for the sick, as will be explained later. The Southern *īwān*, the smallest of the four, was where evidence of more elaborate inscriptions and decorations was found. It was rectangular in shape and had a small basin inside it. Similar to al-Bīmāristān al-Nūrī, this *īwān* may have been where the attending physician would have sat to examine patients, prescribe medications, and give lessons to his students, as indicated in the *waqf* document and in al-Nuwayrī's descriptions.[11] Also, in Shāfiʿ ibn ʿAlī's biography of al-Manṣūr Qalāwūn, he explained that, when inaugurating the bīmāristān, the sultan sat in the southern *īwān* (*al-īwān al-qiblī*) where he verbally announced the consecration of the *waqf*:

> When [the bīmāristān] was completed, the Sultan went to it himself, sat in ... its southern *īwān*, among the emirs of his state, and protectors of his kingdom. A cup of [the bīmāristān's] drink was brought to him, he held it in his hand and said, while the four judges were in attendance, "Witness that I endowed this bīmāristān to those like me or lesser than me" and he gave robes of honor to [the bīmāristān's] attendants.[12]

[8] Ibn Ḥabīb, *Tadhkirat al-Nabīh*, 1: 353.

[9] Al-Nuwayrī, *Nihāyat al-'Arab*, 31: 107.

[10] This occurs in al-Fayyūmī's biography of Jamāl al-Dīn Āqūsh (d. 1335), who supervised the bīmāristān and who was known to visit the mad to check on their conditions. See ʿIsā, *Tārīkh al-Bīmāristānāt fī al-Islām*, 62.

[11] Ibid., 31: 108.

[12] Ibn ʿAlī, Lewicka, *Biography of Qalāwūn*, 407.

Figure 5.1: Floor plan of Qalāwūn Complex

Patients entering the bīmāristān would have seen this space on their left across the water basin. In his biographical dictionary, Ibn Abī Uṣaybiʿah described the process of examination in al-Bīmāristān al-Nūrī: he described how he would accompany Raḍiyy al-Dīn al-Raḥbī or other master physicians, who would sit on a bench; he would examine and prescribe remedies for patients who came to see him but who did not reside in the bīmāristān.[13] In other cases, some relatives or servants of the patient would visit the bīmāristān and describe the symptoms to the attending physician who would prescribe medications. This type of examination, which is reminiscent of what would happen in the market, seems to have been common in many bīmāristāns, with reports from as early as al-

[13] Ibn Abī Uṣaybiʿah, *ʿUyūn al-Anbāʾ*, 4: 328.

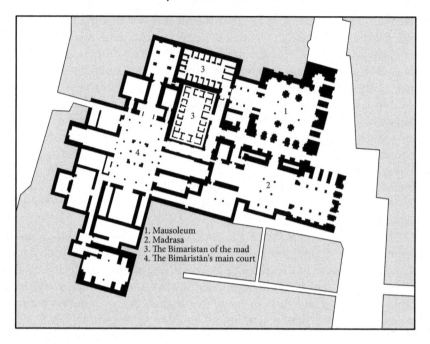

Bīmāristān al-ʿAḍudī,[14] and is also described by al-Rāzī in his hospital practice and by al-Kaskarī in his *Kunnāsh*.

This setting for the examination raises important questions about privacy. On one hand, the setting was largely open, and resident patients and visitors would have heard or seen the examination of other patients. On the other hand, patients were housed in the *iwāns* surrounding the court, all of which were open to the court. The bīmāristān patients and prescription-seekers came from among those who would have sought medical care in the market, where such public explanations of illness and complaints were probably not uncommon. In these contexts, whether in the market or in the bīmāristān, physical examination would not have involved any body parts that could not or should not have been revealed in public.[15] In fact, we have little evidence that such initial examination involved much physical exposure. The columns that separated the *īwāns* from the court were not meant to create an enclosure that provides privacy or isolation but rather to create separate spaces, albeit connected visually. Women patients, whose privacy needed to be protected more, were not housed in these *īwāns* but rather in back halls that were not visible from the courtyard.

This setting may have also caused other problems, such as the possibility of stench spreading from some patient halls or *īwāns* to the courtyard or to other *īwāns*. Sources inform us that stench or bad odors were a concern for the local elites, especially in relation to sites of prayer and to the bīmāristān. For instance, the Mamluk emir Jamāl al-Dīn Āqūsh al-Ashrafī (d. 1335; known as *Nāʾib al-Karak*, the viceroy of al-Karak), who supervised the bīmāristān around 1330, was credited for removing a water basin located close to the complex's portal and used to water animals. People complained that this basin and the animals stopping there to drink caused a stench that one could smell inside the mausoleum, the madrasa, and the bīmāristān. Āqūsh ordered the basin removed and replaced it with a sabil from which people could drink.[16] It is likely that similar concerns would have arisen inside the bīmāristān itself, especially because this open setting would allow for potential bad odors, which might have been caused in the *īwāns* by humidity and moisture along with patients' wastes, to be noticed by other patients, prescription seekers, and visitors, including dignitaries. Physicians

[14] Ibid., 2: 274.

[15] *ʿAwra* signified certain body parts that should not be revealed in public for men and for women. However, it is not clear from the sources whether such rules were observed in relation to medical practice. On similar issues related to examination of female patients, see Pormann, "Female Patients and Practitioners."

[16] Al-Maqrīzī, *al-Khiṭaṭ*, 4: 407.

and medical practitioners must have worried about the stench as well because it would have indicated bad miasms, which were believed to contribute to many afflictions.[17] This may have required consistent and regular cleaning by the janitors and caretakers, and it may explain the *waqf* document's suggestion that the numbers of these janitors and caretakers could change at different times throughout the year. The nāẓir may have hired additional workers when the bīmāristān had or expected more patients during pilgrimage and visitation seasons or during hot and humid seasons.

The bīmāristān also used a number of incenses, such as frankincense and citron seeds; the latter of these was known to alleviate the stench and also to help prevent different diseases, including plague.[18] These incenses and other good-smelling plants, seeds, and roots were hung from the roofs in the different halls and at their entrances. Amulets made of ruby or containing nutmeg may have hung around the courtyard and inside the fever *īwāns*: both were described in Ibn al-Akfānī's writings as useful for fever patients.[19] The Maghrebi traveler Khālid b. ʿĪsá al-Balawī (fl. 1335) also described these ruby amulets in al-Bīmāristān al-Manṣūrī, which he would have seen in the open courtyard and the *īwāns* during his visit.[20] Ibn al-Akfānī also noted other amulets made of river crab's eyes, a wolf's right eye, a rooster's right eye, and dried silkworm, all of which had different therapeutic value and were used and prescribed by physicians like al-Akfānī himself.[21] Although al-Akfānī described amulets that were for individual use and that would hang around a patient's neck or at his or her bed, it is possible that a number of these amulets would have been hung in the *īwāns* for the benefit of all patients. Having individual amulets of these types would have cost huge sums.

After visiting with the attending physician, some patients would have been admitted to the bīmāristān and kept in one of the halls. The majority of patients and prescription seekers would have been given instructions to modify their diets or would have been prescribed specific medications to be prepared by the bīmāristān druggist. The druggist's room, which was used to cook and prepare different medications for the internal patients and prescription-seekers, was located close to the bīmāristān's back entrance

[17] On the concept of contagion and afflictions through miasms, see Stearns, *Infectious Ideas: Contagion in Premodern Islamic and Christian Thought in the Western Mediterranean*.

[18] Ibn Al-Akfānī, *Ghunyat al-Labīb ʿinda Ghaybat al-Ṭabīb*, 78.

[19] Ibid., 80–81.

[20] Al-Balawī described pearls as well. Yet there is no evidence that pearls were thought to have any specific medicinal value. See al-Balawī, *Tāj al-Mafriq fī Taḥliyat ʿUlamāʾ al-Mashriq*.

[21] Ibid., 82–83.

and to a hall dedicated to convalescing male patients. This may have allowed other patients to consult the druggist through the back door without passing through the courtyard. Other patients came in to have their eyes examined and to receive treatment for different eye conditions. The hall for eye patients could have been the long hall parallel to the Eastern *īwān*, with a smaller room at its far end where the oculist would have examined and treated his patients.

The bīmāristān had a third entrance in addition to the main one through the L-shaped corridor and the back one close to the druggist room. This third entrance was located near the oculist hall on the Eastern wall and opened inside the residences of the madrasa students, being as such inaccessible from the street except through the madrasa. This entrance would have allowed students to frequent the bīmāristān more

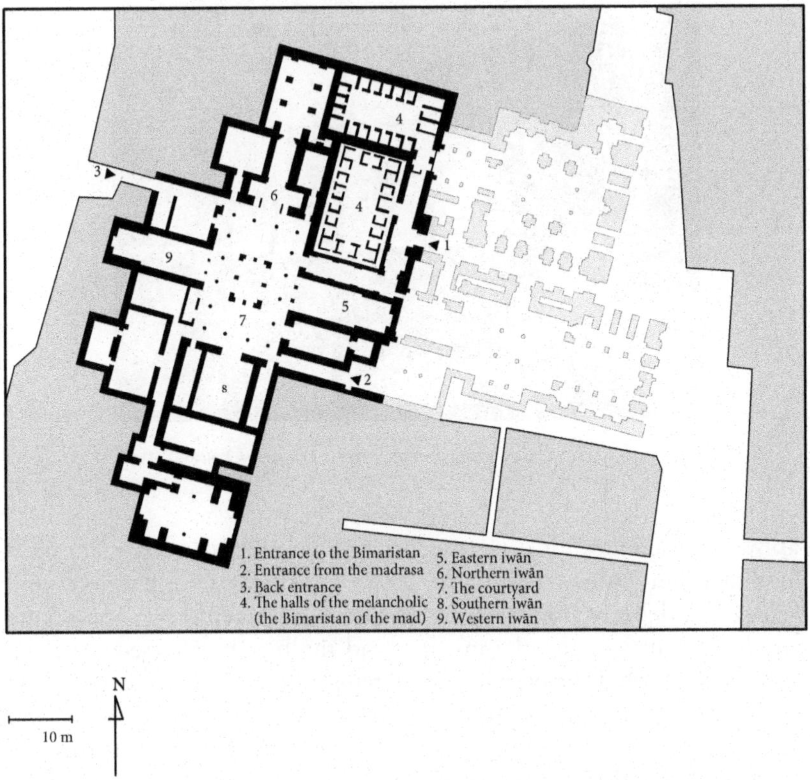

Figure 5.2: Floor plan of Al-Bīmāristān Al-Mansuri

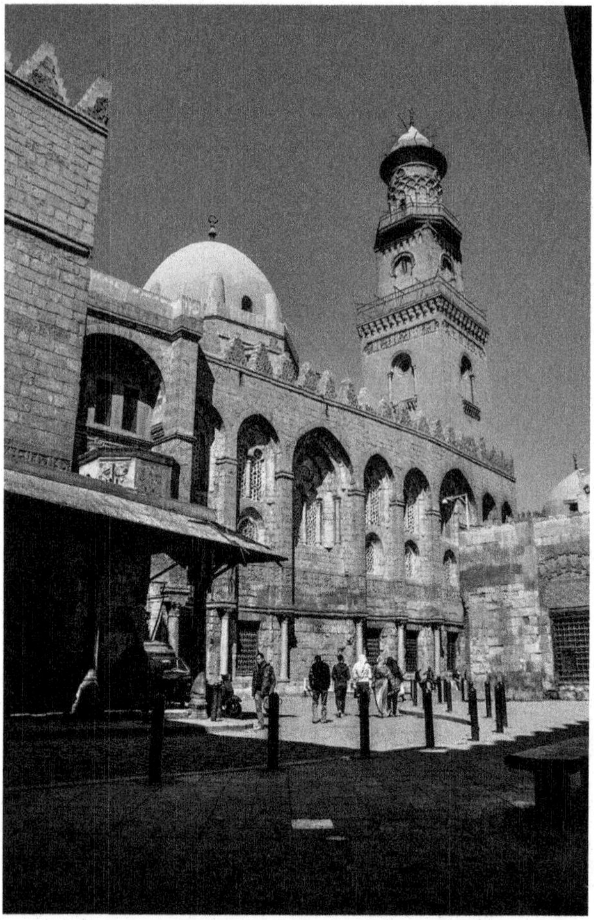

Figure 5.3: The Qalawunid complex from Bayn al-Qaṣrayn street

easily. More significantly, sick students may have received treatment from the bīmāristān without residing in its halls and may have had food and medications delivered to their residences through this entrance. Sources are not clear about whether the madrasa and the bīmāristān used the same kitchen, although descriptions of food items in the *waqf* document for the bīmāristān resembled foodstuffs more commonly used in madrasas and khānaqāhs, thus making it likely that the two shared kitchen. If this was indeed the case, the back entrance to the students' residences would have allowed for the delivery of food to them as well.

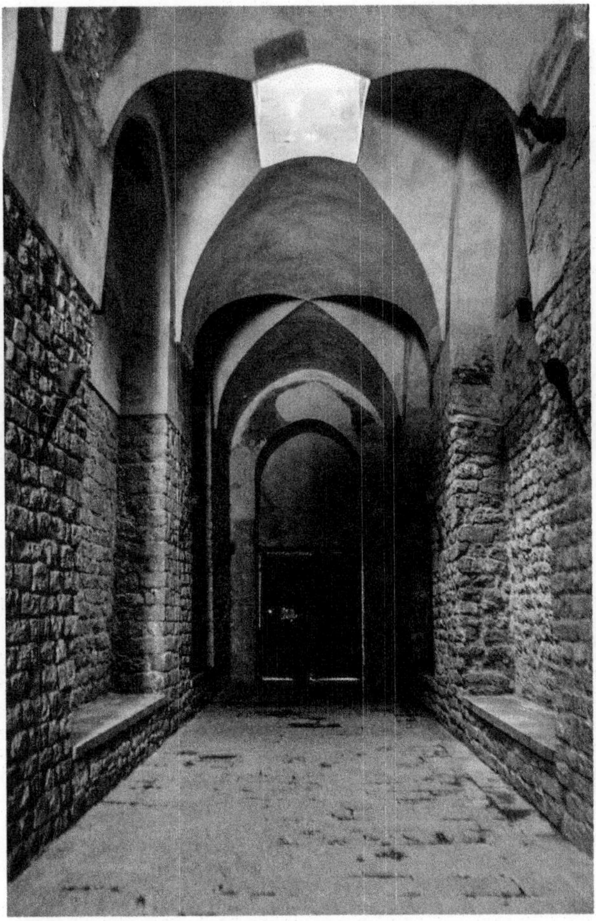

Figure 5.4: The corridor from the street to the bīmāristān (The mausoleum on the right and the madrasa on the left)

Who Were the Bīmāristān Patients?

In his description of the bīmāristān, al-Nuwayrī explained that the sultan did not restrict access to it in anyway and that he insisted on keeping it open to all, at all times, so that no sick person would be turned away.[22] Al-Nuwayrī's statement was repeated in other sources as a sign of the sultan's generosity and also of the huge size of the bīmāristān. This statement echoes the *waqf*

[22] Al-Nuwayrī, *Nihāyat al-'Arab*, 31: 108.

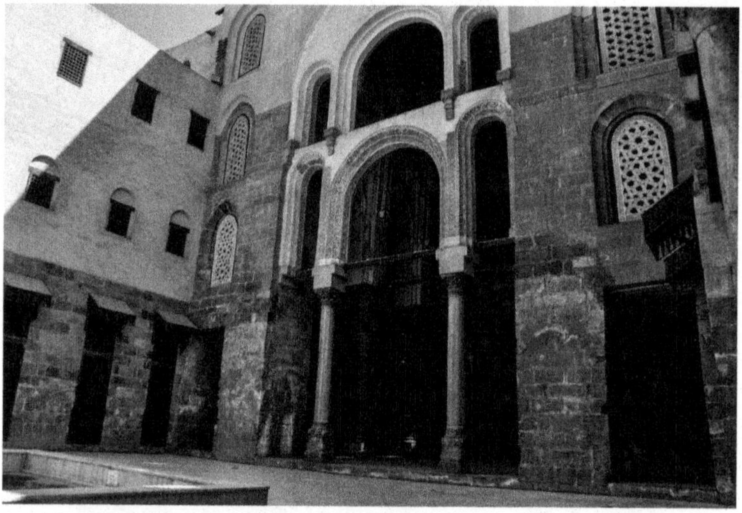

Figure 5.5: An iwan in the madrasa (The Bīmāristān's iwans resembled this)

document, which insisted that no sick man or woman should be turned away from the bīmāristān and that all were to be accommodated.[23] This may have spoken to a known practice of imposing certain admission policies that would restrict the bīmāristān to the acutely sick, who would not stay long in the bīmāristān. One should see this in view of the absence of any evidence for clear discharge criteria or processes that were implemented in al-Bīmāristān al-Manṣūrī or other neighboring bīmāristāns.

The only reported incident of people being actively discharged happened under the supervision of the emir supervisor Jamāl al-Dīn Āqūsh as he was planning to repair and renovate the bīmāristān halls. The bīmāristān stopped admitting new patients, and the existing patients were discharged except for the mad. Although we are not told how this process took place, it appears that the medical or administrative staff in the bīmāristān had some ideas about who should or should not be in the bīmāristān and who could be discharged and sent away. Whether or how these ideas were implemented is unclear. That said, it is possible that physicians or administrators simply ordered patients out without a clear formal process, although there is no positive evidence supporting this claim. Apart from this incident, there is no evidence of other incidents of discharging people. Yet the bīmāristān continued to function, admitting

[23] Ibn Ḥabīb, *Tadhkirat al-Nabīh*, 1: 359.

new patients and not sending newcomers away, suggesting that patients either left out of their own initiative once they improved or were sent away whether formally or informally by the attendants.

On another hand, the bīmāristān's existence as part of a large network of charitable institutions that supported the poor and the needy may have enabled it to survive without being clogged by chronic or incurable patients or flooded by the needy and poor. Many crippled, needy, or poor could have sought help in other charitable institutions, which may have even given better food, smelled better, and offered less risk of getting sick. The bīmāristān's practice of dispensing medications to people in their homes allowed it to help patients without admitting them. It is likely that those capable of caring for themselves, or who had family members to care for them, would have elected to use medications from the bīmāristān and stayed in their houses. In fact, an examination of a number of biographical dictionaries for every mention of the bīmāristān reveals that almost all references to the admitted were to people who had no families or were in very difficult situations, thus leading them to require the family-like care provided in the bīmāristān. These references, however, only focused on times when the bīmāristān played a significant role in a person's life (such as at moments of death and dying) or when a particular episode of illness drastically affected the biographee's life. Other occasions for admission to or interaction with the bīmāristān may not have made their way into these concise biographies. In all cases, a deeper look at the sources can show some of the categories of patients who frequented the bīmāristān.

People with Difficult Conditions

One of the main categories of people attending the bīmāristān may not necessarily have been the poor, but rather people in difficult conditions or approaching death, whether because of accidents or severe and unexpected deterioration due to an existing disease. Al-Dakhwār hinted at the bīmāristān's advantage in these situations by explaining that one of the roles of the bīmāristān was to have stockpiles of ready-made drugs and medications that could be used immediately and without delay.[24] Although the medications themselves may not have been different from others produced in the market, their immediate availability gave the bīmāristān a significant edge, according to al-Dakhwār, who claimed that this was why bīmāristāns were made in the first place. This view may have

24 Al-Dakhwār and Ibn Qāḍī Ba'labak, *Kitāb Sharḥ Tuqaddimuhu al-Ma'rifah lil-Dakhwār.*

been common at the time. For instance, the famous author Zakariyya b. Muḥammad al-Qazwīnī (d. 1283) wrote the following while describing India in his book *Āthār al-Bilād wa Akhbār al-ʿIbād*:

> There, there are serpents, which, if they sting a man, he would be [still] like a dead [person]. The [people] would take him, stretch him on a wooden board and throw him in [a river]. The [river] flows to a place where there is a bīmāristān, which overlooks the river, and which looks out for those stung [by serpents], takes them, and treats them. After a period [of a stay in the bīmāristān], he would return to his people safe and sound.[25]

Al-Qazwīnī's tale, like many of his other anecdotes, was probably apocryphal. What is important for the purpose of this discussion is al-Qazwīnī's view of the bīmāristān's role in providing such emergency intervention for accidents or urgent needs, a role that was entirely comprehensible and believable to his readers. The famous Sufi Ibn al-ʿArabī (d. 1240), who visited the Levant and Egypt in the beginning of the thirteenth century, used the same trope: he depicted the bīmāristān as the site of urgent care when describing what might have been an allegorical story or a mythical anecdote on the miracles of a Sufi saint. In that account, Ibn al-ʿArabī reported that al-Kirmānī (d. 1021; a well-know Sufi but who was still a disciple in Ibn al-ʿArabī's story) was accompanying a Sufi shaykh when the shaykh had severe and sudden abdominal pain. Al-Kirmānī went to the bīmāristān and asked the attending physician to give him medication for the shaykh. In the anecdote, the shaykh ended up inhabiting the body of the bīmāristān attendant and dispensing the medications to al-Kirmānī, eventually teaching the latter a lesson on piety.[26] Regardless of who indeed was the attendant, Ibn al-ʿArabī was clearly convinced that the bīmāristān was a place where one would go in a case of severe emergency, when medications were urgently needed.

The pharmacological formulary *al-Dustūr al-Bīmāristānī*, composed by Ibn Abī al-Bayān (b. 1161) for al-Bīmāristān al-Nāṣirī and also used in al-Bīmāristān al-Manṣūrī, included a number of medications that one should use in cases of urgency. For instance, a powder was prescribed to stop bleeding from wounds; another was used to stop bleeding from arteries. Similarly, the formulary prescribed a medication to be put on rabid dog bites to prevent rabies.[27] Other medications treated burns and other types

[25] Al-Qazwīnī, *Āthār al-Bilād wa Akhbār al-ʿIbād*, 50.
[26] Ibn al-ʿArabī, *al-Futūḥāt al-Makkīyah*, 118.
[27] Ibn Abī al-Bayān and Sbath, *al-Dustūr al-Bīmāristānī [Le Formulaire des Hôpitaux d'Ibn Abil Bayan, Médecin du Bimaristan Annacery au Caire]*, 73.

of injuries.[28] Since all these medications were supposed to be pre-prepared in the bīmāristān and used when the occasion arose, it is likely that the bīmāristān was indeed a site for urgent care, when a pre-prepared medication would be useful. In these situations, the patients were not necessarily poor and may not have resided in the bīmāristān at all.

Travelers

Another group of patients who frequented the bīmāristān and were mentioned in the *waqf* document were travelers, pilgrims, and visitors, those who did not have family or relatives to care for them. As mentioned before, Crusader hospitals exemplified institutions dedicated to the service of pilgrims, and they may have created a significant precedent for similar institutions in the Islamicate context, not least of which are al-Bīmāristān al-Ṣalāḥī built by Ṣalāḥ al-Dīn in Jerusalem, his bīmāristān in Alexandria, and al-Bīmāristān al-Manṣūrī of Hebron. As mentioned earlier, Ibn Jubayr described in more detail the bīmāristān of Alexandria, which was built by Ṣalāḥ al-Dīn. This bīmāristān paid special attention to serving visitors, whether they were passing through, like Ibn Jubayr, or residing there as students at the port's multiple madrasas.[29] The *waqf* document of al-Bīmāristān al-Manṣūrī of Cairo also mentioned travelers and emphasized that the bīmāristān was intended to serve visitors to the city of Cairo, many of whom may have been on their way to the pilgrimage.

Ibn Jubayr's (d. 1217) travelogue provides important information in this regard because it was composed with Maghrebi travelers in mind and intended to provide them with important information about places and sites where they could find help and support. Ibn Jubayr was especially attentive to bīmāristāns, describing some of them in great detail and even asking about them on his travels. When he could not locate a bīmāristān in Homs, he asked one of the older people if it had a bīmāristān "along the custom of cities in these regions? He [the old man] said, with indignation, 'Homs is all a bīmāristān.' "[30] Whereas Ibn Jubayr's question showed his interest, whether personally or as a traveler, in knowing about bīmāristāns, the answer that he received showed that the bīmāristān was not connected primarily to sickness or even simply related to cure and treatment; rather,

28 Ibid., 70.
29 Ibid., 10.
30 Ibn Jubayr, *Riḥlat Ibn Jubayr*, 246.

the bīmāristān was viewed as a site for charity and generosity directed to strangers and visitors. It is only in this charitable sense that we can understand the local man's indignation and his answer that the entire city was a bīmāristān. In all these cases, the bīmāristān seemed to have played a significant role in serving strangers and visitors, those who did not have people to care for them.

Clients of the Charity Network

The bīmāristān served a growing population whose lives were connected to an expanding network of charities in the city, which included bīmāristāns, mosques, madrasas, and khānaqāhs, among others. Although biographical dictionaries mention only a small number of people as having died in the bīmāristān and do not mention any occasional or "unimportant" visits, they provide us with important examples of the role of the bīmāristān in the lives of many people. For many patients, the bīmāristān was part of a larger network of charitable institutions upon which they relied for various needs during different periods of their lives. These individuals, who were mostly poor or without family or relatives, also relied on other institutions within charity networks. They lived in mosques, khānaqāhs, and madrasas and relied for their livelihood on charity or wages given by these same institutions for minor tasks.

For instance, the Damascene chronicler Quṭb al-Dīn al-Yūnīnī, who wrote his chronicle *Dhayl mirʾāt al-Zamān* on the years 697/1297–701/1302, wrote the biography of al-Shaykh Aḥmad al-Zuʿbī who lived in al-Khānqāh al-Ṣalāḥiyyah in Damascus. Al-Zuʿbī did not have a clear profession or stable source of income: he lived his life in the Sufi monastery built by Ṣalāḥ al-Dīn al-Ayyūbī in Damascus, although al-Yūnīnī did not mention that he was a Sufi affiliated to this khānaqāh in particular. The rich Sufi monastery likely provided him with this charitable abode and support in exchange for minor tasks without himself being a Sufi or a member of the monastery. In 706/1306, he fell sick and was taken to the old bīmāristān, known as al-Bīmāristān al-Ṣaghīr, where he passed away.[31] Similarly, Mujāhid al-Manbijī, who also died in al-Bīmāristān al-Ṣaghīr in 708/1308, benefitted from the Damascene charitable network when he was a resident (*mujāwir*) in the Umayyad mosque, meaning that he lived in the mosque and depended on charitable donations from the mosque's *waqf*

[31] Al-Yūnīnī, *Dhayl Mirʾāt al-Zamān*, 2: 1134.

and from the believers. He was sixty years old when he died, and, like al-Zuʿbī, he did not seem to have left a family behind.[32]

Also in Damascus, the historian and *muḥaddith* al-Qāsim b. Muḥammad al-Birzālī (665/1267–739-1339) wrote the biography of "the good shaykh (*al-shaykh al-ṣāliḥ*)" Thābit. Thābit did not have a known last name or even a brief lineage. According to al-Birzālī, he was loved and respected by the many who attended his funeral, although (or perhaps because) he was not interested in people or their affairs but rather was always occupied with prayers, fasting, and Quran recitals (*kāna muwāẓiban ʿalā al-ṣiyām wa al-tilāwah wa al-dhikr, qalīl al-ishtighāl bi-al-nās*). He resided in a mosque all of his life and died in al-Bīmāristān al-Ṣaghīr in 1311.[33] Al-Birzālī also wrote the biography of al-Shaykh Aḥmad al-Ḥarrānī al-Faqīr, a Sufi known for his piety and devotion who lived for years in the Umayyad mosque of Damascus among the Sufis from Aleppo (*al-fuqarāʾ al-ḥalabiyyīn*). He died in the al-Bīmāristān al-Ṣaghīr in Damascus in 1314.[34]

In Cairo, al-Maqrīzī (d. 1442) reported the biography of Rāshid al-Takrūrī, who died in al-Bīmāristān al-Manṣūrī in 796/1394. He was a poor mystic (*majdhūb*) who performed miracles that people believed in (*muʿtaqad*). He spent his life in al-Rāshidah mosque outside the commercial suburbs of Cairo, al-Fusṭāṭ, and died in the bīmāristān. Al-Maqrīzī knew al-Takrūrī and visited him in al-Rashidah mosque but did not report his father's name or his epithet except for al-Takrūrī, which he probably acquired either because he came from Takrūr or because he was black.[35] Similarly, al-Sakhāwī wrote the biography of Rajab b. Yūsuf al-Qāhirī, who was treated in al-Bīmāristān al-Manṣūrī before his death. He attended the lessons of important scholars but was not a scholar himself, and he worked as a servant for a number of scholars and judges. Later in his life, he had to beg from students to survive and served the shrine of the famous Sufi saint al-Layth. Al-Qāhirī fell sick and was carried to the bīmāristān, where his condition improved; he left the bīmāristān only to die a few days later in al-Ẓāhiriyyah madrasa.[36] The bīmāristān appeared to be a normal place for the treatment of someone like Rajab al-Qāhirī. Whereas his education, known piety, and service to important scholars earned him entry into al-Sakhāwī's dictionary, he remained poor throughout his life and relied on begging and the sort of charity given to servants in Sufi shrines. He did not

[32] Ibid., 2: 1228–29.
[33] Al-Birzālī, *al-Wafayāt*, 110.
[34] Ibid., 239.
[35] Al-Maqrīzī, *Durar al-ʿUqūd al-Farīdah fī Tarājim al-Aʿyān al-Mufīdah*, 2: 86.
[36] Al-Sakhāwī, *Al-Dawʾ al-Lāmiʿ li-Ahl al-Qarn al-Tāsiʿ*, 3: 224.

appear to have a family and would not have been able to afford medical care in the market. In this sense, Rajab al-Qāhirī represented one of the paradigmatic patients of the bīmāristān as described and intended by the *waqf* document.[37] For all these individuals and others, the bīmāristān figured naturally in their life histories as part of their reliance on the larger charitable networks that existed in different major cities in the region.

Prescription Seekers

Ibn al-Athīr's (d. 1233) personal experience in Damascus reveals another layer of the normal function of bīmāristāns. When he fell sick, he was told to acquire medications from al-Bīmāristān al-Nūrī. Although he resented the idea at first – he thought one should not crowd the bīmāristān and compete with the poor – he was told that this was a common practice and that even the Ayyubid royalty sought medications from there. One should read Ibn al-Athīr's narrative in light of his biases against the Ayyubids and in favor of the Zangids, which could explain his resentment of what he saw as crowding of the poor or exploitation of the bīmāristān's charitable funds.[38] However, it still testified to what was probably a common practice at the time. In fact, Qalāwūn himself may have made use of al-Bīmāristān al-Nūrī in the same fashion. In the founding accounts of the bīmāristān, Qalāwūn was said to have fallen ill near Damascus and was brought medications from al-Bīmāristān al-Nūrī. The incident motivated his pledge to build the bīmāristān.[39] Although it is difficult to know whether this event actually took place or if Qalāwūn's entourage and regal historians constructed it after the event, its mention and repetition shows that it was not an uncommon practice to seek medications from the bīmāristān. Naturally, Qalāwūn could afford his own medications and

[37] Many other biographies of a similar nature could be found in al-Sakhāwī and others; see Al-Yūnīnī, *Dhayl Mir'āt al-Zamān*, 2: 1300; Al-Sakhāwī, *al-Daw' al-Lāmi' li-Ahl al-Qarn al-Tāsi'*, 2: 72–73; 6: 48.

[38] The same notion of crowding the poor was also expressed by Abū Shāma, who insisted that the bīmāristān was meant only for the poor but that the habit of the people rendered it for all poor and rich: "It has come to me that he [Nūr al-Dīn] did not make it [the bīmāristān] a *waqf* for poor people only, but for all Muslims, rich and poor. I said: I have seen the register of its *waqf*, but saw nothing which specifies that. This is rather talk which has spread on the tongues of people so that, according to God's will, the poor would be crowded out by the rich. It [the *waqf*] rather specifies that whatever important drugs are unavailable [in the markets] should not be withheld from whoever may need them, be they rich or poor . . . and that the bīmāristān is a *waqf* for the poor and displaced. After that it said: and whoever comes to it knowing his illness shall receive medications. It is said that Nūr al-Dīn himself drank from the medication of the bīmāristān, which is in accordance with his *waqf*," translation in Tabba, "The Architectural Patronage of Nur Al-Din, 1146–1174," 231.

[39] Al-Maqrīzī, *al-Khiṭaṭ*, 4: 406.

had his own physicians with him. His physicians, however, may have prescribed a medication that was brought from the bīmāristān because it was already prepared or easier to acquire from there.

Al-Dustūr al-Bīmāristānī's list of medications suggests a similar practice. For instance, among the diseases mentioned in al-Dustūr, one finds treatments for headache and migraine, neither of which would have necessarily required admitting patients. It is possible, however, that these treatments were used to alleviate the pain and discomfort of internal patients while in the bīmāristān. This could also apply to preparations for treating sciatica or back pain. Other medications treated conditions that would not have required admittance into the bīmāristān or have been a concern for its occupants. These included rubs for back pain caused by excessive copulation, along with suppositories for enhancing fertility and for causing or preventing menstruation. They also included oils for stimulating hair growth and dying it black, and dentifrices for whitening teeth, strengthening gums, and treating halitosis. For all these conditions, it appears that the bīmāristān served as a site for distributing medications to people who did not need to be admitted and who suffered from minor conditions or problems. These people might not have belonged to the ranks of the riffraff, paupers, or the extreme poor, but they could have been pilgrims, visitors, students, scholars, and bureaucrats who benefited from the bīmāristān's services. These medications were likely part of the bīmāristān's role in supplying treatment to the sick in their homes, as described in the *waqf* document.[40] In Ibn Abī Uṣaybiʿah's accounts of his and his masters' practice in al-Bīmāristān al-Nūrī, he often described prescription seekers who came to the bīmāristān to complain about specific issues or to describe the ailments affecting their family members or their children in order to acquire the proper medications.[41]

The Mad

Al-Bīmāristān al-Manṣūrī, similar to many other bīmāristāns, contained a specific section for the mad, often called melancholics (*mamrūrīn*) or the disturbed (*mukhtallīn*).[42] In the case of al-Manṣūrī, and as described earlier, this section was entirely separated from the rest of the bīmāristān so that it almost appeared as a discrete bīmāristān. The *waqf* document

[40] Ibn Ḥabīb, *Tadhkirat al-Nabīh*, 1: 367.

[41] For instance, Ibn Abī Uṣaybiʿah's biography of Raḍiyy al-Dīn al-Raḥbī. Ibn Abī Uṣaybiʿah, *ʿUyūn al-Anbāʾ*, 3: 189.

[42] On madness and the treatment of the mad, see Dols, *Majnūn*.

suggested that the melancholics were given food and treatment along with other patients. Also, al-Dustūr offered a number of treatments for the mad, including treatments for melancholy, black bile accumulations (*al-sawdā'*), melancholic obsessions (*al-wuswās al-sawdāwī*),[43] illusions and bad dreams, and mania (*al-junūn al-sab'ī*).[44] These preparations indicate that the mad received specific treatments in the bīmāristān, although their presence did not necessarily mean that they were used on patients kept in the bīmāristān, in particular those who may have been more dangerous or difficult for their families or those who had no families or relatives.

In fact, it appears that the confined mad were usually seen as the most dangerous and deranged and that their appearance was usually in disarray, their words incomprehensible, and their behaviors unexpected. This might be the reason why many sources described, with surprise, the presence of well-groomed, articulate mad kept in bīmāristāns, who were often assumed to be confined because they were victims of conspiracy or malice and were generally seen as an oddity that invited marveling. One of the most famous account testifying to this portrayal is connected to the bīmāristān built by Aḥmad ibn Ṭūlūn (d. 884), who used to visit his bīmāristān and inspect the patients, including the mad, every week. On one of his visits, he was addressed by a chained madman who looked well-groomed and was well-spoken. The young man explained to the emir that he was indeed the victim of intrigue and that he was not mad. Based on his looks and his articulation, the emir ordered him unchained and granted his request for a pomegranate. The patient, however, apparently reverted to his madness, threw the pomegranate at Ibn Ṭūlūn, and almost injured the emir. Ibn Ṭūlūn was reported not to have visited the bīmāristān again.[45] The authenticity of the story is beyond the scope of this discussion. Yet, its continuous repetition proves that the general readership saw an apparent contradiction between a well-spoken, well-groomed young man and their own expectations of what they would find chained in the bīmāristān's ward for the mad. Such contradiction would have explained the emir's actions. This trope of the well-groomed, well-spoken madman recurs frequently in several literary accounts detailing the general perception surrounding the confined mad.[46]

[43] Ibn Abī al-Bayān and Sbath, *Al-Dustūr al-Bīmāristānī [Le Formulaire des Hôpitaux d'Ibn Abil Bayan, Médecin du Bimaristan Annacery au Caire]*, 18–22.

[44] Ibid., 29–50.

[45] Al-Maqrīzī, *al-Khiṭaṭ*, 4: 409–10.

[46] See, for instance, the writings of Abū Ḥayyān al-Tawḥīdī (d. 1023) or Badī' al-Zamān al-Hamadhānī (d. 1007), among many others.

Al-Maqrīzī (d. 1442) reported a number of other anecdotes about those incarcerated in the bīmāristān. In his biography of the physician Shams al-Dīn Muḥammad b. Aḥmad ibn Muḥammad al-Ṣaghīr (d. 1420), the physician reported that he met a well-dressed, handsome young man incarcerated in the bīmāristān. He asked him how and why he had ended up in the mad ward, and the young man replied with two verses of poetry complaining about time and the changes of fortune.[47] Similarly, another biographee, Muḥammad ibn al-Khiḍr al-Shāfiʿī (d. 1438), went to visit a bīmāristān when he first arrived in Cairo from Aleppo. There, he found a chained mad person whose dress he liked. When asked about his conditions, the chained madman also replied in verse about the changes of fortune.[48] In both these cases and others, the incarcerated were seen as people who were victims of bad fortune, misunderstandings, or, sometimes, conspiracies and malice. Those incarcerated in the wards for melancholics must have been in such a wretched condition that the appearance of well-groomed, well-dressed, or handsome men in these wards would attract the attention of visitors who would inquire about their conditions. Although we are never told about the reasons behind their incarceration, we are left with eloquent poetry that spoke to their talent and education and that suggested their fate conspired to land them in these wards.

Confinement in the mad wards of the bīmāristān appeared frequently in anecdotes about Sufis. Ibn al-Sarrāj (d. 1106) narrated a story of the famous Sufi al-Shiblī (d. 946) who entered a bīmāristān and found a (mad) man with one of his hands chained to his neck and the other to a column. When the chained man saw al-Shiblī, he recognized him and said, "O Abū Bakr, ask your God if it was not enough that He filled me with His love that He now put me in chains?!"[49] Al-Ghazālī (d. 1111) reported an anecdote in which al-Shiblī himself was incarcerated (*ḥubisa*) in a bīmāristān where some people went to visit him. Al-Shiblī hurled stones at them saying, "if you love me, withstand my hardships," in reference to what one should do in expressing love and gratitude to God.[50] Although most of these anecdotes occurred in advice and devotional literature, rather than in historiographic or biographical literature (thereby casting doubt on the authenticity of these reports), the repetition of such stories attached to famous Sufis like al-Shiblī shows that the image of a mad saint confined in the bīmāristān due to injustice or lack of understanding was not uncommon.

47 Al-Maqrīzī, *Durar al-ʿUqūd al-Farīdah fī Tarājim al-Aʿyān al-Mufīdah*, 3: 440.
48 Ibid., 3: 357.
49 Al-Sarrāj al-Qāriʾ, *Maṣāriʿ al-ʿUshshāq*, 56.
50 Al-Ghazālī, *Iḥyāʾ ʿUlūm al-Dīn*, 1440.

Some of the mad were confined in the bīmāristān following orders from the courts. In biographical dictionaries, the theme of involuntary incarcerations was most pronounced in the accounts related to the melancholics. In these stories, the bīmāristān was always presented as a form of punishment. Al-Sakhāwī (d. 1497) wrote the biography of ʿAlī Saʿīd b. Ibrāhīm al-Badrashī, a competent and pious student of a number of important scholars who was nevertheless extremely poor and never occupied a stable or well-paying position. The bīmāristān appeared in his life briefly during a period of perturbation (*ikhtilāl*) following a period he had spent in isolation with the famous Sufi sheikh al-Fawwī. During this period of perturbation, he insulted a famous judge and was ordered to be incarcerated in the bīmāristān for a week.[51] Al-Badrashī apparently did not withstand the harsh devotional regime of al-Fawwī and ended up being perturbated and incarcerated. We find another instance of involuntary incarceration in al-Sakhāwī's biography of Aḥmad b. Muḥammad al-Maḥallī (d. 1477), who was incarcerated in the bīmāristān on the orders of the Mamluk Sultan al-Ẓāhir Jaqmaq (r. 1438–1453). Al-Maḥallī, who was promising as a student but never achieved repute, voiced a number of opinions denouncing the statues of lions of Qanāṭir al-Sibāʿ (the Bridge of the Lions built by Baybars I),[52] the treatment of slaves, and the state's tolerance of neighborhoods of prostitutes. The sultan understood that al-Maḥallī wished to demolish Qanāṭir al-Sibāʿ and to ban using slaves in manual work; he therefore decided that al-Maḥallī must be mad and ordered him jailed (*sajanahu*) in the bīmāristān for a period (*waqtan*).[53] In both cases, the confinement was for a limited period of time, although it was not clear whether the period was defined in the confinement orders or assessed by the bīmāristān physicians and attendants.

In the same vein of punishment-like incarceration in the bīmāristān, the literary historian, ʿAlī b. Mūsā b. Saʿīd (d. 1286) wrote about a judge in Erbil in his biographies of the poets of the seventh Hijri century (c. thirteenth century CE):

> It happened that a talkative outspoken man came to him with a case against a youth, who had charming looks and his beard was hardly growing. The judge kept addressing the youth [and did not listen to the complainer]. The man [complainer] said with his lack of tact: "O Judge, I see you favoring this boy and not listening to me!" The judge replied, "It is because

[51] Al-Sakhāwī, *Al-Ḍawʾ al-Lāmiʿ li-Ahl al-Qarn al-Tāsiʿ*, 5: 160.

[52] A famous bridge in Cairo built by al-Ẓāhir Baybars (d. 1277) and adorned by statues of lions, hence the name Qanāṭir al-Sibāʿ (lit. The Bridge of the Lions).

[53] Ibid., 2: 74–75.

> I find truth in his sayings." So the man said, "No, by God! But he charmed you." Some of the people attending [the court] rose to him and were about to attack him, but the judge told them, "no offense should be taken from this man. Take him to the Bīmāristān until he is cured since his brain has dried." He was therefore carried to the Bīmāristān and the case was resolved.[54]

In a case reported by al-Suyūṭī (d. 1505), physicians intervened to replace a death sentence with incarceration in the bīmāristān. In 1416, a man living in the commercial suburb of al-Fusṭāṭ claimed to be a prophet and to have ascended to the heavens, seen God, and talked to him. Some "riffraff (*al-ʿawām*)" believed and followed him, thus prompting action from the authorities. After he was asked to repent and refused, the Maliki judge sentenced him to death "[based] on the testimony of two [men] that he is mentally sound (*ḥāḍir al-ʿaql*)." However, some of "the people of medicine (*ahl al-ṭibb*)" testified that he was mentally disturbed (*mukhtall al-ʿaql*), and he was, therefore, "chained (*quyyida*) in the bīmāristān."[55]

The bīmāristān was used in two different capacities related to punishment and incarceration. On one hand, it was sometimes meant as an actual punishment, in which a person was incarcerated or "jailed" for a predetermined period of time (even as short as one week, as seen before). In these cases, the accusation of madness indicated failure to follow the proper social decorum as opposed to a physical affliction. The fact that the bīmāristān was used in this capacity speaks to how difficult it was to be in the wards of the melancholic and that such residence, no matter how short, involved chaining, jailing, and different forms of hardship. On the other hand, incarceration was sometimes ordered as a result of an actual judgment of madness or mental affliction. The false prophet, who was incarcerated on a judge's order, was sent to the bīmāristān based on the testimonies of physicians and as part of legal proceedings that exempted him from guilt and absolved him from the punishment of death based on his diagnosed madness. In these cases, the incarceration was not defined by a period. Presumably, the person would stay until deemed cured, if ever. This type of incarceration shows that, despite the wretched conditions in the wards of the melancholic, the bīmāristān provided forms of treatment and care, as also indicated in many other sources. Obviously, these two ideal types are only clear extreme cases. The majority of cases would have been somewhere in the middle.

[54] Ibn Saʿīd, *Al-Ghuṣūn al-Yāniʿah fī Maḥāsin Shuʿarāʾ al-Miʾah al-Sābiʿah*, 21.
[55] Al-Suyūṭī, *Tārīkh al-Khulafāʾ*, 510.

One of the most detailed and reliable reports is by al-Maqrīzī (d. 1442) in his biographical dictionary *Durar al-ʿUqūd al-Farīdah* about his own uncle (his mother's maternal uncle) Ismāʿīl b. Aḥmad b. ʿAbd al-Wahhāb b. al-Khuṭabā (d. 803/1401), who worked as a deputy for Cairo's *muḥtasib* for a number of years. Ibn al-Khuṭabā had a slave called Rashīd who served him for a long time. At one point, he became angry with his slave and wanted to punish him. So he asked one of his friends to incarcerate the slave in the bīmāristān "with the mad" for some time as a type of punishment. Some years later, and close to the end of his own life, Ibn al-Khuṭabā showed feeblemindedness (*taghayyar ʿaqluhu*): "When his [feeblemindedness] became [severe and] evident (*fuḍiḥa amruhu*), that slave [Rashīd] went talking and walking with him . . . until they came to Bayn al-Qaṣrayn close to the bīmāristān. [Rashīd] then carried him [by force] and went to the hall of the mad (*qāʿat al-majānīn*). [They took him] and he was incarcerated there for a period." When Ibn al-Khuṭabā's friends would visit him, he would recount how he had caused his slave to be incarcerated and how he, too, ended up incarcerated in the same place: "He would weep and people would weep with him as they knew what he had been and what became of him."[56]

Al-Maqrīzī's anecdote about his uncle shows how the process of incarceration of the mad could work in two different fashions. In the first instance, the slave was incarcerated at the intervention of his master's friend, who presumably had some power that would enable him to order someone's incarceration. With Ibn al-Khuṭabā's position as the deputy *muḥtasib* and his illustrious bureaucratic career, it is not unlikely that he knew the bīmāristān's *nāẓir* or some other important figure in the bureaucracy or in the bīmāristān's medical staff who could facilitate this process. For Ibn al-Khuṭabā, as for his slave and for al-Maqrīzī's readers, incarceration in the bīmāristān, even for a short period, was a terrible punishment. Ibn al-Khuṭabā's own incarceration was different because it did not involve any form of favoritism but presumably followed the regular procedures of incarceration, where family members could incarcerate a member of the family who became evidently sick. Al-Maqrīzī was careful to mention that his uncle's feeblemindedness had become severe and evident to all and that, for this reason, it was easy for his former slave to have him incarcerated. More interestingly, it appears

[56] Al-Maqrīzī, *Durar al-ʿUqūd al-Farīdah fī Tarājim al-Aʿyān al-Mufīdah*, 1: 416–17. Al-Maqrizi's story had a moralizing purpose because it compared the injustice committed by the uncle to the injustice committed against him. This might have led to some exaggeration in the anecdote.

that Ibn al-Khuṭabā and his friends were not immediately able to release him, and he continued to live in the bīmāristān for some time while his friends visited him and wept for him.

"The Needier, then the Less Needy"

To describe the patients, the authors of al-Bīmāristān al-Manṣūrī's *waqf* document used sets of contrasting adjectives to refer to their variability and diversity and to indicate that the bīmāristān was open to everyone, not only the poor. The document explained that the bīmāristān was intended to "treat Muslim patients; [whether] men or women, [whether from] among the wealthy rich (*al-aghniyā' al-muthrīn*) or the needy poor (*al-fuqarā' al-muḥtājīn*), in Cairo, Miṣr [al-Fusṭāṭ] and their suburbs (*ḍawāḥīhimā*); [whether] residents there or visitors from [different] regions or provinces, [regardless of] their different races (*ajnāsihim*) and appearances (*awṣāfihim*), and their afflictions."[57] A few lines later, the document added another series of opposing descriptions in a further attempt to show diversity: "They [patients] come [to the bīmāristān] in groups or individually (*jumū'an wa wiḥdānan*), old and young (*shuyūkhan wa shubbānan*), adults and minors (*bulaghan wa ṣibyānan*), women and boys (*ḥuraman wa wildānan*)."[58] One line later, it described the distribution of medications to patients whether they were "[from] far or near (*al-ba'īd wa al-qarīb*), local or stranger (*al-ahliyy wa al-gharīb*), strong or weak (*al-qawīy wa al-ḍa'īf*), inferior or honorable (*al-danī' wa al-sharīf*), high or base (*al-'alīy wa al-ḥaqīr*), follower or emir (*al-ma'mūr wa al-amīr*), blind or seeing (*al-a'mā wa al-baṣīr*), [those receiving generosity or giving it] (*al-mafḍūl wa al-fāḍil*), celebrated or lazy (*al-mashhūr wa-al-khāmil*), distinguished or obscure (*al-rafī' wa al-waḍī'*), sumptuous or pauper (*al-mutraf wa al-ṣu'lūk*), a king or a slave (*al-malīk wa al-mamlūk*)."[59]

In spite of this emphasis on inclusiveness, whether in the *waqf* document or in al-Manṣūr Qalāwūn's pronouncement during the inauguration ceremony, the bīmāristān's *waqf* document still betrayed that the bīmāristān's primary interest lay in supplying services to the poor in its instructions to the *nāẓir*:

[57] Ibn Ḥabīb, *Tadhkirat al-Nabīh*, 358.

[58] Ibid., I: 359. The term "boys" refers to those commonly known in modern scholarship as beardless boys; it is a reference to the Quranic term, and its placement alongside *ḥuram* is also evidenced that these were viewed as two opposing objects of sexual desire.

[59] Ibid.

> [The nāẓir should favor] the needier then the less needy (*al-aḥwaj fa-al-aḥwaj*) from among the patients, the needy, the weak, the broken-off [from family and kin] (*al-munqaṭi'īn*), the poor and the destitute. [He should] put forward (*yuqaddim*) the needier then the less needy according to what is more beneficial (*bi-ḥasb mā taqḍīh al-maṣlaḥah*) and [to what] increases in [divine] bounty and reward ... The nāẓir of this waqf has to observe devoutness to God (*yurā'ī taqwā Allāh*) ... openly and secretly, and not to favor one with rank (*ṣāḥib jāh*) over the weak, or a powerful [man] over one who is weaker than him, or a kin over a stranger; rather [let him] favor those, on whom spending [wealth] leads to increase in bounty, reward and nearness (*taqrīb*) to the Lord of lords.[60]

The document emphasized the connection between spending on the poor and divine reward, as well as the piety and devoutness (*taqwā*) of the *nāẓir* himself, who would steward the patron's search for divine reward. These pietistic desires were contrasted with favoritism and fear of the powerful, which were seen as contradictory to the fear of God, "the Lord of lords." The document also assumed that both the *nāẓir* and its readers would know the sort of recipients of charity who would lead to a greater divine reward and would thus be knowledgeable of the proper lines of expenditure of charity, as discussed before. This discussion was followed by the proviso, "should expenditure to the designated goals, or to some of them, become difficult, [expenditure] should go to the Muslim poor and destitute whoever they are and wherever they are."[61] By using this regular formula – often used to govern the fate of *waqfs* should their revenue fall short of achieving their original goals – the document identified the main target of the institution as the poor and needy, in spite of its openness to all in moments of abundance.

Neither the document nor the available records and sources, most of which are historiographical, literary, or theoretical, can give us an accurate picture of the patients who frequented the bīmāristān. Moreover, the composition of this patient body must have changed over time in response to varying perceptions of charity, poverty, and propriety and also in relation to environmental, economic, and disease-related crises. For instance, several waves of famines or economic hardships may have rendered more people in need of the bīmāristān's services. Conversely, severe famines affecting all strata of the society may have rendered the bīmāristān itself unable to perform its duties, thereby limiting its role. Periods of epidemic and outbreaks of various diseases may have changed the

60 Ibid., 1: 368.
61 Ibid.

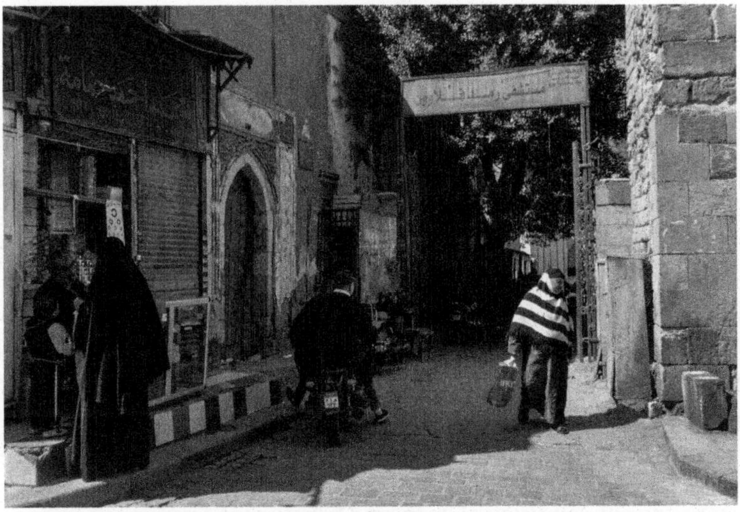

Figure 5.6: "Qalāwūn's Ophthalmology Hospital" (Al-Bīmāristān al-Manṣūrī continues to function today on the same grounds carrying Qalāwūn's name. The Bīmāristān's back entrance now serves as the hospital's main entrance)

population who frequented the bīmāristān, as it may have affected the bīmāristān's own capacities. Seasons of pilgrimage or visitations could have brought more people to the city and therefore more patients or seekers of help to the bīmāristān and to other charitable institutions.

Patient Meets Physician: Medical Encounter and Examination

Most examinations or patient–physician encounters probably started with a complaint from the patient or his or her family. The majority of patients in these cases sought medical help not at the onset of any given illness but rather when new symptoms appeared, when symptoms persisted for an exceedingly long time, or when severe pain began to accompany their conditions. For instance, a female patient suffered from a nosebleed for a number of days but only came to consult al-Rāzī when she developed a headache as well.[62] Another patient had a headache and constipation for five days but came to see the physician because the headache had moved to the forehead.[63] Another man had a severe cough and swelling in his face but only sought consultation when he started having chest pains and

[62] Al-Rāzī, *Kitāb al-Tajārib*, 84.
[63] Ibid., 82.

expirated blood.[64] Other patients came to see the physician because of severe pain shortly after it started.[65] Finally, some patients sought relief of chronic and long-standing conditions such as paralysis or asthma. Many of them had sought medical care before and came with clear ideas about what would or would not work for them.

For the examining physician, there was little difference between symptoms reported by the patient or the prescription-seeker and signs that could be observed by the physician himself. The differentiation appears to have been between three types of signs ('alāmāt) depending on what they indicated: either a state (of health or disease) in the past, the present, or the future. The first was "beneficial to the physician alone, as [interpreting it] will indicate his virtue [in the craft of medicine]." This means that the physician's ability to use these seemingly innocuous signs to describe a patient's health and disease history would show the physician's ability, experience, and knowledge, although it may not be useful in treating the patient's current condition. The second benefited the patient alone because it would help the physician diagnose and treat the patient's current illness. Presumably, it would not help the physician in his career because it was obvious or reported by the patient and therefore detectable by any physician. Finally, the third type, signs indicating a condition or development in the future, would benefit both the patient and the physician because it would help the patient's recovery and prove the physician's worth at the same time.[66] The physician could detect these signs by questioning

[64] Ibid., 176.
[65] See, for instance, a case of a woman who suffered from severe colic and sought the physician only three days later, whereas another sought the physician possibly the next day after suffering severe colics as well (Ibid., 213). Others sought care immediately after feeling dizziness, which may not have been severely painful but was probably sufficiently disruptive (Ibid., 93). Another young man came with severe difficulty in breathing and a feeling of suffocation that apparently started shortly before he sought care (Ibid., 153).
[66] Ibn Al-Nafīs, al-Mūjaz fī al-Ṭibb, 78. Ibn al-Nafīs (d. 1288) summarized this statement and the differentiation between the three types of signs from Ibn Sīnā's al-Qānūn (Avicenna, Kitāb al-Qānūn fī al-Ṭibb, 56). Mujāz al-Qānūn by Ibn al-Nafīs was a popular text since its appearance and well into the eighteenth century. On its authorship, see Fancy, Science and Religion in Mamluk Egypt, 116–20. Fancy casts reasonable doubts on whether Ibn al-Nafīs did indeed write this book based on the fact that the book failed to show Ibn al-Nafīs's distinctive positions in relation to physiology. Fancy suggests that it is possible that al-Mūjaz was authored earlier in Ibn al-Nafīs's career or that the book was largely intended as a practical summary where theoretical discussions were avoided. Regardless of its authorship, Fancy explained, the text was very popular throughout the fourteenth century, contributed to receiving and understanding Ibn Sīnā's work, and became very influential in fashioning medical knowledge and practice at the time. In the context of this discussion, al-Mūjaz is a valuable source on medical practice precisely because of its popularity and also because of its attribution to Ibn al-Nafīs. Although this attribution may not have been accurate, it played a role in the popularity of the book and in legitimizing its contents. I have refrained,

patients, observing their color, their facial features, or their movement, or by examining the three cardinal signs: namely, pulse, urine, and stool.[67] This examination and questioning would need to yield information about the patient's normal complexion and also the changes occurring during the illness, so as to help the physician determine the nature of illness before he prescribed diet modification (*tadbīr*), treatment (*ʿilājāt*), or evacuation (*istifrāgh*). The nature of illness was based on two different aspects: the humoral change that resulted in the illness and the organ or organs affected by such change. As explained by Ibn al-Nafīs, most of the signs indicating the humoral change would have to be reported by the patient or asked about by the physician. These signs included tingling and some heaviness for choleric afflictions, heaviness and redness for sanguine ones, whiteness and decrease in thirst for phlegmatic ones, and dryness with insomnia for melancholic ones. He added, "dreams can also indicate the nature of the substance [causing the imbalance]."[68]

The manner by which a physician was able to detect the different signs in a patient depended on the nature of practice and its site. At one extreme, physicians practicing in courts or with rich clientele had the opportunity to closely observe their patrons: they were able to monitor their health and the changes in their diet carefully. Ibn Abī Uṣaybiʿah's dictionary, as well as al-Qifṭī's and al-Ruhāwī's writings, are full of examples of physicians practicing in the court and of how they became deeply familiar with their patron's health, complexion, pulse, and other signs that appeared necessary for their practice.[69] Al-Rāzī's small collection of cases in *al-Ḥāwī*, which was popular as a source of practical medicine (as seen earlier), also include several examples of his familiarity with the health and history of a specific group of patients.[70] In the first case, al-Rāzī was familiar with the patient's previous incidents of renal affliction; he also knew that the patient's father had a weak bladder.[71] In another case, we are told that he used to monitor the diet of the daughter of a certain al-Ḥusayn ibn ʿAbdawayh and that she

however, from using *al-Mūjaz* to discuss the traditions, practices, and works of al-Dakhwār's circle because authorship is significant in that discussion.

67 Ibn Al-Nafīs, *al-Mūjaz fī al-Ṭibb*, 78–79.

68 Ibid., 79.

69 The historical accuracy of many of these reports is debatable and sometimes even suspicious, and their veracity is beyond the scope of this discussion. What is important for the purpose of this discussion is how Ibn Abī Uṣaybiʿah and his readers perceived the ideals of court practice and imagined it as a practice in which physicians were deeply connected with their patrons and familiar with their conditions. See Moulin, *Le Médecin du Prince: Voyage à Travers les Cultures*.

70 Meyerhof, "Clinical Observations by Rhazes."

71 Meyerhof, "Clinical Observations by Rhazes," AR 1–2. I will use AR to indicate pagination in the Arabic section of Meyerhof's edition and EN to indicate those in his English section.

contracted smallpox when she violated his instructions about drinking milk.[72] His relationship with the family of al-Ḥusayn ibn ʿAbdawayh was apparently strong because he also attended to Ibn ʿAbdawayh's son and knew that his massive body was not due to increased fat or humidity, as other physicians thought, but to increased flesh. It was this knowledge that allowed him to treat the son properly.[73]

Physicians practicing in the bīmāristān were faced with dozens of patients with whom they did not have the opportunity to establish this type of relationship.[74] The bīmāristān appeared clearly in two of al-Rāzī's cases in *al-Ḥāwī*. The first case was of a patient who was one of al-Rāzī's neighbors and suffered from epilepsy (*ṣarʿ*). Al-Rāzī knew that he had been thin (*naḥīf*) since his early youth (*ṣibāhi*), and so al-Rāzī "conjectured (*ḥadastu*)[75] that his affliction was not because of excess phlegm" and prescribed him emetics several times and then a syrup to expel black bile. As a result, the patient did not suffer from any fits until he neglected al-Rāzī's recommendations and ate fish. At the end of the case description, al-Rāzī wrote: "he [the patient] was [administered purgatives] in the bīmāristān but this did not benefit him."[76] Purgatives were used in the bīmāristān probably because his affliction was thought to be caused by excess phlegm or by a combination of phlegm and black bile. These were understood as among the more common causes for epilepsy and would benefit from a purgative. Al-Rāzī's ability to recognize the correct cause of the affliction was due to his intimate knowledge of the patient over a long period of time, something that was not possible for the physicians at the bīmāristān. In the second case, the bīmāristān was not mentioned explicitly but was referred to indirectly when al-Rāzī called his assistant "the reading-out physician (*al-ṭabīb al-muqriʾ*)," a title given to the teaching assistant who helped with lectures delivered in the bīmāristān. In this case, al-Rāzī looked at the patient and saw that his jugulars were full (*mumtaliʾah*), his face reddish and puffy, and his eyes red; therefore he

[72] Ibid., AR 6.

[73] Ibid., AR 7.

[74] It is not clear how many patients would have attended the bīmāristān in any given day. Some reports, that appear to be clearly exaggerated, claimed that al-Bīmāristān al-Manṣūrī received 4,000 patients every day coming to have their eyes treated (Al-Balawī, *Tāj al-Mafriq fī Taḥliyat ʿUlamāʾ al-Mashriq*).

[75] "Conjecture/*ḥadasa*" appeared to be the verb of choice to describe the process of identifying the disease or the cause of affliction based on knowledge of a patient's history and on examining the patient. "Guess/*khammana*" is used occasionally to refer to a similar process, but one based on much less information or evidence.

[76] Meyerhof, "Clinical Observations by Rhazes," AR 8.

ordered the assisting physician to bloodlet him.[77] In this case, al-Rāzī's diagnosis, probably delivered within the bīmāristān, did not rely on any knowledge of the patient's history or even on any questioning of the patient about his condition but depended instead on his appearance and what seemed to be a simpler method of evaluation. In a way, al-Rāzī's diagnosis was similar to the diagnosis and treatment his neighbor received in the bīmāristān.

The bīmāristān was not mentioned again in *al-Ḥāwī* collection of cases. Another collection of cases also attributed to al-Rāzī was arranged and copied in Cairo in 1258 by a physician named Alī b. Ayyūb b. Yūsuf. The collection, known as *Kitāb al-Tajārib (Book of Experiments)*, contained 971 cases and is one of the largest of its kind.[78] Whereas the bīmāristān was mentioned in *al-Ḥāwī* cases explicitly only twice, it was never mentioned explicitly in *al-tajārib*. It is easy to identify, however, two main types of patients in both collections and the diagnostic approach used with each. On one hand, al-Rāzī described patients whom he knew personally, of whose complexions and conditions he had a deep knowledge.[79] Many of these patients were recognizable by name, and their conditions were described in detail along with information on how they progressed through treatment. On the other hand, al-Rāzī gave much briefer descriptions of patients whom he did not know at all and whom he did not question extensively. Whereas the first group represented his personal clientele, mainly dignitaries, distinguished people, or neighbors and personal acquaintances, the second group may have included some of his bīmāristān patients.

With the first group, the epistemological process through which al-Rāzī arrived at conclusions or prescribed treatment relied on detailed narrative construction. Although physical signs and examinations were important, the longer history of the patient's complexion played the most significant role in diagnosis and treatment. In comparison, the second group of cases in *al-Ḥāwī* collection, and all the cases in *al-Tajārib*, seemed to have been diagnosed mainly by examination of different physical signs (including pulse and urine) and with little knowledge of the patients' longer history. For example, al-Rāzī stated that a man "came to me (*jā'anī*)" complaining of palpitations in his heart (*khafaqān fu'ādihi*). The man took al-Rāzī's hand and placed it on his aorta and then showed him his brachial artery

[77] Ibid., AR 19.

[78] Al-Rāzī, *Kitāb al-Tajārib*. This is to be differentiated from another book attributed to al-Rāzī as well, which is called *Jirāb al-Mujarrabāt*, which was a collection of tried and experimented recipes but not of cases. On cases and case histories, see, for instance, Pormann, "Case Notes and Clinicians."

[79] No cases of this description were reported in *al-Tajārib*.

(*al-bāsilaq*) so that he could see that the pulsations were very strong. After some consideration, al-Rāzī prescribed musk-remedy because, he explained, "I estimated that this man's condition in relation to pulse is similar to those with asthma (*rabw*) in relation to breathing. Since [the latters'] chests admit little air, despite the expansion of their chests."[80] That is to say, that little blood arrived in the patient's body despite his violent pulses. Musk-remedy was supposed to improve the quality of his blood. Similarly, al-Rāzī wrote that a woman "came to me (*jāʾatnī*)" with black urine. She "claimed (*zaʿamat*)" that passing this urine relieved some pain that she had in her lower back. "She had urinated this [black urine] for ten days when she came to me and had fever every night." He prescribed a diuretic because he thought this was caused by black bile.[81]

Similarly, he wrote, another man "came to me (*jāʾanī*)" after vomiting about two pounds of blood on excessive drunkenness, and "I found his eyes red and his build plethoric, so I bloodlet him and ordered him to keep on astringents."[82] Finally, a woman who was "brought to me (*jāʾanī bihā*) by Abū ʿĪsā al-Hāshimī al-Naḥḥās" was very fat and paralyzed after labor. "There was no doubt about her condition (*lam yakun fī amrihā labs*) and the signs [of her illness] were clear and obvious (*bal kānat dalaʾil ṣaḥīḥah sādhajah*)." Al-Rāzī gave her strong purgatives and prescribed the Theriac of the Four, but the druggist gave her the wrong preparation. She was nevertheless cured, to the amazement of al-Rāzī and his colleagues.[83] In all these cases, which were narrated using similar verbs and structures, al-Rāzī naturally sought some prior information about the patient's life (the history of the one woman's fever or the other woman's labor and paralysis, etc.).The narrative, however, relied more heavily on the physical manifestations that these patients exhibited and on al-Rāzī's own examinations and observations. As heuristic accounts, these cases served to teach students and young physicians how to observe and understand specific signs rapidly and to prescribe medications that would solve the perceived problem. Unlike the first group of cases, the center of the "medical story" was not located in the complaint's prehistory but rather at the time of complaint itself. It was wrapped within the structure of the ailment, which told its own story as a unique and discrete category.

In short, al-Rāzī's cases exhibit a continuum of approaches to patients' ailments and complaints anchored by two distinctive methods. At one end

80 Ibid., AR 4.
81 Ibid., AR 10.
82 Ibid., AR 9.
83 Ibid., EN 341, AR 8.

of the continuum, we have a patient like ʿAbd Allāh ibn Sawādah, whom al-Rāzī knew intimately and with whose family and history of illnesses al-Rāzī was familiar. In this case, al-Rāzī's ability to construct a disease and a treatment narrative was at its best. Although he ended up hesitating to identify the right disease, this was because he had neglected to ask about a piece of information and his patient did not volunteer the information. The error, therefore, was the result of a lapse in the tightly knit history of his patient. On the other end of the continuum, we have the patient with the puffy face and strong pulse who was immediately prescribed venesection without any discussion of the illness's history or patient's complexion to supplement al-Rāzī's limited observations. In other cases in the *al-Ḥāwī* collection and in *al-Tajārib* (all of which began with variations on the verb *jāʾanī*, or "came to me"), a similar procedure of diagnosis and prescription occurred: al-Rāzī relied more often than not on his own observations and examination of the patient's physical signs, with little attention to the history of illness. Most of the patients coming to the bīmāristān would have been diagnosed through the second method – relying on physical examination and observation. Some would leave with medications or after procedures such as venesection. Others would be admitted, thus allowing the physician, or at times his more experienced colleagues, to visit the patient and monitor the treatment.

In the same way, al-Dakhwār relied on physical examination to diagnose patients in the bīmāristān with no regard to their history of illness. In one anecdote that Ibn Abī Uṣaybiʿah witnessed, al-Dakhwār led young physicians and students in examining patients in the hall of fevers (*qāʿat al-maḥmūmīn*):

> The physicians felt (*jassat*) his [the patient's] pulse and said: "he has weakness (*ḍaʿf*) [in pulse]. Give him chicken soup for strength." He [al-Dakhwār] looked at him and said: "neither his speech nor the look of his eyes indicate (*yaqtaḍī*) weakness." He felt the pulse of his right hand and the pulse of the other hand and said [to the physicians], "feel [plural] (*jissū*) the pulse of his left hand," and we found it strong. He then said, "consider the pulse of his right hand and how it is close to his elbow. The pulsating vessel (*al-ʿirq al-nābiḍ*) had split (*infaraqa*) into two branches (*shuʿbatayn*); one remained [in its original course] and is felt, and the other ascended to the top of radius [bone] and extended to the fingers" and we found this to be true. He said, "In rare (*nādir*) [cases], some people have pulse like this, and it confuses many physicians. They think the pulse is weak but they [are] feeling [only] this branch, which is half the vessel."[84]

[84] Ibid., 4: 327.

Here again, there was very little discussion of the patient's history of diseases, even though such knowledge would be extremely useful for this type of condition. Weakness in pulse could have caused previous episodes of weakness or fainting and might have resulted in impotence or other conditions that would give more credence to the physicians' diagnosis. When objecting to their diagnosis, al-Dakhwār did not rely on such "historical" evidence but rather on immediate observation of the patient's speech, as well as on the color and look of his eyes, which did not corroborate the evidence from his pulse. The physicians' mistake in diagnosis was common and predictable, al-Dakhwār explained, because the condition itself was rare. Al-Dakhwār's detailed observation (and experience), however, enabled him to correct a diagnosis that had mistaken an uncommon condition for a common one.

Ibn Abī Uṣaybiʿah reported a number of accounts about al-Dakhwār's examination of patients "residing (*muqīmīn*) in the bīmāristān." Al-Dakhwār visited patients on days following the initial examination, re-examined them, and modified the remedies that were originally prescribed. In one account, which Ibn Abī Uṣaybiʿah witnessed himself, a patient came (*atā*)[85] to al-Dakhwār with a severe, burning fever (*ḥummā muḥriqah*) and sharp, acidic urine. "[Al-Dakhwār] considered his [the patient's] strength (*iʿtabar quwatahu*) and ordered that he be given ground camphor seeds in a specific amount that he designated in the [patient's] chart (*al-dustūr*), and that he drink it and not have anything else."[86] As shown before, al-Dakhwār's prescription was based on examining the patient's fever and acidic urine, although he had to take into consideration the patient's strength before prescribing a treatment as strong as camphor seeds. Ibn Abī Uṣaybiʿah emphasized that the famous physician designated a specific amount and wrote it down so that no mistakes could be made. "When we came the next day, we found this patient with his fever relieved and his urine free from acidity." The patient was clearly admitted to the hospital, and the physician had the chance to monitor him the next day. In the same manner, al-Dakhwār prescribed a "generous amount of opium" to a patient of mania in the hall of the melancholics (*al-mamrūrīn*). Again, the patient had improved when visited the following day.[87] It seems that al-Dakhwār was well known for "uncommon remedies (*gharāʾib al-mudāwah*), deep consideration in treatment (*al-taqaṣṣī fī al-muʿālajah*), courage (*al-iqdām*) with

[85] Ibn Abī Uṣaybiʿah's description of the bīmāristān patients used the verb "came *atā*," which expresses the same connotation as al-Rāzī's "came to me/us *jāʾanī*" in *al-Ḥāwī* or "came/jāʾa" in *al-tajārib*.
[86] Ibn Abī Uṣaybiʿah, *ʿuyūn al-Anbāʾ*, 4: 326–27.
[87] Ibid., 4: 327.

prescribing medications that would cure in the fastest of times in a manner that excelled and exceeded (*yafūqu*) the people of his time."[88]

In the context of the bīmāristān, physicians had little interactions with their patients beyond examination and possibly later revisits. Physicians were expected to rely on their experience and their practical knowledge to make decisions and treatment recommendations that relied mainly on physical examination. The ability to effectively use uncommon remedies; to deeply, yet quickly, understand patients' conditions; and to prescribe remedies that would work rapidly were all qualities that indicated deep experience and were highly prized in the bīmāristān and elsewhere. Courage in prescribing extreme remedies and trying new regiments may have been possible or even praiseworthy in the bīmāristān but were likely improbable and unwise with more affluent or more powerful clients, as will be seen later.

How Did Physicians Think in the Bīmāristān?

According to Ibn al-Nafīs' instructions in *al-Mūjaz*, treatment was divided into three different types: diet management (*tadbīr*), medications (*dawā '*), and "the work of the hand (*al-'amal bil-yadd*)."[89] As explained earlier, Ibn al-Nafīs and other physicians of al-Dakhwār's circle did not pay much attention to questions of health preservation or to the role of diet in treatment. Similar to al-Rāzī, who was more interested in evacuations either by medications or by other "works of the hand,"[90] Ibn al-Nafīs did not consider diet modification useful except for preserving the patients' power either to receive medications or survive the process of recovery independently. His analysis of diet, spanning only a few lines, focused on explaining that food should be prohibited during crisis (*buḥrān*) and during attacks of fever and colics (*nuwab*). He also explained that chronic ailments required proper feeding early on to avoid weakness at the end of the disease.[91] *Ḥimyah* or healthy diet did not appeal to Ibn

---

[88] Ibid., 4: 326.

[89] Ibn al-Nafīs, *al-Mūjaz fī al-Ṭibb*, 95.

[90] Al-Rāzī's approach was focused on evacuation, and he appeared ready to use aggressive evacuations much earlier than indicated in Galenic writings. His main argument in this regard was in his *Doubts on Galen* (Al-Rāzī, *Kitāb al-Shukūk*), in which he objected to Galen's recommendation to wait for the ripening of humors before evacuation, arguing that evacuation could be used earlier on. Both Ibn Abī Ṣādiq and Ibn al-Nafīs commented on this controversy in their commentaries on the *Aphorisms* and came out on both sides of the controversy, with Ibn Abī Ṣādiq siding with Galen against al-Rāzī (Ibn Abī Ṣādiq al-Nīsābūri, "Sharḥ Fuṣūl Buqrāṭ") and with Ibn al-Nafīs agreeing generally with al-Rāzī, explaining why early evacuation could be useful, and reconciling al-Rāzī with Hippocrates (Ibn al-Nafīs, *Sharḥ Fuṣul Abuqrāṭ*).

[91] Ibn al-Nafīs, *al-Mūjaz fī al-Ṭibb*, 95–96.

al-Nafīs, whether in his discussions in his book *al-Mūjaz* or in the commentary on the *Aphorisms*, where he neglected this aspect almost entirely. Ibn al-Nafīs viewed diet modifications as a tool for treatment in that food, or the lack thereof, did not negatively impact the condition of the patient. Like al-Rāzī, he implied a preference for fasting, explaining: "Food is a friend of nature. But it is also its enemy as it is a friend of disease. Therefore, only what is necessary of it should be used during sickness."[92]

Ibn al-Nafīs' view appears to have been representative of a more general attitude, at least, in the medical circles around the bīmāristāns. The types of foods described in al-Bīmāristān al-Manṣūrī's *waqf* document betrayed a similar approach to nourishment of the sick: that is, little and light feeding during any illnesses except for chronic ones. For this reason, the *waqf* document focused on chicken, young chicks, and soup, all of which were considered light food at the time.[93] Ibn al-Akfānī (d. 1348), who served in a bīmāristān and was said to have helped the *nāẓir* supervise purchases, agreed with Ibn al-Nafīs' view. Writing about what to do when lacking access to physicians, he explained that one could leave the body to deal with diseases by means of its natural powers: "The manner by which a body is left to [its] nature is to leave the patient to his own movements and desires: whenever he feels hungry, he eats the lightest possible food that he is used to, and whenever he is thirsty, he drinks water."[94] If one was taking medications, he explained that "some diseases are quick to end, and the power [of nature] would be mostly preserved without food."[95] Although both Ibn al-Nafīs and al-Akfānī continued to confirm the maxim that "whenever it is possible, [patients should] be treated through arranging their diet and without medications,"[96] their discussion of practice paid little attention to such methods of treatment and offered very little guidance in this regard, especially in comparison to treatment with medications and with "the works of the hand." Ultimately, and in all cases, modifying the diet would only follow after deciding on the nature of the disease and its different stages.

[92] Ibn al-Nafīs, *al-Mūjaz fī al-Ṭibb*, 95.

[93] Ibn Ḥabīb, *Tadhkirat al-Nabīh*, 1: 365. It is not clear whether the *waqf* document authors understood this to be representative of a specific treatment approach or whether they expressed attitudes common in the bīmāristān culture of the time, including al-Bīmāristān al-Nāṣirī. In either case, the specification of these particular foods in the document is a sign of their perceived commonality.

[94] Ibn al-Akfānī, Ghunyat al-Labīb ʿinda Ghaybat al-Ṭabīb, 64.

[95] Ibid., 67.

[96] Ibid.

Ibn al-Nafīs' scheme for diagnosis, explained in *al-Mūjaz*, followed Ibn Sīnā's scheme to a large extent and focused on the identification of the afflicted organ and the nature of the affliction. Recognizing the afflicted organ was the first step in identifying the humoral imbalance, deciding on the medication needed – its strength, dose, and how it should be applied – and deciding whether there would be a need for venesections, cupping, or other procedures. The arrangement of different medical textbooks, such as *al-Ḥāwī*, by organs and bodily regions, from head to toe, was not only a useful and easy organizational tool, but was also connected to the type of medical thinking in which physicians engaged and mimicked the arrangement of a physician's thinking process. Memorizing such books by heart would allow the physician to recall such information at the right time based on the patient's complaint. Ibn al-Nafīs' explanation of different diseases followed this same thinking schemata: identify the afflicted organ, identify the type of humoral imbalance and its degree, and prescribe a treatment to correct the imbalance or treat the symptom, depending on the latter's type and severity. He arranged diseases by organs. In each organ, he started by outlining the signs of different complexions and humoral imbalances, and then he continued with a list of possible afflictions or presentations that one might encounter.[97] For instance, the discussion of chest and lung diseases started by addressing the signs of different complexions that would accompany any given presentation and indicate its origin. This was followed by a list of possible (or common) diseases, their main symptoms and presentations, and their treatments based on their various humoral origins.[98] The same schema was used with all other organs and body regions. After the discussion of diseases connected to organs, Ibn al-Nafīs moved on to talk about diseases that were not specific to any particular organ. In this section, he included fevers[99] and a section on crisis (*al-buḥrān*);[100] tumors, leprosy, and the epidemic (the plague);[101] broken bones, dislocations, and bruises;[102] beautification of hair, including its dyeing;[103] and, finally, poisons and poisoning.[104]

97 Ibn al-Nafīs, *Al-Mūjaz fī al-Ṭibb*, 145.
98 Ibid., 193–96.
99 Ibid., 262–74.
100 Ibid., 275–78.
101 Ibid., 279–86.
102 Ibid., 287–88.
103 Ibid., 289–96.
104 Ibid., 297. Although Ibn al-Nafīs followed *al-Qānūn*'s arrangement faithfully in his *al-Mujāz* (the Summary), his treatment of different topics was not even and did not necessarily reflect the space given to such topics in *al-Qānūn*. For instance, *al-Mūjaz* did not include any section on anatomy,

When encountering a patient, the physician focused primarily on the patient's presentation to discover whether the condition was located in a specific organ, whether it was a non–organ-specific condition, or whether it involved more than one organ. If it appeared to involve more than one organ, he would have to discover which organ the condition affected first – this was where the treatment would start – unless the latter organ was more important (such as the heart or the brain).[105] In all cases, the physician would follow this initial identification with a number of questions intended to ascertain the humoral reason for this condition. In one of the cases in *al-Tajārib*, a young man complained of dizziness and pain in his knees. Al-Rāzī asked him whether he had a bitter taste in his mouth and noticed that the young man had a small cough. The case report differentiated between three aspects of the examination: the patient's complaint, al-Rāzī's questions, and al-Rāzī's observations. The reported complaint, using the verb "*shakā*" (literally, "complained"),[106] allowed the physician to understand that the condition started in the head, as suggested by the dizziness, and may have spread now to the knees. Al-Rāzī, having doubted choleric affliction, asked about bitterness in the mouth and found that that was indeed the case. Before prescribing a treatment, al-Rāzī observed the presence of a light cough that prompted him to prescribe medications for cough and for yellow bile.[107] This schema was repeated in other cases, in which patients presented with similar complaints. In one, a woman complained of dizziness and bitterness in her mouth but had no cough; she was prescribed *ihlīlaj aṣfar* for the yellow bile, which was similar to the prescription given to the young man but without a preparation for cough. An old man, also complaining of dizziness, was asked about the taste in his mouth but did not report bitterness. The patient was then asked whether he slept longer than usual, to which he reported that he had done

and he included a very brief discussion of drugs (*aqrabādhīn* or formulary). Instead, almost half the book was dedicated to diseases, both related to specific organs and generalized conditions. The arrangement of the practical part, including its division into diseases affecting organs followed by diseases affecting the entire body, is reminiscent of *al-Ḥāwī*'s organization because Ibn Sīnā's *al-Qānūn* located these generalized afflictions earlier, before the discussion of organ-specific diseases. This arrangement suggests that *al-Mūjaz* was indeed a book of practical medicine that would have complemented Ibn al-Nafīs' other works on theoretical medicine, such as *Sharḥ al-Qānūn*. If *al-Mūjaz* was indeed seen as a book of practice, this might explain why Ibn al-Nafīs did not engage in any serious discussion of his modifications on Avicennan physiology, as noted by Nahyan Fancy. Fancy, *Science and Religion in Mamluk Egypt*.

105 Avicenna, *Kitāb al-Qānūn fī al-Ṭibb*, 57–58.

106 In other instances, the case reports used the verb "*jā'a bi-* or *atā bi-* (lit. came with)" to indicate the patient's reported complaint.

107 Al-Rāzī, *Kitāb al-Tajārib*, 93.

so and had also experienced a generalized heaviness in his body. Both excessive sleep and heaviness, signs of excess phlegm, helped al-Rāzī make the right diagnosis. Once the absence of bitter taste enabled him to exclude choleric affliction, he followed a different line of inquiry and diagnosis and then prescribed a treatment accordingly.[108]

The first case in al-Rāzī's observations in *al-Ḥāwī* provides an interesting example of his thought process. ʿAbd Allāh ibn Sawādah first complained of a fever recurring every six days; it happened again at smaller and smaller intervals until it afflicted him daily. Al-Rāzī thought that this condition might either be a fever that "wants to turn quartan (*turīd an tanqaliba rabʿan*)" or a renal abscess. But it was not until Ibn Sawādah passed pus in his urine that it became obvious to al-Rāzī that this was a renal abscess. After this, he promised his patient that the fevers would not return, which was indeed the case. The key reason for al-Rāzī's unsure diagnosis was that "[the patient] did not complain to me that his loins resemble a hanging weight when he stood, and I neglected to ask him about it too (*walam yashku illayya anna qaṭanahu shabaha thuql muʿallaq minhu idhā qāma wa aghfaltu anā ayḍan an asʾalahu ʿanhu*)."[109] Al-Rāzī concluded that the abscess must have been small: "After he passed pus in urine (*bāla maddah*), I asked him whether he had felt [a hanging weight in the loins], and he said yes. Were [the abscess] big, he would have complained of this."[110] The absence of the original complaint, and al-Rāzī's failure to ask the proper questions, led to this misdiagnosis. More significantly, al-Rāzī's experience, which he intended to transmit through these cases, enabled him to anticipate a specific complaint given in a particular form (hanging weights from the loins). Such complaint would have allowed him to follow a specific line of thinking that would have led to the right diagnosis.

Other questions were dictated not by the symptoms or signs reported but by the patient's age or sex. Most significantly, al-Rāzī apparently asked almost every female patient about her menses regardless of her complaint. This is understandable because menses affected processes of evacuation as well as the presentations of different diseases. This structured process of questioning aimed not only at probing a patient's longer disease and health history, but also at completing his or her complaint and aiding the physical examination. The standard lines of thinking, which were reflected in standardized lines of questioning, were the reason these cases were useful

[108] Ibid., 93–94.
[109] Meyerhof, "Thirty-Three Clinical Observations by Rhazes," EN 332–33, AR 1–2.
[110] Ibid., EN 333, AR 2.

to students because they were able to follow lines of thinking and deduction and learn how to use their deductive tools. Moreover, these questions show us that these physicians relied on a standardized diagnosis process that had little space for guessing or intuition, although it afforded an important role for experience. At the same time, such a standardized process reduced the physician's ability to adjust to specific patients and flew in the face of the original theoretical maxims of Galenic practice that valued deep consideration of patients' complexions and histories and all but rejected standardized or disease-specific treatments. As such, these methods were more apt for the market – and even more for the bīmāristān – where physicians dealt with many patients who had little power and little knowledge. In contrast, in courts, and with more prestigious clientele, physicians had the time and ability, as required, to carefully consider their patients' history even to a fault. In fact, al-Rāzī's near misdiagnosis of the renal abscess patient was in part due to his deep knowledge of the patient's family history that led him astray (al-Rāzī knew that the patient's father had a weak bladder). Although high-clientele practice represented mostly a minority in general practice, it continued to set the standard and dominate the discursive field.

A Bīmāristānī Pharmacopeia

In his commentary on Hippocrates' *The Acknowledgement* (*Taqdimat al-Maʿrifah*), al-Dakhwār explained that a physician should be ready with the knowledge of different drugs, especially the compound drugs, and the major theriacs and pills. He added that this was why the bīmāristāns were first created: to have a stock of drugs that were well-known and ready to use at any time.[111] Al-Dakhwār's passing reference to bīmāristāns is remarkable because it indicates that, in his view, a major role of these bīmāristāns was to prepare major drugs, especially those that took a long time to make, and to have them readily available for physicians. At the same time, it hinted at what we know from other sources: that the bīmāristān had fewer types of drugs from which to choose. A physician practicing in the bīmāristān needed to be familiar with the limited number of drugs prepared and used in the bīmāristān and from which he was to prescribe.

The major formulary of drugs produced by the Egyptian physician al-Sadīd ibn Abī al-Bayān (b. 1161) clearly emphasized the notion of a

[111] Al-Dakhwār and Ibn Qāḍī Baʿlabak, *Kitāb Sharḥ Tuqaddimuhu al-Maʿrifah lil-Dakhwār 565–628 Ah-1160–1230 AD*, 152.

limited number of available medications. His formulary, *al-Dustūr al-Bīmāristānī*, was a relatively short collection of drugs listing only those used in the bīmāristān.[112] After Ibn al-Bayān composed *al-Dustūr*, this new book rapidly became one of the most significant books in the region despite its small size. The influence of *al-Dustūr* on local medicinal practices in Egypt and the Levant appeared in how frequently other manuals cited it. For instance, the famous herbalist al-Kuḥīn al-'Aṭṭār cited *al-Dustūr* by name on eighty-two different occasions in his famous and well-celebrated formulary *Minhāj al-Dukkān wa Dustūr al-A'yān*.[113] Moreover, *al-Dustūr* was cited even more frequently without reference to the author or book title. In contrast, al-Kuḥīn al-'Aṭṭār cited Ibn al-Tilmīdh's *Aqrabādhīn* at a lesser frequency on par with al-Majūsī and Ibn Jazlah, although neither of the latter two had produced specialized formularies. Finally, *al-Dustūr* was the only formulary produced in a bīmāristān in this region: no comparable text was produced by the physicians of al-Bīmāristān al-Nūrī and al-Bīmāristān al-Manṣūrī, institutions bigger and wealthier than al-Bīmāristān al-Nāṣirī.[114]

Although *al-Dustūr*'s general structure was similar to other formularies, the arrangement of the different chapters and the language and style used to describe the different recipes differed from Sābūr's or Ibn al-Tilmīdh's *Aqrabādhīn*, as well as from al-Kuḥīn's market formulary. Compared to Ibn al-Tilmīdh's and al-Kuḥīn's formularies, both of which circulated at the same time and in the same region as *al-Dustūr*, the latter paid more attention to symptoms and signs in the description of each recipe. It explained the major humoral causes for such symptoms and how the described medication could exert an effect through humoral mechanisms. Conversely, as Leigh Chipman explains, *al-Dustūr* paid little attention to the preparation of drugs and to other concerns of the herbalist or "pharmacists."[115]

---

[112] Ibn Abī al-Bayān and Sbath, *Al-Dustūr al-Bīmāristānī [Le Formulaire des Hôpitaux d'Ibn Abil Bayan, Médecin du Bimaristan Annacery au Caire]*, 17.

[113] Chipman, *The World of Pharmacy and Pharmacists in Mamluk Cairo*, 38. Al-Kuīn's book "Minhāj al-Dukkān" remains very popular among herbalists even today and can be found in many modern popular nonscholarly editions in Cairo.

[114] On the use and popularity of *al-Dustūr*, See also Lev, Chipman, and Niessen, "A Hospital Handbook for the Community: Evidence for the Extensive Use of Ibn Abi 'l-Bayan's al-Dustur al-Bimaristani by the Jewish Practitioners of Medieval Cairo.".

[115] Chipman, *The World of Pharmacy and Pharmacists in Mamluk Cairo*. Chipman argued for differentiating pharmacological writings produced by physicians, such as *al-Dustūr* but also Ibn al-Tilmīdh's *Aqrabādhīn*, from those written by pharmacists, such as al-Kuḥīn's. Seeing that very few writings in the field were produced by pharmacists and herbalists, it seems that Chipman's argument would be better served if limited to al-Kuhīn's writings as opposed to dividing the entire field. That being said, *al-Dustūr* did indeed exhibit little attention to the details of drug making,

Oliver Kahl notes that the structure of the recipes in Ibn al-Tilmīdh's dispensatory is largely consistent: "[T]he individual recipes are built more or less . . . around the same formal skeleton, whose essential parts can be described as follows: name and/or category of the drug, range of its application, list of ingredients with doses, instructions for combining the ingredients, directions for use."[116] In Sābūr's formulary, which was used in al-Bīmāristān al-ʿAḍudī before Ibn al-Tilmīdh's dispensatory replaced it there, every recipe also followed a fixed formula and set order: the name of the medication, the symptoms or indications of prescription and usage, the conditions it could treat, the ingredients, the mixing instructions, and the usage instructions.[117] *Al-Dustūr* followed basically the same structure, but the sections related to the symptoms, and indications occupied more space than in the other formularies and dominated the recipe as a whole.

Not only was the structure more focused on the clinical manifestations and diseases, the division and arrangement of the chapters, as well as of the descriptions of symptoms within every recipe, placed even more emphasis on the practice of drug prescription. Chapters in *al-Dustūr* can be divided into two major categories: those discussing general drugs and those discussing locally acting or specific drugs. Chapters in the first category included drugs that accomplished their effect through specific mechanisms related to the dissolution of certain humors or through the facilitation of evacuation. The mechanism by which these drugs achieved their effects was explained clearly and in a manner that rendered diverse, unmentioned applications possible. For instance, triphala acted on black bile and phlegm, exerting its influence mainly on the stomach, heart, and liver. *Al-Dustūr* explained that it could treat any condition caused by excess humidity or coldness.[118] Similarly, stomachics were said to help digestion by increasing innate heat in the stomach; they were therefore useful in conditions where a lack of innate heat led to problems such as difficulty in digestion due to coldness.[119] The formulary grouped locally acting or specific drugs together, however, because they acted on a specific body part with little attention to their humoral functioning or because they performed a specific role in symptom relief that did not affect the actual

although it had more details than Ibn al-Tilmīdh's writings. See Ahmed Ragab, "Leigh Chipman, the World of Pharmacy and Pharmacists in Mamlūk Cairo," *Speculum* 87, no. (2012).

[116] Ibn al-Tilmīdh and Kahl, *The Dispensatory of Ibn at-Tilmīḏ*, 27–28.

[117] Sahl, *Sabur Ibn Sahl's Dispensatory in the Recension of the Adudi Hospital*, 9.

[118] Ibn Abī Al-Bayān and Sbath, *Al-Dustūr al-Bīmāristānī [Le Formulaire des Hôpitaux d'Ibn Abil Bayan, Médecin du Bimaristan Annacery au Caire]*, 18–23.

[119] Ibid., 23–28.

cause of the condition. For example, the chapters discussing eye medications or mouth and teeth medications included all drugs acting on these specific organs or body parts regardless of the condition affecting them. The text described *lohocs* as useful to treat a cough regardless of its cause, whereas *robs* treated throat problems; *snuffs* cleaned the brain and did not depend on the specific condition present. All of these drugs performed their functions locally and based simply on their specific formation and local effect at the site of administration. Likewise, oils were used to relieve pain at any site in the body and in any condition. Liniments were grouped in one chapter with other medications for abscesses, fistulas, and traumas, presumably due to their local actions when applied.

Al-Dustūr's way of explaining the different indications of each drug differed depending on the nature of the drug itself – whether general and locally acting. For general drugs, the description of these drugs' indications was based on the same schema of diagnosis described in *al-Mūjaz* and other similar texts: the afflicted organs and the nature of affliction as explained in the humoral schema, followed by the type and site of action on which the drug performed. In this way, *al-Dustūr* lent itself to the medical thinking and diagnostic schemes of the physicians reading it, as discussed earlier. Afflictions with black bile or phlegm could be treated by triphala, if these afflictions were caused by conditions in the stomach (such as the relaxation of its upper sphincter allowing vapors to ascend) or the liver. In the same vein, stomachics could help digest these cold and humid humors by increasing innate heat in the stomach. If the black bile or phlegmatic afflictions stemmed from accumulations in the extremities of the body, *hierata* would be the drug of choice. In more chronic afflictions of the same nature, decoctions, presented in the same chapter with *hierata*, might help dissolve these thick humors before they could be expelled. Cachets helped with conditions caused by phlegm and yellow bile, or more generally burned or hot humors, especially those affecting the stomach, liver, and heart. Decoctions could also help when these burned humors were too thick for the body to expel them immediately. Physicians would use syrups to rid the body of any remnants of fever, hot humors, or rottenness. Finally, pastilles could help in removing any blockage in the liver or spleen caused by yellow or black bile accumulations.

For locally acting drugs, the formulary offered little explanation of mechanisms of action, giving the physician few options concerning the use of these drugs on conditions other than the ones described. *Lohochs* and *robs* were used to treat coughs as well as chest and throat discomfort. A physician could also use *robs* in cases of diarrhea because they could function as light feeding, as explained in al-Akfānī. Similarly, one could employ gargles of different kinds to treat different throat conditions. Enemas and suppositories could induce diarrhea, whenever needed, or stop bleeding through their local action. Oils helped with pain anywhere in the body, and different liniments could be used to treat abscesses, fistulas, burns, and injuries. Finally, eye and mouth medications were grouped together because they treated any conditions affecting these organs. In all these cases, *al-Dustūr* was arranged to be read by physicians who followed specific schemes in thinking about their patients and about the medications they chose to prescribe.

Conclusion

The role played by the bīmāristān in a physician's career differed from one region to another, from one bīmāristān to another, and from one physician (or lineage of physicians) to another. In most cases, however, the work in the bīmāristān remained less remunerative and less prestigious than service at the court or serving members of the sociopolitical elite. At the same time, the common presence of bīmāristāns in different cities and urban centers, as they gradually became a favorite project of many physicians and patrons, gave the bīmāristān a more prominent role in the development of medical thought and practice. The institution was, after all, one that relied on learned physicians who professed a commitment to (Galenic) medicine. It also occupied a place within a geography of charity sought by the sick and tired. Nevertheless, practice at the bīmāristān required different arrangements at the practical and epistemological levels, ones that remained connected to those outside the bīmāristān but took into account the special needs of the institution and its major audience.

On one hand, the nature of the practice implied a new practitioner–patient relationship. The practitioners' commitment to their patients was one of good will and charitable intentions and was rooted in the practitioners' ethical and socioprofessional commitments to a community that extended horizontally to include other contemporaneous practitioners and vertically to include professional and intellectual ancestry and offspring. The physicians' commitment to patients in the bīmāristān was not one based on reverence, mutual respect, or even fear, as was the case with the practitioners' relations to sovereigns or rich and powerful patrons and patients, but rather one built on charity and charitable devotion (*iḥtisāb*). On the other hand, the large volume of patients in many hospitals and the rapid turnover of those who sought prescriptions without being admitted posed practical difficulties regarding how practitioners should apply the rules of their art. Physicians needed to know about the patient's complexion and to construct a logical narrative that would explain their affliction. Finally, the physician had at his disposal a limited set of drugs and preparations that were more suitable to the medical practice of the bīmāristān in terms of price and efficiency, adding yet a different type of pressure to the process of diagnosis and prescription.

Yet, throughout the healing process, the bīmāristān patient was, and remained, a stranger, only available for the shortest time possible, one who could not "speak" or comprehend the language of the physician due to a lack of education and low socioeconomic status. When the Baghdadi physician Saʿīd ibn Hibbat Allāh advised a female "prescription-seeker" who sought his help in al-Bīmāristān al-ʿAḍudī to give her sick son cold and wet foods, he did not receive praise but was rather mocked and lamented by an inmate in the hall of the melancholic, no less. The melancholic said: "this is a prescription you can give to one of your students, who works on medicine and knows ... its laws. But for this woman, what would be cold and wet? The [right] way in this [question] is to prescribe for her a specific thing that she could rely on."[120] The melancholic was right, as Saʿīd ibn Hibbat Allāh himself admitted; the woman was simply unable to speak the same language, and he needed to "translate" his medicine into her speech. Furthermore, there was no need to construct an elaborate or even logical narrative that would convince the patient. The physician needed only to know what was wrong and to order its correction.

In this context, observation occupied a more important role in the structure of medical thinking and gained increased significance in the understanding and recognition of diseases. The physician's eyes, hands, and ears became his main tools and surpassed his thinking and ability to ask questions in significance. In this same context, observation facilitated the coming-into-being of the "common" and the "uncommon." These descriptive qualities defined and categorized the objects of observation while simultaneously basing their efficacy on the high volume of patients and the conditions of collective practice in the bīmāristān, the key factors that originally authorized observation. Physicians could recognize what was and was not common, and the master's ability to identify, understand, and treat the uncommon was considered all the more remarkable. The "uncommon" now provided the occasion for the physician to show his skill, replacing the "difficult" and the "life-threatening" in the court practice, where a physician's skill derived from his ability to save the

[120] Ibn Abī Uṣaybiʿah, *Kitāb ʿUyūn al-Anbāʾ*, 2: 274.

patron's life or to treat a condition that no one else could treat. Although these difficult and life-threatening conditions no doubt presented in the bīmāristān practice, the bīmāristān was the sphere of the "uncommon" condition. Even when it was not particularly serious (such as a patient's weak pulse), the treatment of this type of condition was becoming the sign of excellence and ability.

The shift from "dangerous" to "uncommon" conditions as markers of professional excellence indicated a shift in power relations: the ability to evaluate was shifting from the patient to the community of practitioners. Whereas the "dangerous" was a quality best judged by patients and their families, the "uncommon" was based on the collective practice of the community of physicians and its awareness of its own collective and historical experience. This is not to say that the "dangerous" was not a medical category used by the community of medical practitioners, or that the "uncommon" was not also a social category used by patients and their families, or that the "uncommon" entirely replaced "the dangerous" as measures of excellence. Rather, the differing significance of each category in varying practical contexts reflected the difference in the governing epistemologies and perceptions of responsibility. In the court, the physician's worth was best judged by his ability to save his patron's health and life (one recalls the mythical heroics of Banū Bakhtīshūʿs, which consistently involved their saving the lives of caliphs and patrons). The reputation a physician achieved in this context was based on the opinions of his patients and their families above all else. In the bīmāristān, physicians were not accountable to their patients, and the fate of their livelihoods and their reputations did not reside in the hands of their patients. They were accountable to their colleagues. Their glory resided in their ability to solve difficult mysteries in a manner satisfactory primarily to their colleagues and students.

The bīmāristān also relied on collective practice, which included practitioners of the same art or of neighboring arts in the craft of medicine. Collective practice was not a new phenomenon or even an uncommon one. On the contrary, the rule in a court practice was to have many physicians, and the regular practice of patients (or of patienthood) was to seek more than one opinion (sometimes at the same time and to the chagrin of physicians). Al-Rāzī complained of patients seeking more than one opinion in his "aphorisms" and argued that this amounted to their choosing the errors in each physician's opinion: "A patient ought to limit [him- or herself] (*yaqtaṣir*) to one trustworthy physician, as his mistakes compared to his right [doings] are very little (*yasīr jiddan*)," and "whoever sought medical help (*taṭabbab*) with many physicians is about (*yūshik*) to choose the errors of each of them."[121] Yet, al-Rāzī admitted that the presence of other physicians with whom to consult gave each practitioner more courage to implement a difficult or unusual treatment for an important patient. Once, he hesitated in bloodletting one of his patients and in giving him barley water to treat his meningitis (*sirsām*) because there was no other physician with whom to consult; this led eventually to the patient's death.[122] In the court or in the service of wealthy patients, the patient was the main judge over which procedure or treatment should be applied if the physicians disagreed. It was the physician's responsibility to provide a coherent narrative that would justify his diagnosis and his treatment in order to convince his colleagues – but more importantly, to convince his patient. In the bīmāristān, collective practice acquired different dimensions as patients lost their right, ability, and responsibility to arbitrate between their physicians. Instead, it was the bīmāristān's bureaucracy, relying on a hierarchy established *a priori*, that gave one physician precedence over others and that allowed for a smoother and faster process of diagnosis and treatment.

As an institution run by a complex administration, the bīmāristān was governed by a bureaucracy that added more demands to the physician's normal manner of practice. For instance, the bīmāristān required practitioners to use far more writing and paper in their work than they were used to (according to surviving evidence): they were expected to write a document (*dustūr*) for every patient that included the patient's diseases, medications, and progress. These documents served as means of communication with the other practitioners, from herbalists to caretakers and janitors – or indeed anyone who applied the physician's, oculist's, or surgeon's instructions. Some among these were required to fill out other papers to request materials for drug making and for food. Al-Bīmāristān al-Manṣūrī employed a complex system of writing to follow up on all expenses. Al-Nuwayrī, who presided over the bīmāristān himself, described how all requests for *materia medica* needed to be written down and submitted to the bīmāristān's treasurer, who would then authorize the purchase and issue the necessary funds for a procurer. The procurer would in turn obtain the materials and provide receipts for the treasurer. Al-Nuwayrī explained briefly how this system acted to prevent the herbalists or any other practitioner from handling the money and to tightly monitor different expenses.[123] Yet none of these documents survived, and no

[121] Ibid., 3: 27.
[122] Meyerhof, "Clinical Observations by Rhazes," AR 3.
[123] Al-Nuwayrī, *Nihāyat Al-'Arab*, 31: 108.

evidence suggests that physicians or herbalists used them as tools for learning or education. The written paper was a tool of the bureaucracy that imposed significant regulations on medical practice and that demanded a stricter order of management from a largely personalized form of practice. At the same time, it was a temporally limited tool that performed its role almost immediately and ceased to be important for posterity. This probably led to its destruction or reuse.

For a practitioner, life in the bīmāristān was not only about practice but also about education. As a site of medical practice and locus of the medical community, the socioprofessional virtues of studying, reading, and learning helped emphasize the hierarchy that existed outside the bīmāristān and that was highlighted by the institution's bureaucracy. In this framework, al-Manṣūr Qalāwūn's desire to sponsor medical education in a way that would allow more people through the gates of the profession and would break certain monopolies on the practice fitted well with the perceived roles of the bīmāristān – it was also impossible to imagine the bīmāristān without a place for teaching and without a process of learning. Qalāwūn's wishes to expand the profession did not materialize, and, centuries later, the practice of medicine remained within specific families and medical dynasties. Medical education in the bīmāristān did not develop into a system similar to the madrasa or the European schools of medicine, but it served as a site for a pre-existing educational system that relied on the direct relation of master and student. Yet the bureaucratic arrangement of al-Bīmāristān al-Manṣūrī also revealed, established, and affirmed an epistemic hierarchy in which it was important for oculists, surgeons, bone-setters, and blood-letters to attend the medical lessons given by the chief physician. This hierarchy gave the chief physician the authority to organize the medical education and its division into specific groups and allowed him to rule supreme over the realm's medical practice, not only its physicians.

The bīmāristān did not establish or bring into being a distinct type of medical practice because all bīmāristān practitioners also worked elsewhere and were part of the larger scene of practice. The bīmāristān, however, founded a different context that demanded important reconsiderations at the practical, epistemic, and bureaucratic levels. The "bīmāristān's medicine" was more observation-oriented, more efficient in its use of materials and funds, more removed from the patient in language and in practice, and more reliant on physicians' authority and on the collective identity of the community of practitioners. It was rooted in a specific set of sociointellectual virtues and deeply connected with charity and good-doing.

Conclusion

Sanjar al-Jāwilī (d. 1345) was one of the more powerful emirs in the final years of the reign of al-Nāṣir Muḥammad b. Qalāwūn (r. 1293–1342; although that time includes two interruptions totaling three years). In addition to his illustrious military career and his governorships of Gaza and Shoubak, he was also interested in the study of Islamic law and of Arabic. He became known for his erudition – which was uncommon, although not unheard of, among Mamluk emirs.[1] In 1341, al-Nāṣir Muḥammad appointed Sanjar the *nāẓir* of al-Bīmāristān al-Manṣūrī, but, soon enough, Sanjar was criticized for how he managed the bīmāristān. Al-Maqrīzī explained that Sanjar was too strict in handling the bīmāristān's *waqf* and wanted to put limits on the charities funded by the bīmāristān. When the sultan heard about Sanjar's plans, he became very angry and admonished the emir, refusing to listen to his arguments, saying instead that "the bīmāristān is all charity (*al-bīmaristān kuluhu ṣadaqah*)."[2]

This conflict between Sanjar and the sultan, as well as the sultan's clear proclamation, illustrate what the bīmāristān meant to, and what role it performed in, that society. It is not clear which charities al-Maqrīzī was referring to, but clearly – from the lack of any explanation – his fifteenth-century readers would have known what he meant. For al-Maqrīzī and his readers, money for charities was probably still being spent, since the bīmāristān continued to be an important institution in the Mamluk capital through the fifteenth century. It is also clear that "what is spent by the bīmāristān for charity (*mā yuṣraf minhu lil-ṣadaqāt*)" did not refer to the costs associated with hosting patients and feeding and treating them. It might have referred to medication and food sent to the sick poor at their homes but was most likely a more comprehensive or even random list of

[1] Berkey, "A Well-Educated Mamluk," 110–11.
[2] Al-Maqrīzī, *al-Sulūk*, 2: 413.

charity funds – including food and medication, but probably also money – that were spent on the poor, whether or not they were sick. If this was indeed the case, Sanjar's objections were more well-founded than his critics maintained, and his decision to limit such spending would have been rooted in the *waqf* document's conditions. However, it appears that the sultan, and al-Maqrīzī as well, understood this spending as a natural extension of the bīmāristān's role in the society: after all, "the bīmāristān is all charity."

Indeed, there is no doubt that most bīmāristāns of which we are well-informed possessed significant Galenic medical features. For al-Bīmāristān al-Manṣūrī, a Galenic consciousness permeated the *waqf* document as a whole: from its identification of necessary foods to its perception of the hierarchy of medical practitioners and the way it outlined care for the patients. The decrees appointing the chief physician and the bīmāristān lecturer, promulgated only a few days after the inauguration of the bīmāristān, were invested with the same view of medical practice, a view connected to a particular, elite group of Galenic practitioners. Similarly, the story of Islamicate bīmāristāns remains deeply connected to the story of Galenic practitioners in the region, and there is no doubt that these practitioners played a significant role in fashioning these bīmāristāns.[3] However, the medical nature of these bīmāristāns – and the role of medical practitioners inside them – varied from one bīmāristān to another, and, even in the same bīmāristān, from one period to another. Their salient features continued to be their charitable role, as well as their being situated within a growing network of charity in the Islamicate urban environment.

The expanded and regular travel culture, which allowed for significant cultural and scientific exchanges and the remarkable spread of books and ideas across the expanses of Islamdom facilitated by the existence of a number of lingua francas in use throughout the region, has justified the emergence of categories like Islamic medicine or the Islamic hospital in modern historiography, either in relation to or in contradistinction from other antecedent, contemporary, or subsequent practices.[4] In this vein,

[3] See a detailed comparison of Islamicate bīmāristāns and Byzantine institutions in Pormann, "Islamic Hospitals," 339–45.

[4] An example of this in classical scholarship is George Hourani's differentiation between "Islamic" and "non-Islamic" influences in Mu'tazilite thought; see his "Origins of Mu'tazilite Ethical Rationalism." See also Byron and Mary-Jo Good's discussion of "Greco-Islamic" medicine: "The Comparative Study of Greco-Islamic Medicine." A number of scholars discuss the difficulties inherent in using terms like "Islamic" or "Arabic." For instance, Peter Pormann writes: "Whoever undertakes to write about the intellectual history of the Arabic and Islamic world is faced with a number of dilemmas. Should one say 'Islamic medicine'? Can one talk about 'Arabic philosophy'?" In this particular

much of the scholarship on Islamic hospitals deals with all bīmāristāns as one single category, viewing their history as one that can be traced and analyzed as variations of the same model. To their credit, evidence suggests extensive communication among medical, bureaucratic, and scholarly elites, and movement of ideas, traditions, and practices through these communications. Even this book has explored the development of a medical elite around al-Bīmāristān al-Nūrī, which traced its direct origins to the Baghdadi bīmāristān scene.[5] In this context, the conceptual and analytical categories of the "Islamic" (medicine, hospital, tradition) are important to delineate specific fields of study and to inform investigations in the previously mentioned exchanges.

At the same time, employing these categories, as well as their infrastructure of connections and communications, runs the risk of generalization, of obscuring awareness of local and regional specificities in our subject matter.[6] Bīmāristāns were not simply projects of the elite, nor were they strictly medical institutions. They were charitable structures that served specific audiences, most of whom were far less mobile and "worldly" than the medical, political, or bureaucratic elites. The expectations of this audience, which are hard to detect and define from our sources (produced mostly by elites), played a significant role in shaping the effective role and functioning of these institutions and linked them to pre-existing networks and institutions of charity and care. This located each bīmāristān within specific practices of "charity-consumption" to which their audience was accustomed. The bīmāristān, as a patronage project of its founder, needed to address the needs and expectations of its audience, to respond to local perceptions of generosity and magnanimity[7] – and this led to unique regional features and traditions that were not necessarily as portable or mobile as medical and political elites. For this reason, it is important to locate such practices within their regional context.

volume, Pormann uses "oriental" while admitting that it is a choice with its own set of problems: Pormann, "The Oriental," 1. On travel culture, see Touati, *Islam et Voyage*.

5 In the same vein of studying movement and exchanges between areas east and west of Islamdom, see Pormann and Joosse, "Decline and Decadence." For a more famous example – the travels of Ibn Buṭlān and his communications with Ibn Riḍwān in Egypt – see Ibn Buṭlān, *The Medico-Philosophical Controversy*; Sanagustin and Ibn Buṭlān, *Médecine et Société en Islam Médiéval*.

6 See Ahmed, "Mapping the World of a Scholar"; Haarmann, "Regional Sentiment in Medieval Egypt"; Antrim, *Routes and Realms*.

7 On "communal ties" of different charitable and pietistic projects, see Talmon-Heller, *Islamic Piety in Medieval Syria*. See also Bonner, "Rise of the Muslim Urban Poor"; Bonner, Ener, and Singer (eds.), *Poverty and Charity in Middle Eastern Contexts*; Garballeira, "Pauvreté et Fondations Pieuses dans la Grenade Nasride." See also, Singer, *Charity in Islamic Societies*.

In the Levant and Egypt, where this study has focused, bīmāristāns spread rapidly throughout the tenth and eleventh centuries. These institutions appeared to occupy a significant role in the Levantine and Egyptian urban contexts, where one or two bīmāristāns would dominate the entire city, and where massive resources, whether financial or political, would be directed toward the bīmāristān (a patron's central project par excellence). In Baghdad, a city comparable in many respects to Cairo and Damascus, the scene was different from the ninth century onward. A tradition of multiple bīmāristāns with deeper connections to the medical elite dominated the scene; many bīmāristāns co-existed, and even those built by courtiers who had fallen out of favor had a chance at survival. However, this difference in traditions was hardly clear-cut, nor did it arise without communication and connection between these regions, nor did these general features remain static from the ninth through the fourteenth century. For instance, al-Bīmāristān al-ʿAḍudī in Baghdad (built ca. 981) was clearly the largest structure in the Abbasid/Buyid capital and emerged as a central bīmāristān built with the intent to immortalize its founder – much like its later successors in al-Bīmāristān al-Nūrī and al-Manṣūrī. Similarly, there were other, smaller bīmāristāns in Cairo that happened to survive beyond their patrons' periods of prominence. In either case, the historiography of these bīmāristāns must locate them within their own local traditions and precedents while simultaneously taking into account local changes, connections, and communications.

The prologue attempted to highlight differences between the pre-Islamic institutions in Iraq and Iran, on the one hand, and in the Levant and Egypt, on the other, as part of larger differences in the intended populations and relevant patronage structures. The most significant difference lay in the location of the xenodocheion-cum-bīmāristān within its own network of charity. In the Byzantine context, the xenodocheion was part of a larger charitable network sponsored by Church and Empire and was directed toward the main population of the Byzantine urban center. These institutions – each of which differed in size, capacity, and role and thus must be viewed within its own specific charitable context – were part of the larger network of Byzantine charity. In the Sassanid context, a different (Zoroastrian) charitable network existed, including different institutions that had been inherited at different stages under Muslim rule.[8] This network was similarly directed toward the local population of different Sassanid urban centers but did not include bīmāristāns or other institutions of care that paid

[8] See, for instance, Boyce, "The Pious Foundations of the Zoroastrians"; Stewart, "The Politics of Zoroastrian Philanthropy."

special attention to the sick. The institutions that appear the most likely roots of the Islamicate bīmāristān were, in fact, Syriac institutions; these descended from the Byzantine institutions but, unlike them, did not direct their primary attention to the general public but rather to a population of students and clergymen (among others). The difference in audience of these two types of institution (Byzantine and Syriac) mandated a difference in the structures and aims of patronage. Whereas the Byzantine xenodocheion was part of a larger charitable practice sponsored by Church and Empire, the Syriac institution was part of patronage initiatives directed toward physicians by their patrons, with little concern over the institution's value for the general urban community.

Although the continuities between pre-Islamic (Byzantine, Syriac, and Sassanid), and Islamic patronage practices and institutions may be apparent,[9] there is little evidence to suggest that the xenodocheion-cum-bīmāristān was indeed a xenodocheion *turned* bīmāristān. That is to say, there is little evidence to suggest clear, unquestionable, and traceable continuity between these two institutions. In fact, there is little evidence of any such direct institutional continuity, seeing that an institution like the bīmāristān of Gundisapur (oft-cited as a link between these two institutions) was most likely mythical and its story exaggerated, perhaps purposefully, by the Bakhtīshūʿs and their proteges. The continuity, then – rather than being institutional – is one of charitable and patronage practices that took many expressions; these included many sites and establishments that both provided certain forms of medical care and were staffed by Galenists. The waxing and waning of bīmāristāns, then, must be viewed within broader changes in the charitable map, as opposed to being cited as evidence of the decline or rise of a particular institution.

As shown in Part I of this volume, al-Bīmāristān al-Manṣūrī's story begins in this framework of antecedent charitable practices situated within the political history of the Levant and Egypt, where multiple sovereigns used aggressive and ambitious building programs to entrench their rule and emphasize their power. The relative instability of the Egyptian capital's location (despite its remaining in the same region) and the political conditions in the post-Seljuk Levant until the region fell under Mamluk control, may have contributed to the centrality of built patronage in Levantine and Egyptian cities.[10] Be that as it may, the roots of

[9] On patterns of Umayyad patronage and their connections to previous Byzantine practices, see Gibb, "Arab-Byzantine Relations." On the Abbasid patronage and their relations to Sassanid practices and "imperial ideologies," see Gutas, *Greek Thought, Arabic Culture.*

[10] See O'kane, "Monumentality in Mamluk and Mongol Art and Architecture."

al-Bīmāristān al-Manṣūrī lay in the foundations of this built patronage – dating back to Ibn Ṭūlūn – and was deeply connected to the monuments and practices of Nūr al-Dīn Zankī and Ṣalāḥ al-Dīn al-Ayyūbī, including the latter's reappropriation of the Fatimid capital as the Ayyubid-Mamluk capital from which Qalāwūn would rule. Evidence from architectural history, such as the survival of particular decorative patterns and building styles, indicates that Umayyad convention had not been entirely forgotten in the Levant, but was rather revived first by Nūr al-Dīn and then by Mamluk patrons.[11] Such revival/survival suggests the presence of a certain local, artisanal memory that continued virtually uninterrupted, albeit not unchanged, in the region. In this context of Umayyad survival, the accounts of Umayyad bīmāristāns – which are either false or significantly exaggerated – can be understood as part of the construction of regional identity.[12]

The surviving documents from al-Bīmāristān al-Manṣūrī paint a clear image of a prosperous charitable institution that viewed service to the poor as its chief priority. The bīmāristān was to be staffed by physicians and medical practitioners, but the main priorities of spending were directed to the administering bureaucrats and to the costs associated with housing and feeding patients. As mentioned earlier, there is no evidence that the bīmāristān – at least throughout the first three centuries of its existence – ever functioned without medical practitioners or that decisions had to be made to rid the bīmāristān of these practitioners to provide money for housing or feeding patients. However, it is clear that the bīmāristān paid relatively low salaries and was not able to recruit the realm's most talented physicians. This was consistent with Qalāwūn's medical patronage, which was motivated by charity and care for the poor channeled through medicine, rather than directed toward medicine qua practice and profession. Similarly, his interest in providing medical education was most likely motivated by the concern, common among the educated Muslim elites surrounding him, over the small number of Muslim medical practitioners and the corresponding dominance of Christian and Jewish practitioners.

Part II of this volume discussed the medical practice in the bīmāristān. Although there is no evidence that medical practitioners thought of their practice within bīmāristāns as different from their practice outside, there were a number of constraints and traditions that rendered the most effective

[11] See Flood, "Umayyad Survivals and Mamluk Revivals"; Tabba, *Constructions of Power and Piety in Medieval Aleppo*; Tabba, "The Architectural Patronage of Nur Al-Din, 1146–1174."

[12] See Khalek, *Damascus after the Muslim Conquest*; Antrim, *Routes and Realms*.

practices different in different contexts. On one hand – and as is evident from the medical formularies written for bīmāristāns – a bīmāristān would have had relatively few medications, prepared and and kept on hand, in comparison to the variety available in the market place. Chroniclers consistently praised certain bīmāristāns for having many different types of medications, and they also praised patrons for providing expensive and rare medications; this suggests their awareness that many bīmāristāns, and especially those with inadequate funds, had limited medications available. Even with a relatively limited stock, however, bīmāristans played a number of important roles in the lives of their patients. They dispensed drugs and medications to prescription-seekers and provided urgent care in cases of accidents, snake bites, and the like. They also served as sites for the confinement of the mad or disturbed, who usually ended up in bīmāristāns because their relatives had brought them in or because they were being punished by being incarcerated against their will.

The late twelfth century witnessed the rise of a new group of physicians and medical authors who traced their intellectual lineage to Baghdad's most important bīmāristān, al-Bīmāristān al-ʿAḍudī, and it was al-Bīmāristān al-Nūrī that came to serve as a center for this circle of medical practitioners. The teachings of this circle's most prominent members, Muhadhdhab al-Dīn al-Naqqāsh, his students al-Raḥbī I and Ibn al-Muṭrān, the latter's student al-Dakhwār, and finally Ibn al-Nafīs, slowly came to dominate medical practice throughout the entire region. Although not all members of the circle dedicated much of their careers to bīmāristāns, they remained committed to and invested in the bīmāristān as an ideal in medical practice. This is perhaps due to their connections to a well-established bīmāristān practice in Baghdad – a connection that may have resulted in some mythical views about bīmāristāns, as well as a deep idealization of the Baghdad model and charitable medical practice. The rise of this group was accompanied by the rise of a number of texts that were not necessarily as famous in the Levant and Egypt earlier, like the writings of al-Rāzī and of Ibn Sīnā. These became the two dominant authors in the region, with al-Rāzī's writings used mainly for practice and Ibn Sīnā's for theory. Alongside these books, one can detect at that time a renewed interest in the *Aphorisms* and in the *Questions* of Ḥunayn. Interest in the works of the authors of this circle continued to flourish, but Ibn al-Nafīs' writings came to dominate the scene, with his *Mujāz* becoming one of the more important books on medical practice in the following centuries.

Around 1418, the Mamluk Sultan al-Mu'ayyad Shaykh (r. 1412–1421) built a bīmāristān in the eastern part of the capital, close to the citadel. The new bīmāristān was larger than al-Bīmāristān al-Manṣūrī and had a generous *waqf* that was shared with al-Mu'ayyad's new mosque. However, by 1421 (after al-Mu'ayyad Shaykh's death), the new bīmāristān – poised to become the bīmāristān of the capital, effectively replacing al-Bīmāristān al-Manṣūrī – had closed and was then converted to a mosque. Al-Bīmāristān al-Manṣūrī remained the most significant structure of its kind in Cairo under the Mamluks and Ottomans, well into the eighteenth century, when, in 1778, it was renovated by Ottoman general ʿAbd al-Raḥmān Katkhudā. In the third decade of the nineteenth century, and under Mehmet Ali's rule, al-Bīmāristān al-Manṣūrī was renovated again. Mehmet Ali sponsored a medical school and a new hospital in Cairo in 1827, and the old bīmāristān was staffed first with European physicians and then with Egyptian physicians trained in modern European medicine in the new school. Eventually, al-Manṣūrī became a hospital specializing in opthalmology, and it continues to receive patients today, carrying the name of its founder in perpetuity. This volume is the first part of a longer study on al-Manṣūrī and other bīmāristāns in Cairo. The next part of this study will trace the history of this bīmāristān throughout the Ottoman period, analyzing the region's encounter with European medicine, the graduation of new physicians from the new medical school, and the changes that resulted.

ANNEX

Who Built the First Islamic Hospital?

In 1994, Lawrence Conrad published his article "Did al-Walīd I Found the First Islamic Hospital?" in Aram. The article challenged the report – transmitted by many medieval historians, from al-Ṭabarī (838–923) to al-Maqrīzī (d. 1442), among others – that the Umayyad Caliph al-Walīd I (r. 705–715) had built the first known Islamic "hospital" in Damascus. This attribution seemed particularly reasonable: al-Walīd I was one of the more important Umayyad Caliphs, and he undertook Damascus's largest projects of built patronage, including the Umayyad mosque. Al-Walīd I completed the Dome of the Rock, which his father and predecessor, ʿAbd al-Malik b. Marwān's (r. 685–705) had begun constructing in Jerusalem, and he built the Aqsa mosque opposite the Dome. Conrad's meticulous source criticism was the first attempt to analyze both the origins of this account and whether it could be corroborated with sufficient contemporary evidence. His conclusion – that al-Walīd I did not found the hospital – was accepted by other important historians, such as Peregrine Horden[1] and Peter Pormann.[2] Conrad summarizes his conclusions as follows: "There is . . . absolutely no good evidence to recommend al-Walīd as the founder of the first Islamic hospital, or for that matter, for supposing that the origins of this institution are to be sought anywhere in Umayyad domains, or at any time in the Umayyad caliphate."[3] He explains that the only value of these historical accounts is to tell us that bīmāristāns were viewed favorably and that al-Walīd was also well-regarded from the ninth century on.

Conrad is definitely accurate in his assessment that there is no evidence for the existence of "hospitals" under the Umayyads, if one defines a hospital as an institution that boasts high levels of medicalization embodied in service of patients only, that features the service of medical practitioners, and that differs from leprosaria or sites supporting the blind and the disabled. There is no evidence that such institutions existed before the

[1] Horden, "The Earliest Hospitals," 370.
[2] Pormann, "Islamic Hospitals," 353.
[3] Conrad, "Did al-Walid I Found the First Islamic Hospital?," 244.

ninth century or that, even in the ninth century, such a level of assumed medicalization was universally achieved. Moreover, there is no evidence (or reason) for Umayyads to build an institution that would be called a "bīmāristān," given that this type of incorporation of Persian words into Arabic usage appears only later (although there is little evidence for when the word "bīmāristān" was first used). It is also reasonable to assume that had such an institution borne an Arabic name, the name would have had a longer life in the ninth century, at least competing with the Persian cognate. It is, therefore, reasonable to accept the general conclusion that al-Walīd's "bīmāristān" was at best a later identification with an earlier institution, one sensible enough to historians seeking origins and firsts. However, one question remains: did al-Walīd indeed build any sort of establishment that could lend itself to this later identification? This question is answered negatively by Conrad through his analysis of the sources. However, twenty years after Conrad's analysis, and as the historiography of Islamic bīmāristāns has begun to move beyond constricting views of medicalization, it is useful to reconsider his argument.

Conrad builds his argument on one negative assumption (an evidence from silence) and two hypotheses, for which he gives no evidence. On the negative side, he wonders why Ibn ʿAsākir (d. 1174), one of the most important historians of Damascus, did not mention this hospital in his account of al-Walīd or in his accounts of al-Walīd's building projects. Conrad's question is reasonable enough, considering that Ibn ʿAsākir was indeed the leading historian of Damascus and that his huge encyclopedia continues to be a leading source for any study of that city. However, as Pormann notes, "Arguments from silence are notoriously treacherous."[4] Just because Ibn ʿAsākir did not mention the Umayyad *hospital*, it does not necessarily follow that it never existed. In fact, Ibn ʿAsākir also failed to mention al-Bīmāristān al-Ṣaghīr, built by the Seljuk ruler Duqāq ibn Tutush (r. 1095–1104), which was located alongside the Umayyad mosque in the center of the city; evidence suggests that many members of the scholarly elite frequented it and even died there. More significantly, Ibn ʿAsākir did not mention al-Bīmāristān al-Nūrī, built by Nūr al-Dīn Zankī (d. 1175) during Ibn ʿAsākir's lifetime; this is an odd silence, considering that this bīmāristān came to be not only one of the most significant structures in the city, but also the most significant bīmāristān in the Levant.

In Nūr al-Dīn's biography, Ibn ʿAsākir referred briefly to Nūr al-Dīn Zankī's charities for the poor and the mad without identifying his building

[4] Pormann, "Islamic Hospitals," 344.

a bīmāristān even though it was one of the largest in its time. In the same biography, Ibn ʿAsākir mentioned that Nūr al-Dīn built a *dār al-ʿadl* (a house of justice) in every town. Ibn ʿAsākir clearly prioritized religious institutions and government institutions, including mosques, madrasas, and *dūr al-ʿadl* (plural of dār al-ʿadl). He chose to recognize Nūr al-Dīn Zankī's largest establishment only in passing and only after mentioning the emir's charities to scholars and faqīhs, while insisting on mentioning *dār al-ʿadl*, which he saw as a more relevant achievement in the history of the biographee. More significantly, in Ibn ʿAsākir's long introduction to his *History of Damascus*, he enumerated the major landmarks of the city and the establishment that distinguished it from other Islamic metropoles; he focused entirely on mosques and madrasas, failing to mention al-Bīmāristān al-Nūrī. To think that al-Bīmāristān al-Nūrī – one of the most remarkable institutions of its kind, reported on by virtually any traveler to Damascus – was totally neglected by Ibn ʿAsākir allows us to reconsider the author's interests, priorities, and style of writing. Thus, his failure to mention a small infirmary or leprosarium built by al-Walīd I, which had not survived until his time in any case, cannot constitute evidence for the absence of this establishment.

In fact, Ibn ʿAsākir's biography of al-Walīd I was devoid of any mention of his establishments or foundations, including the Umayyad mosque, the Aqsa mosque, and even the renovations to the prophetic mosque, all of which are supported by other historical evidence. The mention of the Umayyad mosque was limited to the book's introductory chapters, which introduced the city and its main landmarks. Conrad's argument concerning the absence of references to al-Walīd's *hospital* is therefore misleading and fails to take into account either Ibn ʿAsākir's lack of interest in bimāristāns in general or his reluctance to mention any of al-Walīd's achievements except in the context of identifying Damascus's main mosque. In fact, though, Ibn ʿAsākir did actually refer to the old Umayyad bīmāristān, but not in his discussion of al-Walīd I. Rather, he noted it in passing in his biography of ʿAmr b. al-ʿĀṣ (d. 664), an important political and military figure during the caliphates of ʿUmar I, ʿUthmān, and, most notably, under the Umayyads (being himself an Umayyad). Ibn ʿAsākir explained that ʿAmr owned a number of houses in Damascus either before or immediately after the Muslim conquest, and that one of them is the one known as "the first bīmāristān."[5] Although it is not clear what he meant by "the first bīmāristān," he was likely referencing what appeared to be a

[5] Ibn ʿAsākir, *Tārīkh Madinat Damashq*, 46: 109.

common story among Damascenes about the existence of an old Umayyad bīmāristān. In addition to "the first bīmāristān," Ibn ʿAsākir referred to "a house of the blind," which may have been functioning in Damascus as early as 722,[6] and a hospice (dār al-ḍiyāfah),[7] which housed the poor and needy and which also dates to the Umayyad period. This may have been the hospice attributed by al-Maqrīzī to being built by al-Walīd I, along with the bīmāristān.

Other historians who spent long spans of their life in Damascus consistently agreed on the story of al-Walīd I building a bīmāristān. Take for example Ibn Kathīr (d. 1373), who quoted al-Madāʾinī (c. 752–839), writing that "For the people of the Levant, al-Walīd ibn ʿAbd al-Malik was their best caliph: he built (*banā*) mosques in Damascus, established (*waḍaʿa*) minarets, gave people [charity], and gave to the lepers (*aʿṭā al-majdhūmīn*) and told them 'do not beg people' (*lā tasʾalū al-nās*), and gave every crippled (*muqʿad*) a servant, and every blind (*ḍarīr*) a guide, and conquered in his reign many great conquests."[8] Similarly, Ibn al-ʿImād (1623–1679), who spent time in Damascus as well, reported how Damascenes believed that the old bīmāristān of their town was built by Muʿawiyah.[9] In all cases, it appears that a long-standing local memory perpetuated the narrative about the presence of an older (or first) bīmāristān built by the Umayyads, which Ibn ʿAsākir thought was built on one of Amr b. al-ʿĀṣ's properties in the city.

In addition to this argument from silence, Conrad traces the origins of the account of al-Walīd's hospital to al-Ṭabarī reporting from Ṣāliḥ ibn Kaysān:

> Sāliḥ ibn Kaysan said: al-Walīd wrote to ʿUmar about smoothing the [mountain] passes (*fī tashīl al-thanāyā*), and digging wells in Medina, and his letters went forth to the provinces of the same, and al-Walīd wrote to to Khālid b. ʿAbd Allāh of the same. [Ṣāliḥ] said: And [al-Walīd] restricted the lepers from circulating among the people and provided for them allowances, which used to be provided for them (*wa ḥabasa al-majdhūmīn ʿan an yakhrujū ʿalā al-nās wa ajrā ʿalayhim arzāqan wa kānat tajrī ʿalayhim*).[10]

[6] Ibid., 37: 244.
[7] Ibid., 51: 167.
[8] Ibn Kathīr, *Al-Bidāyah wa al-Nihāyah*, 12: 609–10. Conrad quotes the same passage from al-Ṭabarī but mistakenly claims that Ibn Kathīr, another Damascene historian, did not mention any of these accounts of the leprosarium or hospice. Conrad, "Did al-Walid I Found the First Islamic Hospital?," 244.
[9] Ibn al-ʿImād, *Shadharāt al-Dhahab fī Akhbār man Dhahab*, 3: 407.
[10] Al-Ṭabarī, *Tārīkh al-Rusul wa al-Mulūk*, 6: 437. This is the same text used by Conrad, although not his translation. Conrad provided this translation: "Muḥammad b. ʿUmar said: Ibn Abī Sabra told

Conrad first argues that the account concerns Medina and Mecca alone, since Ibn Kaysān spent most of his life in Medina, and since the governors mentioned in the quote are ʿUmar b. ʿAbd al-ʿAzīz (who was the governor of Medina at the time) and Khālid b. ʿAbd Allāh (who was governor of Mecca).[11] Then, he argues that although these events were reported by al-Ṭabarī in the context of the year 707, they may have happened in 710, close to al-Walīd's pilgrimage.[12] Based on these two hypotheses, he argues that al-Walīd ordered the governors of Medina and Mecca to incarcerate the lepers because he anticipated that they would flood the holy cities when the caliph arrived in what must have been a very crowded pilgrimage season. "Providing for them" was not a real act of charity, Conrad argues, but rather a necessity of their being incarcerated, and so it follows that the report does not indicate any kind of permanent establishment or effort to help the lepers.

In his first hypothesis, Conrad misreads the text, which actually included two different reports separated by the repetition of the verb "said" (*qāla*); this verb was used to distinguish the second report – which stood as independent in subject and possibly even in time – from the first, even though both reports share the same chain of transmission. The first report included three different orders issued by al-Walīd. One was to ʿUmar b. ʿAbd al-ʿAzīz, to further facilitate the access to Medina and provide facilities for the pilgrims and visitors. The second was to governors of different provinces "with the same" orders; that is, to facilitate the already-defined routes of pilgrimage and visitation to Medina and to provide at least water for the pilgrims. The third was to the governor of Mecca to do the same. Here, it is important to note that the repetition of al-Walīd's name in the report signified a different act of ordering that was not directly connected to the previous act, which included orders to both ʿUmar, the governor of Medina, and the other governors of the provinces. Within the context of the year 707, when al-Walīd started his major project of renovating the prophetic mosque in Medina, these orders seem natural; the process of renovation included facilitating the routes and providing more supplies to visitors to the prophetic city, who were

me: Sāliḥ ibn Kaysān told me: al-Walīd wrote to ʿUmar [ordering him] to facilitate the crossing of the mountain passes and to dig wells in Medina, and his letters to similar effect went forth to the provinces, including one to Khālid b. ʿAbd Allāh. [Ṣāliḥ] said: And [al-Walīd] restricted the lepers from circulating among the people and [ordered that] they be provided with allowances, so these were provided to them."

[11] Conrad, "Did al-Walid I Found the First Islamic Hospital?," 229–30.

[12] Ibid., 231–32.

expected to increase in numbers after the renovations. It appears that al-Walīd, after having second thoughts and possibly at a later date, decided to extend these services to Mecca, a city that had fallen out of Umayyad favor after supporting a rebellion against al-Walīd's father.

The second report, which starts with another "[Ibn Kaysān] said (*qāla*)," did not mention any orders issued by al-Walīd to any governor or deputy. Instead, the report attributed the acts to al-Walīd himself, departing from the previous narrative process and suggesting that the acts relating to the lepers may have been enforced by al-Walīd himself, mostly in his own immediate environ: Damascus, where he effectively ruled without intermediary. Here, it is important to remember the overall context of these reports, which was the discussion of al-Walīd's good acts (*dhikr mā ʿamila al-Walīd min al-maʿrūf*). These acts included his facilitating the roads for pilgrims, his providing water for them, and his care for the lepers. The mention of the lepers in this context further emphasizes that al-Ṭabarī and his informants thought of this as an act of charity to the lepers; the reference to the giving of charities and stipends, then, was not seen as an act of public organization, where lepers were incarcerated to prevent them from begging.

Conrad's argument that the entire report happened in Medina because Ibn Kaysān left Medina only briefly is problematic. Although Ibn Kaysān did indeed spend most of his life in Medina, he was the one entrusted with supervising the constructions in the prophetic mosque, which brought him in direct contact with al-Walīd and his aides.[13] More importantly, al-Walīd sent for Ibn Kaysān and brought him to Damascus to tutor his [al-Walīd's] son, thus allowing Ibn Kaysān to spend time in Damascus.[14] Therefore, it stands to reason that Ibn Kaysān was well-informed about the Damascene court. Moreover, there is no reason to assume that Ibn Kaysān reported only what he saw or knew personally. In fact, he did report on Mecca, as well as on the other provinces, in this same account. He was also one of the sources who reported on the communications between al-Walīd and the Byzantine emperor concerning al-Walīd's plans to renovate the prophetic mosque.[15] Historians are confident that such events and communications with the Byzantine emperor happened at a time when Ibn Kaysān was in Medina, working for its governor, ʿUmar b. ʿAbd al-ʿAzīz.

[13] Ibn al-Jawzī, *Al-Muntaẓam fī Tārīkh al-Mulūk wa al-Umam.*
[14] Ibn ʿĀshūr, *Tarājim al-Aʿlām.*
[15] Al-Ṭabarī, *Tārīkh al-Rusul wa al-Mulūk*; Gibb, "Arab-Byzantine Relations."

Conrad also argues that these events did not happen in 707. But he does not present any proof of his proposed date (710). Instead, he rightly explains that medieval chroniclers like al-Ṭabarī did not always have good information on when specific events took place, may have received many reports that were simply undated, and that they would normally place these accounts alongside other related events. In this case, 88 AH/707 CE seemed a good choice to al-Ṭabarī because it included al-Walīd's renovations in Medina. Conrad writes: "Once released from the obligation to find some context in the year 88 AH/707 CE in particular, our attention is drawn to possibly relevant developments in adjacent years. One thus finds that in 91 AH/710 CE, al-Walīd made what was his first and only pilgrimage as caliph to Mecca and Medina."[16] However, there is no reason to "release" oneself from connecting these events to the year 707 as al-Ṭabarī had placed them. The simple fact that al-Ṭabarī, along with other historians, occasionally placed events in a wrong annalistic location does not necessarily indicate that these particular events did not happen in that specific location. Moreover, there are relevant developments happening in 707; namely, the beginning of al-Walīd's constructions in Medina, which would be concluded in 710 (when he would make his visit), that would justify these events.

The report simply discussed a number of pietistic and charitable endeavors that al-Walīd undertook in the context of this particular year, when he started to renovate the Prophetic mosque, his most appreciated endeavor for Abbasid authors such as al-Ṭabarī. Yet the report was not concerned with the building but with al-Walīd's charities and, particularly, his spending on the poor, whether through facilitating their pilgrimage or by providing for the lepers. In this context, two reports originating with Ibn Kaysān were transmitted by al-Ṭabarī: one related to pilgrims and the other related to lepers, with little indication as to whether the two were indeed related or not. Modern editors placed the two reports in one paragraph, adding punctuation markings that were not part of the original text. More importantly, Ibn Kaysān added that the lepers had been provided for before, although we have no mention of such care before al-Walīd.[17] There is also no evidence, apart from Conrad's interpretation of

[16] Conrad, "Did al-Walid I Found the First Islamic Hospital?," 232.

[17] Conrad chose to replace "and [charities] had been provided for them before (wa kānat tajrī ʿalayhim)" with "So [charities] were provided for them (fakānat tajrī ʿalayhim)." The second formulation occurred in one of the manuscripts used for the edition cited by Conrad but was not chosen by the editors because it was at variance with the more complete manuscripts.

this report, that Medina had such facilities or charities for lepers during the Umayyad period.

Al-Madāʾinī (d. ca. 830) repeated the same report from Ibn Kaysān but added the crippled and the blind to the lepers. This can help us better understand al-Walīd's initiative, which was in no way an institution of specialized medical care but rather a charitable place that housed (or supported) the crippled and the blind, as well as the lepers incarcerated there. Therefore, and in the context of Ibn ʿAsākir's reports about "the first bīmāristān" built on ʿAmr b. al-ʿĀṣ' property, the house of the blind, and the hospice (also reported on by al-Maqrīzī), it appears that al-Walīd I and/or other Umayyad rulers may have established some forms of houses and charities for the lepers, the blind, and the crippled. These would have been similar in many ways to Byzantine structures of charity that probably already existed in Damascus, the capital of Byzantine Syria. These institutions of care were not similar to the bīmāristāns known from the ninth century, except in their charitable nature, and they may not have had any serious or stable administrative structures. Both later historians and Damascene locals, however, identified the earlier Umayyad institutions as bīmāristāns and linked them to al-Walīd, whose efforts in this regard might have been more pronounced than others.

In reconsidering Lawrence Conrad's question, "Did al-Walīd I found the first Islamic hospital?," the answer is probably "No." This is simply because bīmāristāns, in their ninth-century iterations, did not exist at the time. However, al-Walīd I and possibly other Umayyad rulers likely created charities that inherited and competed with Byzantine charities for lepers, the blind, and the crippled; these charities were probably established in the Umayyad capital as well as in other urban main centers. These institutions maintained a level of continuity in charitable care from the Byzantine through the Umayyad period, later inherited by more specialized, ninth-century institutions – including the bīmāristān.

Bibliography

ʿAbd Allāh, Maḥmūd Sayyid. *Madāfin Ḥukkām Miṣr al-Islāmīyah bi-Madīnat al-Qāhirah*. Alexandria: Dār al-Wafāʾ li-Dunyā al-Ṭibāʿah wa al-Nashr, 2004.

Abrahams, I. "An Eighth-Century Genizah Document." *The Jewish Quarterly Review* 17, no. 3 (1905): 246–430.

Ahmed, Shahab. "Mapping the World of a Scholar in Sixth/Twelfth Century Bukhāra: Regional Tradition in Medieval Islamic Scholarship as Reflected in a Bibliography." *Journal of the American Oriental Society* (2000): 24–43.

Al-Aṣbahānī, Aḥmad b. ʿAbd Allāh Abū Naʿīm. "Al-Ṭibb al-Nabawī." Dār al-Kutub: Ṭibb Ṭalʿat, no.: 480.

Al-ʿAṭṭār al-Isrāʾīlī, Abū al-Munā b. Abī al-Naṣr. *Minhāj al-Dukkān wa Dustūr al-Ayān fi Amāl wa Tarākīb al-Adwiyah al-Nāfiʿah lil-Abdān*. Edited by Muḥammad Raḍwān Muhannā. Cairo: al-Jumhurrīyah al-Miṣrīyah, 1970.

Allouche, Adel. "The Establishment of Four Chief Judgeships in Fatimid Egypt." *Journal of the American Oriental Society* 105, no. 2 (1985): 317–20.

Alpini, Prosper. *Histoire Naturelle de l'Égypte, 1581–1584*. Edited by R. de Fenoyl, Serge Sauneron, and Marcelle Desdames, Collection des Voyageurs Occidentaux en Égypte. Cairo: Institut Français d'Archéologie Orientale du Caire, 1979.

Alston, Richard. *The City in Roman and Byzantine Egypt*. London: Routledge, 2002.

Amin, Muhammad. "Un Acte de Fondation de Waqf par une Chrétienne (Xe Siècle H., XVIe S. Chr:)." *Journal of the Economic and Social History of the Orient* 18, no. 1 (1975): 43–52.

Amr, Samir S. "Ibn al-Nafis: Discoverer of the Pulmonary Circulation." *Annals of Saudi Medicine* 27, no. 5 (2007): 385–87.

Al-Andalusī, Ṣāʿid b. Aḥmad, Louis Cheikho, and Régis Blachère. *Kitāb Ṭabaqāt al-Umam*. Vol. 1, Publications of the Institute for the History of Arabic-Islamic Science. Frankfurt am Main: Institute for the History of Arabic-Islamic Science at the Johann Wolfgang Goethe University, 1999.

Antrim, Zayde. *Routes and Realms: The Power of Place in the Early Islamic World*. New York: Oxford University Press, 2012.

Ayalon, David. *The Mamlūks: The Organization and Structure of a Moslem Military Society in the Middle Ages, Selected Reading Passages for the Lectures of Prof. D. Ayalon*. Jerusalem: Hebrew University, 1961.

Ayalon, David. *Outsiders in the Lands of Islam: Mamluks, Mongols and Eunuchs.* London: Variorum Reprints, 1988.

Bacharach, Jere L. "Marwanid Umayyad Building Activities: Speculations on Patronage." *Muqarnas* 13 (1996), 27–42.

Bagnall, Roger S. *Egypt in the Byzantine World, 300–700.* New York: Cambridge University Press, 2007.

Al-Balāṭunusī. *Taḥrīr al-Maqāl fī mā Yaḥil wa Yaḥrum min Bayt al-Māl.* al-Manṣura: Dār al-Wafā', 1989.

Al-Balawī, 'Abd Allāh b. Muḥammad. *Sīrat Aḥmad ibn Ṭūlūn.* Damascus: al-Maktabah al-'Arabīyah fī Dimashq, 1939.

Al-Balawī, Khālid b. 'Īsā. *Tāj al-Mafriq fī Taḥliyat 'Ulamā' al-Mashriq.* Edited by al-Ḥasan al-Sā'iḥ. Rabat: Ṣundūq Iḥyā' al-Turāth al-Islāmī, 1980.

Baqué, Valérie. "Du Bimaristan à l'Asile Moderne: Mise en Place de l'Institution et de la Médecine Psychiatriques en Égypte, 1882/1930." Ph.D. Thesis, Université de Provence, 1995.

Bar, Hebraeus. *The Chronography of Gregory Abû'l Faraj, the Son of Aaron, the Hebrew Physician, Commonly Known as Bar Hebraeus: Being the First Part of His Political History of the World.* Edited by E. A. Wallis Budge. London: Oxford University Press, 1932.

Bareket, Elinoar. *Fustat on the Nile: The Jewish Elite in Medieval Egypt.* Boston: Brill, 1999.

Barḥadbeshabbā, Arbāyā, and Addai Scher. *Cause de la Fondation des Écoles.* Paris: Firmin-Didot, 1908.

Becker, Adam H. *Fear of God and the Beginning of Wisdom: The School of Nisibis and Christian Scholastic Culture in Late Antique Mesopotamia.* Philadelphia: University of Pennsylvania Press, 2006.

Becker, Adam H. *Sources for the History of the School of Nisibis.* Liverpool: Liverpool University Press, 2008.

Becker, C. H. "Badr al-Djamālī." *Encyclopaedia of Islam, Second Edition.* Edited by P. Bearman, Th. Bianquis, C. E. Bosworth, E. van Donzel, W. P. Heinrichs. Brill Online, 2014. http://referenceworks.brillonline.com/entries/encyclopaedia-of-islam-2/badr-al-d-j-ama-li-SIM_1018

Behrens-Abouseif, Doris. *The Citadel of Cairo: Stage for Mamluk Ceremonial.* Cairo: l'Institut Français d'Archéologie Orientale, 1988.

Behrens-Abouseif, Doris. *Islamic Architecture in Cairo: An Introduction.* New York: Brill, 1989.

Behrens-Abouseif, Doris. "The Abd al-Rahman Katkhuda Style in 18th Century Cairo." *Annales Islamologiaues* 26 (1992): 117–26.

Behrens-Abouseif, Doris. "The Façade of the Aqmar Mosque in the Context of Fatimid Ceremonial." *Muqarnas* 9 (1992): 29–38.

Berkey, Johnathan. "'Silver Threads among the Coal': A Well-Educated Mamluk of the Ninth/Fifteenth Century." *Studia Islamica* 73 (1991): 109–25.

Al-Birzālī, al-Qāsim b. Muḥammad. *Al-Wafayāt lil-Birzālī.* Kuwait: Gharrās lil-Nashr wa al-Tawzī' wa al-Di'āyah wa al-I'lān, 2005.

Blair, Sheila S. "The Mongol Capital of Sulṭāniyya, 'the Imperial.' " *Iran* 24 (1986): 139–51.

Bloom, Jonathan M. "The Mosque of al-Ḥākim in Cairo." *Muqarnas* 1 (1983): 15–36.

Bloom, Jonathan M. "The Mosque of the Qarafa in Cairo." *Muqarnas* 4 (1987): 7–20.

Bonner, Michael. "Definitions of Poverty and the Rise of the Muslim Urban Poor." *Journal of the Royal Asiatic Society* 6, no. 3 (1996): 335–44.

Bonner, Michael David, Mine Ener, and Amy Singer (eds.) *Poverty and Charity in Middle Eastern Contexts*. Albany: State University of New York Press, 2003.

Borgolte, Michael, and Tillmann Lohse. *Stiftungen in Christentum, Judentum und Islam vor der Moderne: Auf der Suche Nach Ihren Gemeinsamkeiten und Unterschieden in Religiösen Grundlagen, Praktischen Zweckenund Historischen Transformationen*. Berlin: Akademie, 2005.

Boyce, Mary. "The Pious Foundations of the Zoroastrians." *Bulletin of the School of Oriental and African Studies* 2 (1968): 270–89.

Brentjes, Sonja. "The Study of Geometry According to Al-Sakhāwī (Cairo, 15th C) and Al-Muhibbī (Damascus, 17th C)." *Acta Historica Leopoldina* 54 (2008): 323–41.

Brodman, James. *Charity and Welfare: Hospitals and the Poor in Medieval Catalonia*. Philadelphia: University of Pennsylvania Press, 1998.

Brown, Peter Robert Lamont. *Authority and the Sacred: Aspects of the Christianisation of the Roman World*. New York: Cambridge University Press, 1995.

Buell, Paul D. "How Did Persian and Other Western Medical Knowledge Move East, and Chinese West? A Look at the Role of Rashid al-Din and Others." *Asian Medicine* 3, no. 2 (2007): 279–95.

Cahen, Claude. "Réflexions sur le Waqf Ancien." *Studia Islamica* 14 (1961): 37–56.

Chipman, Leigh. *The World of Pharmacy and Pharmacists in Mamluk Cairo*. Leiden: Brill, 2010.

Chipman, Leigh, and Efraim Lev. "Syrups from the Apothecary's Shop: A Genizah Fragment Containing One of the Earliest Manuscripts of Minhaj al-Dukkan." *Journal of Semitic Studies* 51, no. 1 (2006): 137–68.

Chipman, Leigh, and Efraim Lev. "Arabic Prescriptions from the Cairo Genizah." *Asian Medicine* 6 (2010): 75–94.

Cohen, Mark R. *Poverty and Charity in the Jewish Community of Medieval Egypt*. Princeton, NJ: Princeton University Press, 2005.

Conrad, Lawrence I. "Did al-Walid I Found the First Islamic Hospital?" *Aram* 6 (1994): 225–44.

Constantelos, Demetrios J. *Byzantine Philanthropy and Social Welfare*. New Brunswick, NJ: Rutgers University Press, 1968.

Cooperson, Michael. *Classical Arabic Biography: The Heirs of the Prophets in the Age of Al- Ma'mun*. Cambridge: Cambridge University Press, 2000.

Corbet, Eustace K. "The Life and Works of Aḥmad Ibn Ṭūlūn." *Journal of the Royal Asiatic Society of Great Britain and Ireland* (1891): 527–62.

Cotton, Hannah. *From Hellenism to Islam: Cultural and Linguistic Change in the Roman Near East*. Cambridge/New York: Cambridge University Press, 2009.

Crecelius, Daniel. "The Organization of Waqf Documents in Cairo." *International Journal of Middle East Studies* 2, no. 3 (1971): 266–77.

Crecelius, Daniel. "Incidences of Waqf Cases in Three Cairo Courts: 1640–1802." *Journal of the Economic and Social History of the Orient* 29, no. 2 (1986): 176–89.

Crecelius, Daniel. "Problems of ʿAbd al-Raḥmān Katkhudāʿs Leadership of the Qazdughli Faction." In *The Mamluks in Egyptian and Syrian Politics and Society*, edited by Michael Winter and Amalia Levanoni, 373–86. Leiden: Brill, 2004.

Creswell, K. A. C., Marguerite Gautier-Van Berchem, and Félix Hernández. *Early Muslim Architecture: Umayyads, Early ʿAbbāsids & Ṭūlūnids*. Oxford: The Clarendon Press, 1932.

Daiber, Hans. "Abū Ḥātim ar-Rāzī (10th Century AD) on the Unity and Diversity of Religions." In *Dialogue and Syncretism: An Interdisciplinary Approach*, edited by Jerald D. Gort, Hendrik M. Vroom, Rein Fernhout, and Anton Wessels, 87–104. Amsterdam/Grand Rapids, MI: Editions Rodopi/Wm. B. Eerdmans Publishing, 1989.

Al-Dakhwār, Muhadhdhab al-Dīn ʿAbd al-Raḥīm, and Badr al-Dīn Muẓaffar ibn Qāḍī Baʿlabak. *Kitāb Sharḥ Tuqaddimuhu al-Maʿrifah lil-Dakhwār 565-628 AH-1160-1230 AD*. Edited by Māhir ʿAbd al-Qādir Muḥammad ʿAlī. Alexandria: Dār al-Maʿrifah al-Jāmiʿīyah, 2000.

Daneshgar, Majid. "Abū Ḥātim al-Rāzī: The Proofs of Prophecy: A Parallel English-Arabic Text (Review)." *Journal of Shiʿa Islamic Studies* 5, no. 4 (2012): 498–500.

Al-Dawādār, Baybars al-Manṣūrī. *Zubdat al-Fikrah fī Tārīkh al-Hijrah [History of the Early Mamluk Period]*. Edited by D. S. Richards. Berlin: Das Arabissche Buch, 1998.

Denoix, Sylvie, Aḥmad b. ʿAlī Maqrīzī, and Ibrāhīm b. Muḥammad Ibn Duqmāq. *Décrire le Caire Fustāṭ-Miṣr d'après Ibn Duqmāq et Maqrīzī: L'Histoire d'une Partie de la Ville du Caire d'après Deux Historiens Égyptiens des Xive-Xve Siècles*. Cairo: L'Institut Français d'Archéologie Orientale du Caire, 1992.

Al-Dhahabī, Muḥammad b. Aḥmad. *Al-Tārīkh al-Kabīr: Aw Tārīkh al-Islām wa Ṭabaqāt al-Mashāhīr al-A wa Ṭabaqāt al-Mashāhīr al-Aʿlām*. Cairo: Maṭbaʿat Dār al-Kutub, 1973.

Al-Dhahabī, Muḥammad b. Aḥmad. *Al-Ṭibb al-Nabawī*. Riyadh: Maktabat Nizār Muṣṭafā al-Bāz, 1996.

Dols, Michael W. "The Leper in Medieval Islamic Society." *Speculum* 58, no. 4 (1983): 891–916.

Dols, Michael W. "The Origins of the Islamic Hospital: Myth and Reality." *Bulletin of the History of Medicine* 61, no. 3 (1987): 367–90.

Dols, Michael W. *Majnūn: The Madman in Medieval Islamic Society*. Edited by Diana E. Immisch. Oxford: Oxford University Press, 1992.

Drijvers, Han J. W. *The School of Edessa: Greek Learning and Local Culture*. Leiden: Brill, 1995.

Dunlop, D. M., G. S. Colin, and Bedi N. Sehsuvaroglu. "Bīmāristān." *Encyclopaedia of Islam, Second Edition*. Edited by P. Bearman, Th. Bianquis, C. E. Bosworth, E. van Donzel, and W. P. Heinrichs. Brill Online, 2014. http://referenceworks.brillonline.com/entries/encyclopaedia-of-islam-2/bi-ma-rista-n-COM_0123

Durand-Guédy, David. "Private Letters, Official Correspondence: Buyid Inshā' as a Historical Source." *Journal of Islamic Studies* 13, no. 2 (2002): 125–54.

El-Leithy, Tamer. "Sufis, Copts and the Politics of Piety: Moral Regulation in Fourteenth-Century Upper Egypt." In *Le Développement du Soufisme en Égypte à l'Époque Mamelouke*, edited by Richard McGregor, Adam Sabra, and Mireille Loubet, 75–119. Cairo: L'Institut Français d'Archéologie Orientale du Caire, 2006.

El-Leithy, Tamer. "Living Documents, Dying Archives: Towards a Historical Anthropology of Medieval Arabic Archives." *Al-Qantara* 32, no. 2 (2011): 389–434.

Escovitz, Joseph H. "The Establishment of Four Chief Judgeships in the Mamluk Empire." *Journal of the American Oriental Society* 102, no. 3 (1982): 529–31.

Fancy, Nahyan. "The Virtuous Son of the Rational: A Traditionalist's Response to Falāsifa." In *Avicenna and His Legacy*, edited by Tzvi Y. Langermann, 219–47. Turnhout: Brepols Publishers, 2010.

Fancy, Nahyan. *Science and Religion in Mamluk Egypt: Ibn Al-Nafis, Pulmonary Transit and Bodily Resurrection (Culture and Civilization in the Middle East).* London: Routledge, 2013.

Fattal, Antoine. *Ibn Tulun's Mosque in Cairo [La Mosquée d'Ibn Touloun Au Caire].* Beirut: Impr. Catholique, 1960.

Al-Fayrūzābādī al-Shīrāzī, Muḥammad b. Ya'qūb, and 'Abd Allāh ibn 'Abbās. *Tanwīr al-Miqbās min Tafsīr Ibn 'Abbās.* Translated by Mokrane Guezzou. Amman: Āl al-Bayt Institute for Islamic Thought, 2007.

Fernandes, Leonor. "The Foundation of Baybars al-Jashankir: Its Waqf, History, *and Architecture.* "Muqarnas 4 (1987): 21–42.

Fernandes, Leonor. "Mamluk Politics and Education: The Evidence from Two Fourteenth Century Waqfiyya." *Annales Islamologiaues* 23 (1987): 87–98.

Fernandes, Leonor. "On Conducting the Affairs of the State: A Guideline of the Fourteenth Century." *Annales Islamologiaues* 24 (1988): 81–91.

Fleisher, Jeffrey. "Rituals of Consumption and the Politics of Feasting on the Eastern African Coast, AD 700–1500." *Journal of World Prehistory* 23, no. 4 (2010): 195–217.

Flood, F. B. "Umayyad Survivals and Mamluk Revivals: Qalawunid Architecture and the Great Mosque of Damascus." *Muqarnas* 14 (1997): 57–79.

Flood, Finbarr B. "The Medieval Trophy as an Art Historical Trope: Coptic and Byzantine 'Altars' in Islamic Contexts." *Muqarnas* 18 (2001): 41–72.

Freimark, P. "Muḳaddima." *Encyclopaedia of Islam, Second Edition.* Edited by P. Bearman, Th. Bianquis, C. E. Bosworth, E. van Donzel, and W. P. Heinrichs. Brill Online, 2014. http://referenceworks.brillonline.com/entries/encyclopaedia-of-islam-2/muk-addima-SIM_5453

Frenkel, Miriam, and Yaacov Lev (eds.) *Charity and Giving in Monotheistic Religions.* Studien zur Geschichte Und Kultur Des Islamischen Orients. Berlin/New York: Walter de Gruyter, 2009.

Frenkel, Yehoshu'a. "Political and Social Aspects of Islamic Religious Endowments ('Awqāf'): Saladin in Cairo (1169–73) and Jerusalem (1187–93)."

Bulletin of the School of Oriental and African Studies, University of London 62, no. 1 (1999): 1–20.

Galenus. *Kitāb Jālinūs fī Firaq al-Ṭibb lil-Muta'alimīn Naql Abī Zayd Ḥunayn Ibn Isḥāq al-'Ibādī.* Edited by Muḥammad Salīm Sālim. Cairo: General Egyptian Book Organization, 1978.

Galinsky, Judah D. "Jewish Charitable Bequests and the Hekdesh Trust in Thirteenth-Century Spain." *The Journal of Interdisciplinary History* 35, no. 3 (2005): 423–40.

Gannagé, Emma. "Médecine et Philosophie à Damas à l'Aube Du XIIIème Siècle: Un Tournant Post-Avicennien?" *Oriens* 39, no. 2 (2011): 227–56.

Garballeira, Ana Maria. "Pauvreté et Fondations Pieuses dans la Grenade Nasride: Aspects Sociaux et Juridiques." *Arabica* 52, no. 3 (2005): 391–416.

Al-Ghazālī, Abū Ḥāmid. *Iḥyā' 'Ulūm al-Dīn.* Cairo: Mu'assasat al-Ḥalabī, 1967.

Gibb, H. A. R. "Arab-Byzantine Relations under the Umayyad Caliphate." *Dumbarton Oaks Papers* 12 (1958): 221–33.

Good, Byron, and Mary-Jo Delvecchio Good. "The Comparative Study of Greco-Islamic Medicine: The Integration of Medical Knowledge into Local Symbolic Contexts." In *Paths to Asian Medical Knowledge*, edited by Charles Leslie and Allan Young, 257–88. Los Angeles: University of California Press, 1992.

Gordon, Stewart. *Robes and Honor: The Medieval World of Investiture.* New York: Palgrave, 2001.

Gorke, Andreas. "The Historical Tradition about al-Hudaybiya: A Study of Urwa B. al-Zubayr's Account." In *The Biography of Muhammad: The Issue of Sources*, edited by Harald Motzki, 276–97. Leiden: Brill, 2000.

Grey, Cam. *Constructing Communities in the Late Roman Countryside.* Cambridge: Cambridge University Press, 2011.

Guest, A. R. "The Foundation of Fustat and the Khittahs of that Town." *Journal of the Royal Asiatic Society of Great Britain and Ireland* (1907): 49–83.

Gutas, Dimitri. *Greek Thought, Arabic Culture: The Graeco-Arabic Translation Movement in Baghdad and Early 'Abbāsid Society (2nd–4th/8th–10th Centuries).* London/New York: Routledge, 1998.

Gutas, Dimitri. "The Heritage of Avicenna: The Golden Age of Arabic Philosophy, 1000–ca. 1350." In *Avicenna and His Heritage: Acts of the International Colloquium Leuven – Louvain-La-Neuve September 8–September 11, 1999*, edited by Jules Janssens and Daniel De Smet, 81–98. Leuven: Leuven University Press, 2002.

Haarmann, Ulrich. "Regional Sentiment in Medieval Egypt." *Bulletin of the School of Oriental and African Studies* 43, no. 1 (1980): 55–66.

Haarmann, Ulrich. "Rather the Injustice of the Turks than the Righteousness of the Arabs: Changing 'Ulama' Attitudes towards Mamluk Rule in the Late Fifteenth Century." *Studia Islamica* no. 68 (1988): 61–77.

Ḥajjī, Ḥayāt Nāṣir. *Al-Sulṭān al-Nāṣir Muḥammad Ibn Qalāwūn wa Niẓām al-Waqffiahdih: Ma'a Taḥqīq wa-Dirāsat Wathīqat Waqf Suryāqūs.* Kuwait: Maktabat al-Falāḥ, 1983.

Hamarneh, Sami. "Development of Hospitals in Islam." *Journal of the History of Medicine and Allied Sciences XVII*, no. 3 (1962): 366–84.

Ḥāmid, Maḥmūd, and ʿAzzah Ismāʿīl. *Al-Nāṣir Muḥammad Ibn Qalāwūn*. Cairo: al-Maktab al-ʿArabī lil-Maʿārif, 1997.

Al-Ḥanbalī al-ʿUlaymī, Mujīr al-Dīn. *Al-Uns al-Jalīl bi-Tārīkh al-Quds wa al-Khalīl*. Edited by Adnan Yūsuf Abū Tibbānah. Amman: Dandīs, 1999.

Al-Harawī, ʿAlī Ibn Abī Bakr, and Josef W. Meri. *A Lonely Wayfarer's Guide to Pilgrimage: Alī Ibn Abī Bakr al-Harawī's Kitāb al-Ishārāt ilā Maʿrifat al-Ziyārāt*. Princeton, NJ: Darwin Press, 2004.

Al-Harithy, Howyda N. "Urban Form and Meaning in Baḥrī Mamlūk Architecture." Ph.D. Thesis, Harvard University 1992.

Al-Harithy, Howyda N. "The Concept of Space in Mamluk Architecture." *Muqarnas* 18 (2001): 73–93.

Al-Harithy, Howyda N. *Kitāb Waqf al-Sulṭān al-Nāṣir Ḥasan Ibn Muḥammad Ibn Qalāwūn ʿalā Madrasatihi bi-l-Rumaylah*. Beirut: Dār al-Nashr al-Kitāb al-ʿArabī, 2001.

Harrak, Amir. *The Acts of Mār Māri the Apostle*. Atlanta: Society of Biblical Literature, 2005.

Harvey, Steven. "Did Maimonides' Letter to Samuel Ibn Tibbon Determine Which Philosophers Would Be Studied by Later Jewish Thinkers?" *The Jewish Quarterly Review* 83, no. 1 (1992): 51–70.

Hathaway, Jane. "The Wealth and Influence of an Exiled Ottoman Eunuch in Egypt: The Waqf Inventory of Abbas Agha." *Journal of the Economic and Social History of the Orient* 37, no. 4 (1994): 293–317.

Henderson, John. *The Renaissance Hospital: Healing the Body and Healing the Soul*. New Haven, CT/London: Yale University Press, 2006.

Hennequin, Gilles. "Waqf et Monnaie dans l'Égypte Mamluke." *Journal of the Economic and Social History of the Orient* 38, no. 3 (1995): 305–12.

Herzfeld, Ernst. "Damascus: Studies in Architecture: I." *Ars Islamica* 9 (1942): 1–53.

Hirschler, Konrad. *Medieval Arabic Historiography: Authors as Actors*. London: Routledge, 2006.

Hoffman, Birgitt. "Rasiduddin Fadlallah as the Perfect Organizer: The Case of the Endowment Slaves and Gardens of the Rabʿ-i Rasidi." *Serie Orientale Roma* 73 (1995): 287–96.

Horden, Peregrine. "The Earliest Hospitals in Byzantium, Western Europe and Islam." *Journal of Interdisciplinary History* 35, no. 3 (2005): 361–89.

Horden, Peregrin. *Hospitals and Healing from Antiquity to the Later Middle Ages*. Aldershot/Burlington: Ashgate Variorum, 2008.

Hourani, George F. "Islamic and Non-Islamic Origins of Muʿtazilite Ethical Rationalism." *International Journal of Middle East Studies* 7, no. 1 (1976): 59–87.

Hume, Edgar Erskine. *Medical Work of the Knights Hospitallers of Saint John of Jerusalem*. Baltimore: Johns Hopkins Press, 1940.

Humphreys, R. Stephen. "The Expressive Intent of the Mamluk Architecture of Cairo: A Preliminary Essay." *Studia Islamica*, no. 35 (1972): 69–119.

Hunter, Erica C. D. "The Transmission of Greek Philosophy via the 'School of Edessa.'" In *Literacy, Education and Manuscript Transmission in Byzantium and Beyond*, edited by Catherine Holmes and Judith Waring, 225–42. Leiden: Brill, 2002.

Ibn ʿAbd al-Ẓāhir, Muḥyī al-Dīn. *Tashrīf al-Ayyām wa al-ʿUṣūr fī Sīrat al-Malik al-Manṣūr*. Edited by Murād Kāmil and Muḥammad ʿAlī Najjār. Cairo: Wizārat al-Thaqāfah wa al-Irshād al-Qawmī al-Idārah al-ʿĀmmah lil-Thaqāfah, 1961.

Ibn ʿAbd al-Ẓāhir, Muḥyī al-Dīn. *Al-Rawḍ al-Zāhir fī Sīrat al-Malik al-Ẓāhir*. Edited by ʿAbd al-Ẓāhir al-Khuwaytar. Riyadh: al-Khuwayṭir, 1976.

Ibn Abī al-Bayān, Abū al-Faḍl Dāwūd b. Sulaymān. *Al-Dustūr al-Bīmāristānī [Le Formulaire des Hôpitaux d'Ibn Abil Bayan, Médecin du Bimaristan Annacery au Caire]*. Edited by Paul Sbath. Cairo: L'Institut Français d'Archéologie Orientale, 1933.

Ibn Abī Ṣādiq al-Nīsābūri, Abū al-Qāsim ʿAbd al-Raḥmān b. ʿAlī, "Sharḥ Fuṣūl Buqrāṭ," Houghton Library, Harvard University: MS Arab, No. SM4272.

Ibn Abī Ṭāhir Ṭayfūr, Aḥmad. *Tārīkh Baghdād*. Beirut: Dār al-Kutub al-ʿIlmīyah, 2009.

Ibn Abī Usaybiʿah, Muwaffaq al-Dīn Aḥmad. *ʿUyūn al-Anbāʾ fī Ṭabaqāt al-Aṭibbāʾ*. Edited by ʿAmmār al-Najjār. Cairo: Egyptian General Book Organization, 2001.

Ibn al-Akfānī, Muḥammad b. Ibrāhīm *Ghunyat al-Labīb ʿinda Ghaybat al-Ṭabīb*. Edited by Ṣāliḥ Mahdī ʿAbbās. Baghdad: Wizārat al-Taʿlīm al-ʿĀlī wa al-Baḥth al-ʿIlmī, Jāmiʿat Baghdād, Markaz Iḥyāʾ al-Turāth al-ʿIlmī al-ʿArabī, 1989.

Ibn al-ʿArabī, Muḥammad b. ʿAlī. *Al-Futūḥāt al-Makkīyah*. Beirut: Dār al-Kutub al-ʿIlmīyah, 1999.

Ibn ʿAsākir, ʿAlī Ibn al-Ḥasan. *Tārīkh Madīnat Dimashq: wa-Dhikr Faḍlihā wa Tasmiyat man Ḥallahā min al-Amāthil aw Ijtāza bi-Nawāḥīhā min Wāridīhā wa-Ahlihā*. Amman: Dār al-Bashīr, 1980.

Ibn ʿAsākir, ʿAlī Ibn al-Ḥasan. *Tārīkh Madīnat Dimashq: Al-Zuhrī Abū Bakr Muḥammad Ibn Muslim Ibn ʿUbayd Allāh Ibn ʿAbd Allāh Ibn Shihāb al-Zuhrī al-Qarshī*. Beirut: Muʾassasat al-Risālah, 1982.

Ibn ʿAsākir, ʿAlī Ibn al-Ḥasan. *Tārīkh Madīnat Dimashq*. Edited by Muḥḥib al-Dīn al-Amrawy. Beirut: Dār al-Fikr, 1995.

Ibn ʿAlī, Shāfi. *Šāfiʿ Ibn ʿAlī's Biography of the Mamluk Sultan Qalāwūn*. Edited by Paulina B. Lewicka. Warsaw: Dialog, 2000.

Ibn ʿĀshūr, Muḥammad. *Tarājim al-Alʿlām*. Tunis: al-Dār al-Tūnisīyah lil-Nashr, 1970.

Ibn Buṭlān. *Daʿwat al-Atibbāʾ: Ṣafaḥāt min al-Adab al-Ṭibbī al-ʿArabī*. Edited by ʿIzzat ʿUmar. Damascus: Dār al-Fikr, 2003.

Ibn Buṭlān. *The Medico-Philosophical Controversy between Ibn Butlan of Baghdad and Ibn Ridwan of Cairo: A Contribution to the History of Greek Learning among the Arabs*. Edited by Joseph Schacht and Max Meyerhof. Cairo: Egyptian University, Faculty of Arts, 1937.

Ibn Faḍl Allāh al-ʿUmarī, Aḥmad b. Yaḥyá. *Masālik al-Abṣār fī Mamālik al-Amṣār*. Edited by Muḥammad ʿAbd al-Qādir Khuraysāt, ʿIṣām Muṣṭafá Hazāyimah, and Yūsuf Aḥmad Banī Yāsīn. Al-ʿAyn, UAE: Markaz Zāyid lil-Turāth wa al-Tārīkh, 2001.

Ibn al-Furāt, Muḥammad b. ʿAbd al-Raḥim. *Tārīkh Ibn al-Furāt*, Publications of the Faculty of Arts and Sciences. Beirut: al-Maṭbaʿah al-Amīrkānīyah, 1936.

Ibn Ḥabīb al-Ḥalabī, Badr al-Dīn al-Ḥasan b. ʿUmar. *Tadhkirat al-Nabīh fī Ayyām al-Manṣūr wa Banīh*. Edited by M. M. Amīn and S. A. F. ʿAmmār. Cairo: Egyptian General Book Organization, 1976.

Ibn Ḥabīb al-Ḥalabī, Badr al-Dīn al-Ḥasan b. ʿUmar. *Wathāʾiq Waqf al-Sulṭān al-Nāṣir Muḥammad Ibn Qalawūn*. Cairo: al-Hayʾah al-Miṣrīyah al-ʿĀmmah lil-Kitāb, 1982.

Ibn Hishām. *Al-Sīrah al-Nabawiyyah*. Edited by Taha Abdel Raouf Saad. Beirut: Dār al-Jīl, 1987.

Ibn al-ʿImād, ʿAbd al-Ḥayy b. Aḥmad. *Shadharāt al-Dhahab fī Akhbār man Dhahab*. Beirut: al-Maktab al-Tijārī lil-Ṭibāʿah wa al-Nashr wa al-Tawzīʾ. 1966.

Ibn Iyās. *Badāʾial-Zuhūr fī Waqāʾiʿ al-Duhūr*. Edited by Muḥammad Muṣṭafā. Cairo: al-Hayʾah al-Miṣrīyah al-ʿĀmmah lil-Kitāb, 1982.

Ibn Jamāʿah, Badr al-Dīn Muḥammad b. Ibrāhīm. *Taḥrīr al-Aḥkām fī Tadbīr Ahl al-Islām*. Qatar: Dār al-Thaqāfah, 1988.

Ibn al-Jawzī, Abū al-Faraj ʿAbd al-Raḥmān b. ʿAlī. *Al-Muntaẓam fī Tārīkh al-Mulūk wa al-Umam*. Edited by Muṣṭafā ʿAbd al-Qādir Aṭā and Ibrāhīm Shams al-Dīn. Beirut: Dār al-Kutub al-ʿIlmīyah, 1992.

Ibn Jubayr Muḥammad b. Aḥmad. *Riḥlat Ibn Jubayr fī Miṣr wa Bilād Al-a Bilād Al-ʿArab wa al-ʿIrāq wa Al-Shām wa Siqillīyah ʿAṣr al-Ḥurūb al-Ṣalībīyah*. Cairo: Maktabat Miṣr, 1955.

Ibn Kathīr, Ismāʿīl b. ʿUmar. *Al-Bidāyah wa al-Nihāyah*. Cairo: Dār ʿĀlam al-Kutub, 2003.

Ibn al-Nadīm, Mohammed b. Isḥaq. *Al-Fihrist*. Beirut: Khayat, 1964.

Ibn al-Nafīs, ʿAlī b. Abī al-Ḥazm. *Sharḥ Fuṣul Abuqrāṭ*. Edited by Yusuf Zaidan. Cairo: Nahdit Misr, 2008.

Ibn al-Nafīs, ʿAlī b. Abī al-Ḥazm. *Kitāb Sharḥ Tashrīḥ al-Qānūn*. Edited by Salmān Qaṭāyah and Paul Ghaliyunji. Cairo: al-Hayʾah al-Miṣrīyah al-ʿĀmmah lil-Kitāb, 1988.

Ibn al-Nafīs, ʿAlī b. Abī al-Ḥazm. *Kitāb Mūjaz al-Qānūn*. Calcutta: Education Press, 1828.

Ibn al-Nafīs, ʿAlī b. Abī al-Ḥazm. *Al-Mūjaz fī al-Ṭibb*. Beirut: Dār al-Kutub al-ʿIlmīyah, 2004.

Ibn al-Nafīs, ʿAlī b. Abī al-Ḥazm. *Al-Muhadhdhab fī al-Kuḥl al-Mujarrab*. Edited by Muḥammad Ẓāfir Wafāʾī, and Muḥammad Rawwās Qalʿaʾjī. Riyadh: M. Ẓ. al-Wafāʾī, 1994.

Ibn Qayyim al-Jawzīyah, Muḥammad b. Abī Bakr. *Al-Ṭibb al-Nabawī*. Edited by Muḥammad Fatḥī Abū Bakr. Cairo: Al-Dār al-Miṣrīyah al-Lubnānīyah, 1989.

Ibn Saʿīd, ʿAlī b. Mūsā. *Al-Ghuṣūn al-Yāniah fī Maḥāsin Shuarāʾ al-Miʾah al-Sābi-Miʾah al-Sābiʿah*. Cairo: Dār al-Maʿārif, 1967.

Ibn Sa'īd, 'Alī b. Mūsā. *Al-Mughrib fī Ḥulā al-Maghrib*. Edited by Zakī Muḥammad Ḥasan, Shawqī Ḍayf, and Sayyidah Ismā'īl Kāshif. Cairo: Fouad I University, 1953.

Ibn Shaddād, Yūsuf. *The Life of Saladin*. Edited by Charles William Wilson and C. R. Conder. London: Committee of the Palestine Exploration Fund, 1897.

Ibn al-Shiḥnah, Muḥibb al-Dīn Muḥammad b. Muḥammad, and Muḥammad b. 'Abd al-Raḥmān Batrūnī. *Tārīkh Ḥalab*. Edited by Keiko Ohta. Tokyo: Institute for the Study of Languages and Cultures of Asia and Africa, 1990.

Ibn Sīnā. *Kitāb al-Qānūn fī-l-Ṭibb*. Romae: Typographia medicae, 1593.

Ibn al-Tilmīdh, Hibat Allāh b. Ṣā'id, and Oliver Kahl. *The Dispensatory of Ibn at-Tilmīdh: Arabic Text, English Translation, Study and Glossaries*. Leiden/Boston: Brill, 2007.

Ibn Ṭūlūn, Shams al-Dīn Muḥammad b. 'Alī. *Al-Manhal al-Rawī fī-l-Ṭibb al-Nabawī*. Edited by Aziz Beg. Riyadh: Dār 'Ālam al-Kutub, 1995.

Ibn al-Ukhuwwah, Muḥammad b. Muḥammad. *Maālim al-Qurba fī Aḥkām al-Ḥisbah of Ḍiyāal-Dīn Muḥammad Ibn Muḥammad al-Qurashī al-Shāfi'ī Known as Ibn al-Ukhuwwa*. Edited by Reuben Levy. Cambridge/London: Printed by the Cambridge University Press for the Trustees of the "E. J. W. Gibb Memorial," 1938.

'Īsá, Aḥmad. *Tārīkh al-Bīmāristānāt fī al-Islām*. Damascus: Jam'īyyat al-Taḍāmun al-Islāmī, 1939.

Al-Iṣfahānī, 'Imād al-Dīn Muḥammad b. Muḥammad. *Al-Fatḥ al-Qussī fī-l-Fatḥ al-Qudsī*. Cairo: Dār al-Manār, 2004.

Israeli, Isaac, and Muḥammad Ṣabbāḥ. *Kitāb al-Aghdhīyah wa al-Adwīyah*. Beirut: Mu'assasat 'Izz al-Dīn, 1992.

Jackson, Sherman A. "The Primacy of Domestic Politics: Ibn Bint al-A'azz and the Establishment of Four Chief Judgeships in Mamlûk Egypt." *Journal of the American Oriental Society* 115, no. 1 (1995): 52–65.

Jacquart, Danielle, and Françoise Micheau. *La Médecine Arabe et l'Occident Médiéval*. Paris: Maisonneuve et Larose, 1996.

Johansen, Baber. *The Islamic Law on Land Tax and Rent: The Peasants' Loss of Property Rights as Interpreted in the Hanafite Legal Literature of the Mamluk and Ottoman Periods*. London/New York: Croom Helm, 1988.

Jomier, J. "al-Fusṭāṭ." *Encyclopaedia of Islam, Second Edition*. Edited by P. Bearman, Th. Bianquis, C. E. Bosworth, E. van Donzel, and W. P. Heinrichs. Brill Online, 2014. http://referenceworks.brillonline.com/entries/encyclopaedia-of-islam-2/al-fust-a-t-SIM_2409

Al-Kindī, Muḥammad b. Yūsuf. *Al-Wulāh wa al-Quḍāh*. Beirut: Dār al-Kutub al-'Ilmī, 2003.

Kedar, Benjamin Z. "A Note on Jerusalem's Bīmāristān and Jerusalem's Hospital." In *The Hospitallers, the Mediterranean and Europe*, edited by Karl Borchardt, Nikolas Jaspert, and Helen Nicholson, 7–11. Aldershot: Ashgate, 2007.

Khafipoor, Hani. "A Hospital in Ilkhanid Iran: Toward a Socio-Economic Reconstruction of the Rab'-i Rashīdī." *Iranian Studies* 45, no. 1 (2011): 97–117.

Khalek, Nancy A. *Damascus after the Muslim Conquest: Text and Image in Early Islam*. Oxford/New York: Oxford University Press, 2011.
Khemir, Sabiha. *The Palace of Sitt al-Mulk and Fatimid Imagery*. Lodon: University of London, 1990.
Khusraw, Nāṣir-i. *Nāṣer-e Khosraw's Book of Travels [Safarnāma]*. Edited by W. M. Thackston. Albany, NY: Bibliotheca Persica, 1986.
Klein-Franke, Felix; Ming Zhu, and Dai Qi. "The Passage of Chinese Medicine to the West." *The American Journal of Chinese Medicine* 29, no. 3–4 (2001): 559–65.
Klein-Franke, Felix, and Ming Zhu. "Rashīd ad-Dīn as a Transmitter of Chinese Medicine to the West." *Le Muséon* 109, no. 3 (1996): 395–404.
Kraus, Paul. "Raziana II: Extrait du Kitāb Aʿlām Al-Nubuwwa d'Abū Ḥātim al-Rāzī." In *Muḥammad Ibn Zakarīyā Ar-Rāzī (D. 313/925): Texts and Studies*, edited by Fuat Sezgin, Māzin Amāwī, Carl Ehrig-Eggert, and E. Neubauer. Frankfurt am Main: Institute for the History of Arabic-Islamic Science at the Johann Wolfgang Goethe University, 1999.
Kuban, Doğan. *Muslim Religious Architecture*. Leiden: Brill, 1974.
Lambton, Ann. "Awqāf in Persia: 6th–8th/12th–14th Centuries." *Islamic Law and Society* 4, no. 3 (1997): 298–318.
Lev, E., L. Chipman, and F. Niessen. "A Hospital Handbook for the Community: Evidence for the Extensive Use of Ibn Abi 'l-Bayan's al-Dustur al-Bimaristani by the Jewish Practitioners of Medieval Cairo." *Journal of Semitic Studies* 53, no. 1 (2008): 103–18.
Lev, Yaacov. "The Social and Economic Policies of Nūr al-Dīn (1146–1174): The Sultan of Syria." *Der Islam* 81 (2004): 218–42.
Lev, Yaacov. "The Ethics and Practice of Islamic Medieval Charity." *History Compass* 5, no. 2 (2007): 603–18.
Levanoni, Amalia. "Food and Cooking during the Mamluk Era: Social and Political Implications." *Mamluk Studies Review* 9, no. 2 (2005): 201–22.
Lewicka, Paulina. *Food and Foodways of Medieval Cairenes: Aspects of Life in an Islamic Metropolis of the Eastern Mediterranean*. Leiden: Brill, 2011.
Lewicka, Paulina. *Medicine for Muslims? Islamic Theologians, Non-Muslim Physicians and the Medical Culture of the Mamluk Near East*. Bonn: Annemarie Schimmel Kolleg Working Papers, 2012.
Lindsay, James E. *Daily Life in the Medieval Islamic World*. Westport, CT: Greenwood Press, 2005.
Little, Donald P. "Coptic Conversion to Islam under the Baḥrī Mamlūks, 692–755/1293–1354." *Bulletin of the School of Oriental and African Studies* 39, no. 3 (1976): 552–69.
Little, Donald P. "Notes on Mamluk Madrasahs." *Mamluk Studies Review* 6 (2002): 9–20.
Luttrell, Anthony. "The Hospitallers in Twelfth-Century Constantinople." In *The Experience of Crusading*, edited by Jonathan Simon Christopher Riley-Smith, Marcus Graham Bull, Norman Housley, P. W. Edbury, and Jonathan Phillips, 225–32. Cambridge: Cambridge University Press, 2003.

Macdonald, A. A., Michael W. Twomey, and G. J. Reinink. *Learned Antiquity: Scholarship and Society in the near East, the Greco-Roman World, and the Early Medieval West*. Leuven/Dudley, MA: Peeters, 2003.

Macevitt, Christopher Hatch. *The Crusades and the Christian World of the East: Rough Tolerance*. Philadelphia: University of Pennsylvania Press, 2008.

Mackenzie, Neil D. *Ayyubid Cairo: A Topographical Study*. Cairo: American University in Cairo Press, 1992.

Maimonides, Moses. *Moses Maimonides' Two Treatises on the Regimen of Health: Fī Tadbīr al-Ṣiḥḥah, and Maqālah fī Bayān ba'ḍ al-A'rāḍ wa al-Jawāb 'anhā*. Edited by Ariel Bar-Sela. Philadelphia: American Philosophical Society, 1964.

Makdisi, George. "Muslim Institutions of Learning in Eleventh Century Baghdad." *Bulletin of the School of Oriental and African Studies* 24, no. 1 (1961): 1–56.

Makdisi, George. "The Scholastic Method in Medieval Education: An Inquiry into Its Origins in Law and Theology." *Speculum* 49, no. 4 (1974): 640–61.

Al-Manṣūrī, Baybars. *Al-Tuḥfah al-Mulūkīyah fī al-Dawlah al-Turkīyah*. Edited by A. Ṣāliḥ Ḥimdān. Cairo: Al-Maṣrīyah al-Lubnānīyah, 1987.

Manzano-Moreno, Eduardo. "Oriental "Topoi" in Andalusian Historical Sources." *Arabica* 39, no. 1 (1992): 42–58.

al-Maqrīzī, Aḥmad b. 'Alī. *Itti'āẓ al-Ḥunafā bi-Akhbār al-A'immah Al-Fāṭimīyīn al-Khulafā*. Cairo: Dār al-Fikr al- 'Arabī, 1948.

al-Maqrīzī, Aḥmad b. 'Alī. *Kitāb al-Sulūk li-Ma'rifat Duwal al-Mulūk*. Edited by M. M. Ziyādah and S. A. F. Āshūr. Cairo: National Library Press, 1972.

al-Maqrīzī, Aḥmad b. 'Alī. *Kitāb al-Mawā'iẓ wa al-I'tibār bi-Dhikr al-Khiṭaṭ wa al-Āthār*. Cairo: General Organization for Culture Centers, 1999.

al-Maqrīzī, Aḥmad b. 'Alī. *Durar Al-'Uqūd al-Farīdah fī Tarājim al-A'yān al-Mufīdah*. Edited by Maḥmūd Jalīlī. Beirut: Dār al-Gharb al-Islāmī, 2002.

Mathews, Karen Rose. "Mamluks and Crusaders: Architectural Appropriation and Cultural Encounter in Mamluk Monuments." In *Languages of Love and Hate: Conflict, Communication, and Identity in the Medieval Mediterranean*, edited by Sarah Lambert and Helen Nicholson, 177–200: Turnhout: Brepols Publishers, 2012.

Mayer, Wendy. "Patronage, Pastoral Care and the Role of the Bishop at Antioch." *Vigiliae Christianae* 55, no. 1 (2001): 58–70.

McVaugh, Michael R. "Bedside Manners in the Middle Ages." *Bulletin of the History of Medicine* 71, no. 2 (1997): 201–23.

Meyerhof, Max. "Thirty-Three Clinical Observations by Rhazes." *Isis* 23, no. 2 (1935): 321–72.

Miller, Timothy S. "Knights of Saint John and the Hospitals of the Latin West." *Speculum* 53, no. 4 (1978): 709–33.

Miller, Timothy S. "Byzantine Hospitals." *Dumbarton Oaks Papers* 38 (1984): 53–63.

Al-Minūfī, al-Isḥāqī. *Akhbār al-Uwal fī man Taṣrrafa fī Miṣr min Arbāb al-Duwal*. Cairo: General Organization for Culture Centers, 1998.

Morgan, D. O. "Rashīd al-Dīn Ṭabīb." 2012.

Mottahedeh, Roy. "Some Islamic Views of the Pre-Islamic Past." *Harvard Middle Eastern and Islamic Review* 1 (1994): 17–26.

Moulin, Anne Marie. *Le Médecin du Prince: Voyage à Travers les Cultures*. Paris: Odile Jacob, 2010.

Mourad, Suleiman Ali, and James E. Lindsay. *The Intensification and Reorientation of Sunni Jihad Ideology in the Crusader Period.* Leiden: Brill, 2012.

Mouton, Jean-Michel. *Damas et sa Principauté sous les Saljoukides et Les Bourides (468–549/1076–1154): Vie Politique et Religieuse.* Cairo: L'Institut Français d'Archéologie Orientale, 1994.

Munajjid, Ṣalāḥ al-Dīn. *Bīmāristān Nūr Al-Dīn.* Dimashq: [s.n.], 1946.

Naaman, Erez. "Sariqa in Practice: The Case of al-Ṣāḥib Ibn ʿAbbād." *Middle Eastern Literatures* 14, no. 3 (2011): 271–85.

Naghawi, ʿAïda. "Umayyad Filses Minted at Jerash." *Syria* 66, no. 1/4 (1989): 219–22.

Northrup, Linda. *From Slave to Sultan: The Career of al-Manṣūr Qalāwūn and the Consolidation of Mamluk Rule in Egypt and Syria (678–689 A.H./1279–1290 A.D.).* Stuttgart: F. Steiner, 1998.

Northrup, Linda. "Qalawun's Patronage of the Medical Sciences in Thirteenth-Century Egypt." *Mamluk Studies Review* 5 (2001): 119–40.

Al-Nuʿaymī, ʿAbd al-Qādir b. Muḥammad. *Al-Dāris fī Tārīkh al-Madāris.* Beirut: Dar al-Kutub al-ʿIlmīyah, 1990.

Nutton, V. "'The Birth of the Hospital in the Byzantine Empire' by Timothy S. Miller. Essay Review." *Medical History* 30, no. 2 (1986).

Al-Nūwayrī, Shihāb al-Dīn Aḥmad. *Nihāyat al-ʿArab fī Funūn al-Adab.* Edited by Fahīm M. Shaltūt. Cairo: Dār al-Kutub, 1998.

O'kane, Bernard. "Monumentality in Mamluk and Mongol Art and Architecture." *Art History* 19, no. 4 (1996): 499–522.

Pahlitzsch, Johannes. "Christian Pious Foundations as an Element of Continuity between Late Antiquity and Islam." In *Charity and Giving in Monotheistic Religions*, edited by Miriam Frenkel and Yaacov Lev, 125–51. Berlin: Walter de Gruyter, 2009.

Park, Katharine, and Lorraine Daston. "Introduction: The Age of the New." In *The Cambridge History of Science Volume 3: Early Modern Science*, edited by Katharine Park and Lorraine Daston, 1–20. Cambridge: Cambridge University Press, 2008.

Pehro, Irmeli. *The Prophet's Medicine: A Creation of the Muslim Traditionalist Scholars.* Helsinki: Kokemaki, 1995.

Petry, Carl F. "Travel Patterns of Medieval Notables in the Near East." *Studia Islamica* no. 62 (1985): 53–87.

Pormann, Peter E. *The Oriental Tradition of Paul of Aegina's Pragmateia*, Studies in Ancient Medicine, V. 29 and Index. Leiden/Boston: Brill, 2004.

Pormann, Peter E. "Case Notes and Clinicians: Galen's Commentary on the Hippocratic Epidemics in the Arabic Tradition." *Arabic Sciences and Philosophy* 18, no. 2 (2008): 247–84.

Pormann, Peter E. "Medical Methodology and Hospital Practice: The Case of Fourth-/Tenth-Century Baghdad." In *In the Age of al-Farabi: Arabic Philosophy in the Fourth–Tenth Century*, edited by Peter Adamson, 95–118. London: Warburg Institute, 2008.

Pormann, Peter E. "Female Patients and Practitioners in Medieval Islam." *Lancet* 373, no. 9675 (2009): 1598–99.

Pormann, Peter E. "Islamic Hospitals in the Time of al-Muqtadir." In *Abbasid Studies II: Occasional Papers of the School of Abbasid Studies, Leuven, 28 June–1 July 2004*, edited by John A. Nawas, 337–81. Leuven: Uitgeverij Peeters en Departement Oosterse Studies, 2010.

Pormann, Peter E., and N. Peter Joosse. "Decline and Decadence in Iraq and Syria after the Age of Avicenna?: ʿAbd al-Latif al-Baghdadi (1162–1231) between Myth and History." *Bulletin of the History of Medicine* 84, no. 1 (2010): 1–29.

Pormann, Peter E., and Emilie Savage-Smith. *Medieval Islamic Medicine*. Edinburgh: Edinburgh University Press, 2007.

Pruitt, Jennifer A. *Fatimid Architectural Patronage and Changing Sectarian Identities (969–1021)*. Ph.D. Thesis, Harvard University, 2009.

Al-Qadi, Wadad. "Biographical Dictionaries as the Scholars' Alternative History of the Muslim Community." In *Organizing Knowledge: Encyclopedic Activities in the Pre-Eighteenth Century Islamic World*, edited by Gerhard Endress, 23–75. Leiden: Brill, 2006.

Al-Qālaqashandī, Aḥmad b. ʿAlī. *Kitāb Ṣubḥ al-Aʿshā fī Ṣināʿat al-Inshā*. Edited by Muṣṭafā Musā. Cairo: General Egyptian Book Organization, 2006.

Al-Qazwīnī, Zakarīyā b. Muḥammad. *Āthār al-Bilād wa Akhbār al-ʿIbād*. Beirut: Dār Ṣādir, 1960.

Al-Qifṭī, ʿAlī b. Yūsuf. *Tārīkh al-Ḥukamāʾ*. Leipzig: Dieterich'sche Verlagsbuchhandlung, 1903.

Al-Quḍāʿī, *Tārīkh al-Quḍāʿī: Kitāb ʿUyūn al-Maʿārif wa Funūn Akhbār al-Khalān Akhbār al-Khalāʾif*. Mecca: Umm al-Qurā University, 1995.

Rabbat, Nasser. *The Citadel of Cairo*. Geneva: Aga Khan Trust for Culture, 1989.

Rabbat, Nasser. "Al-Azhar Mosque: An Architectural Chronicle of Cairo's History." *Muqarnas* 13 (1996): 45–67.

Rabbat, Nasser. "Architects and Artists in Mamluk Society: The Perspective of the Sources." *Journal of Architectural Education (1984-)* 52, no. 1 (1998): 30–37.

Raby, Julian. "Nur Al-Din, the Qastal al-Shuʿaybiyya, and the 'Classical Revival.'" *Muqarnas* 21 (2004): 289–310.

Al-Rahim, Ahmed H. "Avicenna's Immediate Disciples: Their Lives and Works." In *Avicenna and His Legacy*, edited by Tzvi Y. Langermann. Turnhout: Brepols Publishers, 2010.

Ragab, Ahmed. "Epistemic Authority of Women in the Medieval Middle East." *HAWWA: Journal of Women of the Middle East and the Islamic World* 8, no. 2 (2010): 181–216.

Ragab, Ahmed. "Leigh Chipman, the World of Pharmacy and Pharmacists in Mamlūk Cairo. (Sir Henry Wellcome Asian Series, 8.) Leiden and Boston: Brill, 2010. Pp. ix, 318; tables. $154. ISBN: 978-9004176065." *Speculum* 87, no. 1 (2012): 196–97.

Ragib, Yusuf. "Deux Monuments Fatimides au Pied du Muqattam." *Revue des Etudes Islamiques Paris* 46, no. 1: 91–118.

Ragib, Yusuf. "Un Oratoire Fatimide au Sommet du Muqattam." *Studia islamica* 65: 51–67.

Ragib, Yusuf. "Les Premiers Monuments Funèraires de l'Islam." *Annales Islamologiaues* 9 (1970): 21–36.

Ragib, Yusuf. "Les Mausolées Fatimides du Quartier d'al-Masāhid." *Annales Islamologiaues* 17 (1981): 1–30.

Ragib, Yusuf. "Les Pierres de Souvenir: Stèles du Caire de La Conquét Arabe à la Chute Des Fatimides." *Annales Islamologiaues* 35 (2001): 321–83.

Ragib, Yusuf. "Al-Sayyida Nafīsa, sa Légende, son Culteet son Cimetière." *Studia Islamica*, no. 44 (1976): 61–86.

Rapoport, Yossef. "Legal Diversity in the Age of Taqlid: The Four Chief Qadis under the Mamluks." *Islamic Law and Society* 10, no. 2 (2003): 210–28.

Raymond, Andre. "Les Constructions de l'Emir ʿAbd al-Raḥmān Katkhudā au Caire." *Annales Islamologiaues* 11 (1972): 235–51.

Al-Rāzī, Abū Bakr Muḥammad b. Zakāriyyā. *Kitāb al-Shukūk lil-Rāzī ʿalā Kalām Fāḍil al-Aṭibbāʾ Jālinūs*. Edited by Muṣṭafā Labīb ʿAbd al-Ghanī. Cairo: Dār al-Kutub, 2005.

Al-Rāzī, Abū Bakr Muḥammad b. Zakāriyyā. *Kitāb al-Tajārib: Maʿa Dirāsah fī Manhaj al-Baḥth al-ʿIlmī ʿinda al-Rāzī*. Edited by Khālid Aḥmad Ḥarbī. Alexandria: Dār al-Wafāʾ li-Dunyā al-Ṭibāʿah wa al-Nashr, 2006.

Al-Rāzī, Abū Ḥātim Aḥmad b. Ḥamdān. *Aʿlām al-Nubūwah fī al-Radd ʿalā al-Mulḥid Abū Bakr al-Rāzī*. Edited by George Ṭarābīshī. Beirut: Dār al-Sāqī, 2003.

Richards, D. S. "Saladin's Hospital in Jerusalem; Its Foundation and Some Later Archival Material." In *The Frankish Wars and Their Influence on Palestine: Selected Papers Presented at Birzeit University's International Academic Conference Held in Jerusalem,* March 13–15, 1992, 70–83. Beirzeit: Beirzeit University, 1994.

Richardson, Kristina L. *Difference and Disability in the Medieval Islamic World: Blighted Bodies*. Edinburgh: Edinburgh University Press, 2012.

Riley-Smith, Jonathan. *The Knights Hospitaller in the Levant, c.1070–1309*. London: Palgrave Macmillan, 2012.

Rizq, ʿĀṣim Muḥammad. *Aṭlas al-ʿImārah al-Islāmīyah wa al-Qibṭīyah*. Cairo: Maktabat Madbūlī, 2003.

Robinson, Chase F. *Islamic Historiography,* Themes in Islamic History. Cambridge/New York: Cambridge University Press, 2003.

Rosenthal, Franz. *A History of Muslim Historiography*, 2nd rev. ed. Leiden: E. J. Brill, 1968.

Rosenthal, Franz. "An Eleventh-Century List of the Works of Hippocrates." *Journal of the History of Medicine and Allied Sciences* 28, no. 2 (1973): 156–65.

Ruffini, Giovanni. *Social Networks in Byzantine Egypt*. Cambridge/New York: Cambridge University Press, 2008.

Sabra, A. I. "The Appropriation and Subsequent Naturalization of Greek Science in Medieval Islam: A Preliminary Statement." *History of Science* 25, no. 3 (1987): 223–43.

Sabra, Adam. *Poverty and Charity in Medieval Islam: Mamluk Egypt 1250–1517*. Cambridge: Cambridge University Press, 2000.

Sabra, Adam. "Public Policy or Private Charity? The Ambivalent Character of Islamic Charitable Endowments." In *Stiftungen in Christentum, Judentum und Islam vor der Moderne: Auf der Suche Nach Ihren Gemeinsamkeiten und Unterschieden in Religiösen Grundlagen, Praktischen Zwecken und Historischen Transformationen*, edited by Michael Borgolte and Tillmann Lohse, 95–108. Berlin: Akademie, 2005.

Sabra, Adam Abdelhamid. *Poverty and Charity in Medieval Islam: Mamluk Egypt, 1250–1517*. Cambridge: Cambridge University Press, 2000.

Sābūr Ibn Sahl. *The Small Dispensatory*. Edited by Oliver Kahl. Leiden: Brill, 2003.

Sābūr Ibn Sahl. *Sabur Ibn Sahl's Dispensatory in the Recension of the Adudi Hospital*. Edited by Oliver Kahl. Leiden: Brill, 2008.

Al-Ṣafadī, Khalīl b. Aybak. *Kitāb al-Wāfī bi-l-Wafayāt*. Leipzig: Deutsche Morgenländische Gesellschaft in Kommission bei F. A. Brockhaus, 1931.

Al-Sakhāwī, Muḥammad b. ʿAbd Al-Raḥmān. *Al-Ḍawʾ al-Lāmiʿ li-Ahl al-Qarn al-Tāsiʿ*. Cairo: Maktabat al-Qudsī, 1935. (Republished Beirut: Dār Maktabat al-Ḥayah, 1960.)

Sanagustin, Floréal, and Ibn Buṭlān. *Médecine et Société en Islam Médiéval: Ibn Butlān ou La Connaissance Médicale au Service de la Communauté: Le Cas de l'Esclavage*. Paris: Geuthner, 2010.

Al-Sarrāj al-Qāriʾ, Jaʿfar b. Aḥmad. *Maṣāriʿ al-ʿUshshāq*. Beirut: Dār Ṣādir, 1970.

Savage-Smith, Emilie. "Galen's Lost Ophthalmology and the Summaria Alexandrinorum." *Bulletin of the Institute of Classical Studies* 45, no. S77 (2002): 121–38.

Sayyid, Ayman Fuʾād. *La Capitale de l'Égypte jusqu'à l'Époque Fatimide al-Qāhira et al-Fusṭāṭ: Essai de Reconstitution Topographique*. Beirut: Orient-Institut der Deutschen Morgenländischen Wissenschaft; Stuttgart: in Kommission bei Franz Steiner Verlag, 1998.

Al-Sayyid Marsot, Afaf. "The Political and Economic Functions of the Ulama in the 18th Century." *Journal of the Economic and Social History of the Orient* 16, no. 2 (1973): 130–54.

Schein, Sylvia. "Latin Hospices in Jerusalem in the Late Middle Ages." *Zeitschrift des Deutschen Palästina-Vereins (1953-)* 101, no. 1 (1985): 82–92.

Scher, Addai. *Histoire Nestorienne Inédite: (Chronique de Séert)*. Paris: Firmin-Didot, 1908.

Schofield, Phillipp R. "The Social Economy of the Medieval Village in the Early Fourteenth Century." *The Economic History Review* 61, no. 1 (2008): 38–63.

Shaham, Ron. "Christian and Jewish "Waqf" in Palestine during the Late Ottoman Period." *Bulletin of the School of Oriental and African Studies* 54, no. 3 (1991): 460–72.

Al-Shujāʿī, Shams al-Dīn. *Tārīkh al-Malik al-Nāṣir Muḥammad Ibn Qalāwūn al-Ṣāliḥī wa-Awlādih*. Edited by Barbara Schäfer. Weisbaden: Dār al-Nashr Frānz Shtāynar, 1978.

Al-Shayzarī, ʿAbd al-Raḥmān b. Naṣr. *Book of al-Muḥtasib Entitled Kitāb Nihāyat al-Rutbah fī Ṭalab al-Ḥisbah*. Edited by al-Sayyid al-Bāz al-Arīnī and M. M. Ziada. Cairo: Association of Authorship, 1946.

Sheehan, Peter. *Babylon of Egypt: The Archaeology of Old Cairo and the Origins of the City*. Cairo: American University in Cairo Press, 2010.

Sijpesteijn, Petra M. *Shaping a Muslim State: The World of a Mid-Eighth Century Egyptian Official*. Oxford: Oxford University Press, 2013.

Singer, Amy. "Serving up Charity: The Ottoman Public Kitchen." *The Journal of Interdisciplinary History* 35, no. 3 (2005): 481–500.

Singer, Amy. *Charity in Islamic Societies*. Cambridge: Cambridge University Press, 2008.

Sourdel, D. "Bukhtshūʿ." *Encyclopaedia of Islam, Second Edition*. Edited by P. Bearman, Th. Bianquis, C. E. Bosworth, E. van Donzel, and W. P. Heinrichs. Brill Online, 2014. http://referenceworks.brillonline.com/entries/encyclopaedia-of-islam-2/buk-h-ti-s-h-u-SIM_1514

Stearns, Justin K. *Infectious Ideas: Contagion in Premodern Islamic and Christian Thought in the Western Mediterranean*. Baltimore: Johns Hopkins University Press, 2011.

Stewart, Sarah. "The Politics of Zoroastrian Philanthropy and the Case of Qasr-e Firuzeh." *Iranian Studies* 45, no. 1 (2012): 59–80.

Stilt, Kristen Ann. "The Muḥtasib, Law, and Society in Early Mamluk Cairo and Fustat (648–802/1250–1400)." Ph.D. Thesis, Harvard University, 2004.

Al-Suyūṭī, Jalāl al-Dīn ʿAbd al-Raḥmān. *Tārīkh al-Khulafāʾ*. Cairo: Dār Miṣr, 1969.

Al-Suyūṭī, Jalāl al-Dīn ʿAbd al-Raḥmān. *Al-Raḥmah fī-l-Ṭibb wa al-Ḥikmah*. Tunis: Dār al-Maʿrifah, 1989.

Al-Suyūṭī, Jalāl al-Dīn ʿAbd al-Raḥmān. "Al-Inṣāf fī Tamyīz al-Awqāf." In *Rasāʾil Ḥawal Al-Waqf*, edited by Muḥammad Shawqī Makkī, 263–83. Riyadh: al-Narjis, 1999.

Al-Suyūṭī, Jalāl al-Dīn ʿAbd al-Raḥmān. "Al-Wajh al-Nāḍir fīmā Yaqbiḍuhu al-Nāẓir." In *Rasāʾil Ḥawal al-Waqf*, edited by Muḥammad Shawqī Makkī, 283–89. Riyadh: al-Narjis, 1999.

Swelim, M. Tarek. *The Mosque of Ibn Ṭūlūn: A New Perspective*. Ph.D. Thesis, Harvard University, 1994.

Al-Ṭabarī, Abū Jaʿfar Muḥammad b. Jarīr. *Tārīkh al-Rusul wa al-Mulūk*. Edited by Muḥammad Abū al-Faḍl Ibrāhīm. Cairo: Dār al-Maʿārif, 1968–69.

Al-Ṭabarī, Abū Jaʿfar Muḥammad b. Jarīr. *Tafsīr al-Ṭabarī: Jāmiʿ al-Bayān ʿan Taʾwīl Āy al-Qurʾān*. Edited by ʿAbd Allāh b. ʿAbd al-Muḥsin al-Turkī. Cairo: Hajr, 2001.

Tabbaa, Yasser. "The Architectural Patronage of Nur Al-Din, 1146–1174." Ph.D. Thesis, New York University, 1982.

Tabbaa, Yasser. *Constructions of Power and Piety in Medieval Aleppo*. University Park: Pennsylvania State University Press, 1997.

Talmon-Heller, Daniella. *Islamic Piety in Medieval Syria: Mosques, Cemeteries and Sermons under the Zangids and Ayyūbids (1146–1260)*. Leiden: Brill, 2007.

Taylor, Christopher S. "Reevaluating the Shiʿi Role in the Development of Monumental Islamic Funerary Architecture: The Case of Egypt." *Muqarnas* 9 (1992): 1–10.

Taylor, Christopher S. "Saints, Ziyāra, Qiṣṣa, and the Social Construction of Moral Imagination in Late Medieval Egypt." *Studia Islamica*, no. 88 (1998): 103–20.

Taylor, Christopher Schurman. *In the Vicinity of the Righteous: Ziyāra and the Veneration of Muslim Saints in Late Medieval Egypt*. Boston: Brill, 1999.

Touati, Houari. *Islam et Voyage au Moyen Âge: Histoire et Anthropologie d'une Pratique Lettrée*. Paris: Seuil, 2000.

Al-Ulaymī, ʿAbd al-Raḥmān b. Muḥammad. *Al-Uns al-Jalīl bi-Tārīkh al-Quds wa al-Khalīl*. Negev: al-Wahbīyah, 1866.

Uthmān, MuḥammadAl-JāmiAl-Jāmiʿ al-Aqmar. Dirāsah Āthārīyah Madhhabīyah. Alexandria: Dār al-Wafāʾ li-Dunyā al-Ṭibāʿah wa al-Nashr, 2012.

Vajda, Georges. "Les Lettreset les Sons de la Langue Arabe d'après Abū Ḥātim al-Rāzī." *Arabica* 8, no. 2 (1961): 113–30.

Veen, Marijke Van Der. "When Is Food a Luxury?" *World Archaeology* 34, no. 3 (2003): 405–27.

Walker, Paul E. "Fatimid Institutions of Learning." *Journal of the American Research Center in Egypt* 34 (1997): 179–200.

Wiesehöfer, Josef (Kiel). "Gundeshapur." *Brill's New Pauly*. Antiquity volumes edited by Hubert Cancik and Helmuth Schneider. Brill Online, 2014. www.paulyonline.brill.nl/entries/brill-s-new-pauly/gundeshapur-e500280

William, Archbishop of Tyre. *A History of Deeds Done beyond the Sea*. Vol. 35, Records of Civilization, Sources and Studies, no. 35. New York: Columbia University Press, 1943.

Williams, Caroline. "The Cult of ʿAlid Saints in the Fatimid Monuments of Cairo Part I: The Mosque of al-Aqmar." *Muqarnas* 1 (1983): 37–52.

Williams, Caroline. "The Cult of ʿAlid Saints in the Fatimid Monuments of Cairo Part II: The Mausolea." *Muqarnas* 3 (1985): 39–60.

Williams, John Alden. "Urbanization and Monument Construction in Mamluk Cairo." *Muqarnas* 2 (1984): 33–45.

Al-Yaʿqūbī, Aḥmad b. Abī Yaʿqūb. *Tārīkh al-Yaʿqūbī*. Beirut: Dār Ṣādir, 1960.

Al-Yūnīnī, Mūsā b. Muḥammad. *Dhayl Mirʾāt al-Zamān: Tārīkh al-Sanawāt, 697–711 H/1297–1312 M*. Edited by ʿAbbās, Ḥamzah Aḥmad. Abu Dhabi:

Abu Dhabi: Hay'at Abū Ẓaby lil-Thaqāfah wa al-Turāth, al-Mujamma' al-Thaqāfī, 2007.

Zaborowski, Jason R. "Arab Christian Physicians as Interreligious Mediators: Abū Shākir as a Model Christian Expert." *Islam and Christian–Muslim Relations* 22, no. 2 (2011): 185–96.

Zacharias, Bishop of Mytilene. *The Syriac Chronicle Known as That of Zachariah of Mitylene*. Edited by E. W. Brooks and F. J. Hamilton. New York: AMS Press, 1979.

Al-Zuhrī, Muḥammad b. Muslim. *Al-Maghāzī al-Nabawīyah*. Dimashq: Dār al-Fikr, 1980.

Index

Lightning Source UK Ltd.
Milton Keynes UK
UKOW04n0855191017
311256UK00008B/178/P

9 781107 109605